Image Processing with MATLAB®

Applications in Medicine and Biology

Image Processing with MATLAB®

Applications in Medicine and Biology

Omer Demirkaya

Musa Hakan Asyali

Prasanna K. Sahoo

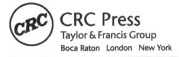

CRC Press
Taylor & Francis Group
Boca Raton London New York

CRC Press is an imprint of the
Taylor & Francis Group, an **informa** business

CRC Press
Taylor & Francis Group
6000 Broken Sound Parkway NW, Suite 300
Boca Raton, FL 33487-2742

© 2009 by Taylor & Francis Group, LLC
CRC Press is an imprint of Taylor & Francis Group, an Informa business

International Standard Book Number-13: 978-0-8493-9246-7 (Hardcover)

Library of Congress Cataloging-in-Publication Data

Image processing with MATLAB : applications in medicine and biology / Omer
    Demirkaya ... [et al.].
        p. ; cm.
    Includes bibliographical references and index.
    ISBN 978-0-8493-9246-7 (alk. paper)
    1. Imaging systems in medicine. 2. MATLAB. I. Demirkaya, Omer. II. Title.
    [DNLM: 1. MATLAB. 2. Diagnostic Imaging. 3. Image
Processing, Computer-Assisted--methods. 4. Image Interpretation,
Computer-Assisted--methods. 5. Software. WN 180 I308 2008]

R857.O6I456 2008
616.07'54--dc22   2008044163

Visit the Taylor & Francis Web site at
http://www.taylorandfrancis.com

and the CRC Press Web site at
http://www.crcpress.com

Dedicated by

Ömer Demirkaya

to his parents Nehabat and Mehmet

and

his wife Semra, and children Meryem, Hatice and Abdullah,

and

Musa Hakan Asyalı

to his parents, Kiraz and Yaşar Asyalı

and

his wife Elçin and daughters Ahsen Nur and Ayşe Nur,

and

Prasanna Sahoo

in memory of his mother Sairendry

and

to his wife Sadhna and son Amit

Contents

Preface

Imaging, mainly due to its impact on medicine and biology, has been selected as one of the greatest achievements of the twentieth century by the National Academy of Engineering. In the last several decades, medical imaging systems have advanced in quantum leaps. There have been substantial improvements on their characteristics such as sensitivity, resolution and acquisition speed. Multislice, 320-slice currently, computer tomography (CT) scanners, for instance, allow the visualization of the entire coronary tree, even atherosclerotic plaques within the coronaries with extremely high accuracy and detail. Similar advances have occurred in the other medical imaging modalities such as magnetic resonance imaging (MRI) and positron emission tomography (PET).

Substantial effort has been put into the integration of different modalities. These systems are also called hybrid systems. The integration of CT and PET scanners has enabled physicians to localize biochemical activity (functional) with a high degree of certainty in the human body. As a result of the significant advances in small animal imaging, a new research discipline known as molecular imaging, which can be defined as in-vivo imaging of biochemical or molecular activity in an organ, is emerging. In-vitro molecular imaging has already been contributing to the advancement of the study of genome and efficacy of new drugs. With the help of imaging, now biologists can get a snapshot of almost the entire genomic activity (expression or disexpression of genes) within a diseased tissue in a matter of days. It will not be long before physicians can visualize, in-vivo, the biochemical processes triggered by a disease. All of this may soon result in a paradigm shift in healthcare. It may open up the possibility of designing drugs as per a patient's individual genetic profile (i.e., personalized medicine).

Advanced techniques of image processing and analysis find widespread use in biology and medicine. In medical and biological fields, image data are ubiquitously used in clinical as well as scientific studies to infer details regarding the process under investigation whether it be a disease process or a biochemical pathway. Today, perhaps, health care institutions alone produce the largest amount of image data which are used in diagnosis and treatment of patients. Information provided by medical images has become an indispensable part of today's patient care. As the number of images produced increases, utilization, and handling of image data are becoming an increasingly formidable task for engineers, scientists, and medical physicists.

There are two main issues that concern the field of image processing and analysis applied to medical applications.

- Improving the quality of the acquired image data
- Extraction of information (i.e., feature) from medical image data in a robust, efficient and accurate manner

Image enhancement techniques such as noise filtering, contrast, and edge enhancement; and image restoration techniques that focus on removing degradations in images, all fall within the former category, whereas image analysis methods deal primarily with the latter issue.

The shear size of images in medical applications has been increasing rapidly with the advent of imaging technologies; hence, transfer and storage issues are also challenging tasks. The main goal of developing efficient image data compression techniques is to address these two issues.

Unlike the images produced in industrial applications, the images generated in medical and biological applications are complex and vary substantially from application to application. In addition, as one can imagine, the field of image processing and analysis has to tackle a diverse and complex set of problems. Because this is such a vast subject, we focus on certain topics that we consider important in the fields of medicine and biology.

Some concepts in image processing and analysis are theory-laden and may be difficult for the beginners to grasp. Explaining complex topics in image processing through examples and MATLAB algorithms is the principle aim of this book. While working on this book, we tried to strike a balance between theory and practice. We wanted to keep it neither too shallow nor too complex so readers from diverse fields could benefit without difficulty. Image processing techniques in general are ad-hoc in the sense that they are optimized and tailored to solve a particular problem in hand, although they are based on solid mathematical theories. That is, they are not applicable to wide range of applications or situations. This lack of generalizability often forces scientists and researchers to resort to the method of trial-and-error. The algorithms provided in this book will help scientists and researchers to quickly identify the most effective method of solution for a particular problem at hand.

This book will help readers understand advanced concepts through algorithms applied to real-world problems in medicine and biology. The examples and exercises included in every chapter will make the book suitable for use as a textbook for students at the senior undergraduate or graduate level, who are studying image processing and analysis for the first time; or a reference book for researchers, scientists, and biologists in the related fields.

In addition to fundamental topics in image processing and analysis, the book covers new areas such as nonlinear diffusion filtering (NDF) or partial differential equation (PDE) based image filtering, and relatively advanced topics such as segmentation methods based on Markov Random Field (MRF) modeling. Statistical and stochastic modeling in image processing is also emphasized in this book.

In the past, computation times and memory demand for 3-D algorithms were unrealistic, but with the advent of computer (or CPU) technology, processing time and memory needs in 3-D are no longer a prohibitive factor. Therefore, we discussed the applications for 3-D volumetric images. We tried to expand the techniques (algorithms) to 3-D whenever we could.

Finally, the reader with a moderate level of calculus, linear algebra, and probability and statistics background will find this book reasonably easy to follow.

The content of this book can be summarized as follows:

Chapter 1 discusses major imaging modalities in diagnostic radiology. They include CT, MRI, gamma camera, and single photon emission tomography (SPECT) systems, and PET.

In Chapter 2, we discuss fundamental image processing techniques. We have presented basic but useful as well as advanced image processing and analysis techniques with MATLAB codes or functions. Most of these techniques are not available in the image processing toolbox; hence are unique. Some of these techniques have also been used in the subsequent chapters of the book.

Chapter 3 covers the theory of probability and statistics on which some image processing and analysis methods are built. This chapter will help the readers build a background that may help them follow the other chapters such as Chapters 6 and 7.

Chapter 4 introduces the 2-D Fourier Transform with unique examples. We also briefly discuss the tomographic image reconstruction method, filtered back projection, as it is one of the medical applications in which the Fourier transform is used.

Chapter 5 deals with nonlinear diffusion filtering as well as some of the partial differential equation (PDE) based image denoising techniques. This relatively recent class of filters has found many applications in medical imaging because of their superior performance in removing noise and preserving the edge sharpness.

Chapter 6 discusses most of the intensity-based image segmentation methods. It discusses the thresholding techniques based on between-class variance, the Kullback function, and the entropy. We also discuss K-means, fuzzy C-means clustering, and mixture modeling-based techniques and their application to image segmentation.

Chapter 7 discusses the image segmentation method based on MRF modeling. In this approach, we model the spatial dependency of the intensities in a local neighborhood. The conditional density of the intensities and the MRF local dependency model are combined under the Bayesian framework, where the MRF model is viewed as a priori. This formulation leads to the maximum a posteriori (MAP) estimate of the true image (i.e., the image not deteriorated by the noise and the imaging system). We have discussed both the deterministic and probabilistic methods of finding the MAP estimate.

Chapter 8 discusses deformable models and their application to image segmentation. The theory of both parametric and geometric deformable models has been covered.

Chapter 9 talks about the fundamental image analysis methods that are applicable to wide range of problems. These methods include, for example, regions properties, boundary analysis, curvature analysis, and line and circle detection using Hough transform.

Chapters 10, 11, and 12 include three applications of image processing and analysis. Through these applications, we wish that the reader will also gain the experience that one requires to tackle a problem at hand.

Our initial aim was to develop this book as a reference or guide for the graduate students and/or researchers (i.e., professionals developing image processing applications and algorithms in the field), where they can have access to a reasonably large library of image processing methods. In many cases, the ideas offered by others may be a good starting point. For instance, the MATLAB Central's file exchange, available at http://www. mathworks.com/matlabcentral/fileexchange offers a unique resource where people in the field, from students to the professional, can contribute to and benefit from a rich pool of ideas. The files and demos presented there constitute precursors upon which many serious applications can be developed. As a group of scientists who are working on biomedical signal and/or image processing, bioinformatics, and biostatistics, with some years of experience, we thought that the time has come to share our experience with others in the form a book. Similar to the MATLAB Central File exchange's function, we hope that the ideas and implementations (sample codes) that we present in this book will inspire researchers and students with diverse backgrounds.

After we had started this book project, it turned out that the wealth and depth of subjects covered also makes it suitable to be used as a textbook. We humbly suggest that this book could be used as the main or supplementary textbook for senior undergraduate and graduate level courses in image processing in general. Especially, image processing courses offered in biomedical sciences and/or life-sciences may benefit more from this book, as almost the entire example applications are from those fields.

When this book is used as a "reference book," the communication between the reader and the book is one-way, the book simply serves as a static supply of information and example uses on some image processing methods for the interested readers. Whereas in the "textbook" mode of use, we are planning to make this book a living book where users (instructors and students) can interact with us, i.e., with the developers through a Web site dedicated solely to this book, www.biomedimaging.org. We will supplement our book with more example applications and sample end-of-chapter questions through its Web site. In this context, we kindly ask you (both reference and textbook users of this book) to visit our web-site and contribute to this project with your comments, suggestions for improvements and by sending/sharing your sample applications.

MATLAB® is a registered trademark of the MathWorks, Inc. and is used in this book with permission. For product information, please contact:

> The MathWorks, Inc.
> 3 Apple Hill Drive
> Natick, MA 01760-2098 USA
> Tel: 508 647 7000
> Fax: 508-647-7001
> E-mail: info@mathworks.com
> Web: www.mathworks.com

Disclaimer

The MATLAB algorithms, scripts, and image data in this book and on its website are provided "AS IS" without any warrenty of any sort. The authors and the publisher make no warranties, express or implied that the algorithms and scripts are error-free nor guarantee the accuracy, completeness, usefulness, or adequacy available at or through these algorithms and scripts.

They should not be relied on for solving a problem whose incorrect solution may result in damage to a person. You can use these algorithms in such a manner at your own risk. The authors and the publisher of the book disclaim all the liability for consequential damages resulting from the use of the algorithms and scripts in this book and on its Web site.

Acknowledgments

We would like to thank Dr. Ersin Bayram for contributing the Deformable Model chapter and the MRI section of Chapter 1. We are thankful to Mr. Kostas Chantziantoniou for contributing to the Computer Tomography section in Chapter 1. We would also like to thank Edward D. Carroll and John Schneider for proofreading some chapters and for pointing out places where the text was unclear.

We are very thankful to the MathWorks, Inc. for supporting us with free-of-charge MATLAB licenses through their book program.

Finally, the authors are very thankful to Michael Slaughter, senior editor, Andrea Dale, editorial assistant, Susan Horwitz, project editor, and Elise Oranges, proofreader from the Taylor & Francis Group. This book would not have been possible in its present form without the help of these people.

1

Medical Imaging Systems

CONTENTS

1.1   Introduction

In this chapter, we discuss the major medical imaging modalities used in diagnostic imaging. These modalities generate an image of the body either through the detection of photons or the use of electromagnetic waves. Let us recall the dual nature of light. The duality theory asserts that light has the properties of both waves and particles. This duality is also applicable to the photons that are involved in our imaging modalities. Figure 1.1 shows the positions of these imaging modalities in the electromagnetic

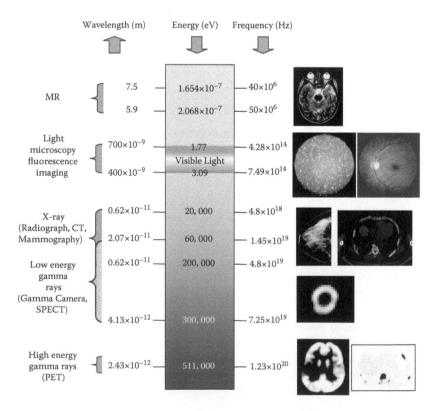

FIGURE 1.1
Positions of the imaging methods in the electromagnetic spectrum.

spectrum. The relation between the frequency (or wavelength) and energy of the photon is given by

$$E = hv \tag{1.1}$$

where E is the energy, $h = 4.136 \times 10^{-15}$ eV* is the Planck's constant, and v is the frequency. The frequency of the wave is given by $v = c/\lambda$, where $c = 299792458\ ms^{-1}$ is the speed of the light in vacuum, and λ is the wavelength. This means that the product of the wavelength and frequency is always constant and is equal to the speed of light in vacuum. For example, the frequency and the wavelength of a 20 keV x-ray photon can be calculated using the following script:

```
E = 20000; % 20 KeV
h = mipconstants('plank','ev');
c = mipconstants('light speed');
% frequency in 1/s or Hz
>> v = E/h
v =
4.8356e+018
% Compute the wavelength in m
>> lambda = c/v
lambda =
6.1997e-011
```

Note that our function `mipconstants` returns some fundamental constants, taken from reference [1], used in physics. Any of the three characteristics of the photons can be computed using these relations. For other constants, the reader can refer to the function itself.

Light microscopy and fluorescence imaging involve light photons from the range of the spectrum known as visible light. These methods are widely used in in vitro imaging of cellular and subcellular structures. Magnetic resonance (MR) imaging employs radio frequency (RF) or short waves to produce images of the body. The x-ray spectrum can be divided into two regions: soft (low-energy) and hard (high-energy) x-ray regions. To image soft tissue, low-energy x-ray photons are used because high-energy x-ray photons will penetrate through the tissue without much attenuation. For instance, mammography imaging uses low-energy x-rays, whereas computer tomography (CT) uses high-energy x-ray photons. Low-energy and high-energy gamma rays are also involved in diagnostic imaging of the human body. Gamma cameras, single photon emission tomography (SPECT), and positron emission tomography (PET) all produce images through the detection of gamma rays. Note that the energy spectrum of gamma rays overlaps that of the x-ray. The difference between gamma

---

* Electron volt is a unit of energy. One electron volt is 1.6×10^{-19} J. It is the amount of energy gained by an electron moving across a potential difference of 1V.

rays and x-rays is the source of the radiation. X-rays are produced as a result of the movement of electrons from one shell to another, or alternatively, acceleration or deceleration of electrons, whereas gamma rays are produced as a result of a nuclear decay process.

In the subsequent sections, we will discuss the basic physics, the instrumentation, image formation, and some of the important characteristics of CT, MR, SPECT, and PET imaging modalities, such as noise and image resolution.

1.2 Computed Tomography

X-ray radiation has been used in medicine to diagnose patients for well over 100 years, and it is the penetrating power characteristic of x-ray photons that is being utilized to generate patient images. X-ray photons are often produced by x-ray tubes when focused emitted electrons from a cathode filament are accelerated at high potential differences toward a rotating anode, typically between 20 and 140 kV_p (depending on the radiology imaging modality and examination procedure), and then are stopped as they interact with atoms of the anode (usually made of tungsten) at the focal spot region. Because the emitted x-ray photons undergo x-ray absorption and scattering interaction processes in tissue, not all of the incident x-ray photons will pass through the patient (the beam is said to be attenuated) to expose the imaging receptor (radiographic film or digital detector). The degree of photon attenuation that does occur depends on the incident x-ray photon energy, the atomic number, and the thickness, as well as the physical and electronic densities of the interacting material. Air, because of its low x-ray linear attenuation coefficient, is imaged as black; bone, because of its much higher x-ray linear attenuation coefficient (arising from its higher atomic number, and physical and electronic densities), is imaged as white; whereas soft tissue is often presented in between these two extremes as shades of gray. The resulting image (see Figure 1.2) is a 2-D representation of the total x-ray attenuation that occurred when the incident photons in the collimated x-ray beam interacted with the various material atoms in the exposed patient volume.

X-ray computer tomography (CT), from its first clinical application in 1972, has often been referred to as the most important invention in diagnostic radiology since the discovery of x-rays in 1895. The primary advantages CT has over conventional or digital radiography are threefold:

1. A sequential CT examination study comprises a set of 2-D cross-sectional images instead of a single 2-D image rendered by the compression of a 3-D body structure volume onto a 2-D image plane (where over- and underlying tissues and structures are superimposed, as seen in Figure 1.2), thus resulting in reduced conspicuity and subject contrast.

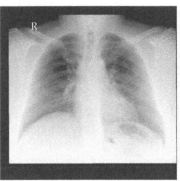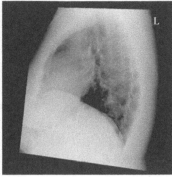

FIGURE 1.2
Computed radiography views acquired when performing a chest x-ray examination. Left: Posterior–anterior (PA) view. Right: Lateral view. R and L on the images refer to the right side of the PA view and lateral projection, respectively.

2. The volume of data can be reformatted (see Figure 1.3) in various planes (sagittal, coronal, and axial) or even as volumetric (3-D) representations (e.g., multiplanar reformation, maximum intensity projection, perspective volume rendering, and virtual colonoscopy) of structure.

3. The sensitivity of CT to subtle differences in x-ray attenuation (typically around 0.5% in contrast differences) is at least a factor of 16 higher than that normally achieved by film/screen radiography systems due to an improved (lower) scatter-to-primary ratio, resulting from a much narrower, finely collimated CT x-ray beam profile that reduces scatter photon contributions and the use of detectors of higher x-ray absorption efficiency.

In sequential CT, 2-D images (or slices) are typically acquired in a 512 × 512 image matrix with 16-bit resolution. The picture element (or pixel),

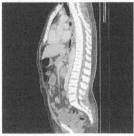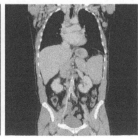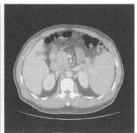

FIGURE 1.3
Various 2-D display views that can be attained from a CT examination. Left: Sagittal. Middle: Coronal. Right: Axial.

after digitization, is set to a value called Hounsfield Unit (HU) or CT number, and is defined as

$$\text{CT Number (HU)} = C \cdot \frac{\mu_p - \mu_w}{\mu_w} \tag{1.2}$$

where C is an integer constant, called *contrast scale*, and has been standardized to 1000; μ_p is the calculated pixel mean x-ray attenuation coefficient; and μ_w is the mean x-ray attenuation coefficient of water, which is determined from the periodic scanner calibrations of water or water-equivalent phantoms. Because x-ray attenuation coefficients are affected by x-ray beam energy, proper calibration of the CT scanner x-ray tube generator is important for accurate and reproducible CT number calculations. In the earlier formulation, the CT numbers of air and water are −1000 and 0, respectively, and both typically can have CT number accuracy on the order of 3 HU.

Because 2-D slices also have a depth (along the scanner z-axis or long patient axis) equal to the slice thickness (acquisition parameter), the image pixel for all practical purposes is a volume element (or voxel). The physical size of each pixel on the displayed image depends on the display field-of-view (DFOV) and reconstruction image matrix size. For a common matrix size of 512 × 512, the pixel size is computed from

$$\text{Pixel Size} = \frac{\text{DFOV}}{512} \tag{1.3}$$

Typical DFOV settings are 16, 20, and 50 cm for pediatric, head, and whole-body acquisition protocols, respectively, which attain corresponding physical pixel sizes of 0.31, 0.39, and 0.98 mm.

The 2-D images are reconstructed using a filtered backprojection technique, in which the image data set is acquired from multiple fan-beam projections at various angles around the object to be imaged, as per the Radon theory methodology (see Chapter 4). For a detailed discussion of CT image reconstruction, the reader can consult [2]. Filters with mnemonic names such as standard, smooth, detail, and bone are selectable during examination prescription and are chosen to deliver the best compromise between image resolution and noise for the region of anatomy being imaged.

In third-generation CT scanner geometry, the patient lies on an examination table that can be moved through the scanner gantry, and the x-ray tube and detector array, which are mechanically fixed directly opposite to the x-ray tube, rotate in synchrony around the patient at some fixed radius from the gantry center of rotation (see Figure 1.4).

Sequential 2-D images are reconstructed from multiple x-ray projections (or views) acquired by rapidly rotating the x-ray tube 360° around

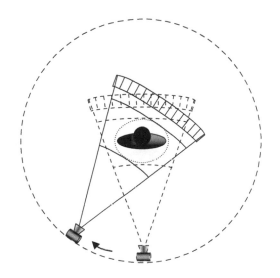

FIGURE 1.4
Third-generation CT scanner geometry design.

the patient and exposing a detector subsystem (or array) with transmitted (attenuated) x-ray radiation. At specific x-ray tube angles, the intensity of the transmitted x-ray photons at each element of the detector array is measured, and the data from all elements on the detector array data are combined to form a single view or projection. From approximately 1000 views and 800 rays/view, the sinogram is constructed, the image reconstruction is performed, the mean x-ray attenuation coefficient value of tissue at each voxel, the position on the image is computed, a CT number is assigned to the voxel, and the 2-D image is displayed on a monitor screen at some DFOV, which is often different from the scan-field-of-view (SFOV), which pertains to the area of the patient that was physically exposed by x-ray radiation during the CT scan. The 512 × 512 acquired CT images are often displayed as an image series on workstation monitors using 1024 × 1024 matrices by means of image interpolation (see Figure 1.5).

Because the human body comprises fluids and tissue that can vary in their x-ray attenuation properties, a single CT image (depending on the cross section being imaged) can have voxels whose CT numbers range from −1000 (air) to 2000 HU (dense cortical bone), or to as high as 4000 HU, and this would require on the order of 3000 or more gray levels to differentiate all the types of tissue/fluids on a single image. As a human observer can only discern up to a maximum of 60 to 80 gray levels at any one time, the displayed CT image is windowed. Windowing, whose schematic is shown in Figure 1.6, is performed by assigning the total monitor display intensity (usually 256 gray levels) to the CT number range of interest (L to U region); voxels with CT values below the lower window (L)

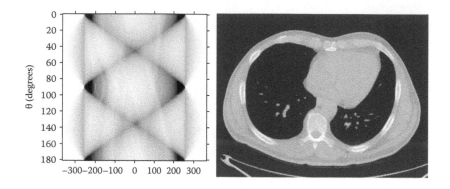

FIGURE 1.5
The image on the right shows the CT slice at the chest level. The image on the left is the sinogram generated using the MATLAB function radon, which assumed that the center of the image is at the center of rotation and used a total of 180 views over 180°.

setting will be displayed as black, and voxels with CT values above the upper window (U) setting, as white. The procedure of windowing, which is interactively performed by the CT operator at the console with a mouse or a trackball, requires the assignment of two parameters: the window level (WL), and the window width (WW). The WL is chosen to correspond approximately to the mean CT number of the tissue structure of interest, and the WW is chosen to determine the display contrast (dynamic range) of the image. As the WW is reduced, the CT number range represented by each gray level is also reduced, and thus, improvements in display contrast visibility are attained. For the display of very small x-ray attenuation differences, as given in a brain image, for example, a narrow WW is chosen (see Figure 1.7 [left]), whereas for the display of large differences in

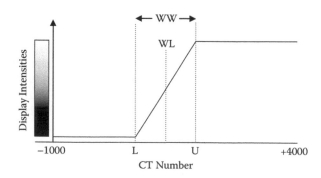

FIGURE 1.6
The concept of how window width and center (or level) is used to manipulate the display contrast of a CT image.

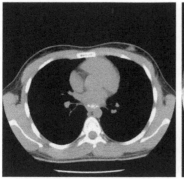 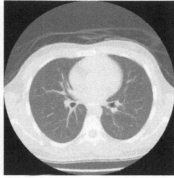

FIGURE 1.7
These two images are of the same image section viewed at different window (WL and WW) settings. Left: Chest/abdomen window (WL:56, WW: 342) image reveals structures within the mediastinum, but no lung parenchyma can be seen. Right: Lung window (WL: −498, WW: 1465) image reveals the details of the lung parenchyma at the expense of the mediastinum.

x-ray attenuation, as presented by the lungs or the mediastinum in a chest image, a wide WW (see Figure 1.7 [right]) is chosen.

The following MATLAB function can perform the windowing or mapping illustrated in Figure 1.6. The reader can try different windowing parameters on the CT image provided by the image database. Note that the output image will have intensities in the range 0–255.

```
function oimg = mipmapCTwindow(img,wl,ww)
% Calculate the CT number limits
L = wl - ww/2;
U = wl + ww/2;
img = double(img);
% Clip the intensities outside the display range.
img(img < L) = 0;
img(img > U) = 255;
minL = -min(img(:));
% Add the intercept
img = img + minL;
mxL = max(img(:));
% Calculate the slope
slope = 255/mxL;
% Carry out the mapping
% and convert to 8-bit unsigned integer
oimg = uint8(slope*img);
```

The continuous drive by manufacturers and the medical community to optimize image quality, minimize x-ray radiation exposure to the patient, minimize image artifacts (objects seen on images generated by the reconstruction process and/or patient movement that are not present in the anatomy), and minimize study acquisition times have led to the following pivotal technology implementations, which all modern CT scanners use today: Third-generation scanner geometry (as shown in Figure 1.4, where the x-ray tube and detector array rotate around patient in synchrony), ¼ detector width offset relative to gantry center of rotation (this offset doubles the reconstruction sampling density in third-generation scanners), low-voltage slip rings (a technology that allows for the passage of electrical power and projection data to the rotating components in the gantry without fixed connections, thus allowing for continuous x-ray tube rotation), and a multiple ceramic detector array (which allows for the acquisition of more than one image per complete rotation of the x-ray tube). With these major technologies (and some not mentioned here), CT scanners today can be operated in numerous acquisition modes and can typically attain (depending on the manufacturer) voxel dimensions of 0.35 mm for all three axes (isotropic), table scan speeds of 18 cm/s, as many as 256 (RSNA 2007, annual meeting) images per tube rotation, and x-ray tube rotation time on the order of 0.4 s. In the following section, we will discuss the four most common CT acquisition modes.

1.2.1   Scout Images

A scout (or topogram) image is acquired to assist the CT technologist in planning the patient protocol and to establish the target organ location. Scout images are typically generated by first selecting an x-ray tube orientation with respect to the patient or table long axis (typically 0°, 90°, 180°, or 270°), and then translating the table at constant speed through the gantry opening while the x-rays are being delivered. The x-ray tube and detector array do not rotate around the patient during the acquisition, and the resulting image looks like a regular x-ray radiograph (see Figure 1.8).

In modern CT scanners, scout images are also used as low-exposure prescan x-ray attenuation maps of the patient, which during the scan are used to drive automatic exposure control (AEC) algorithms that adjust (or modulate) the x-ray tube current as the patient thickness (and hence total x-ray attenuation) changes with respect to the x-ray tube/detector array orientation in the same axial plane and along the patient long axis, thus reducing patient radiation exposure and image quality variations. Even more advanced AEC techniques are being developed and implemented so that image quality variations are minimized between different patients.

1.2.2   Axial Sequences

In axial (or step-and-shoot) acquisitions, the x-ray tube continuously rotates around the patient, and the table travel is adjusted so that its movement goes through a series of starts and stops throughout the entire scan, always stopping at some predefined z-axis travel increment. Slice

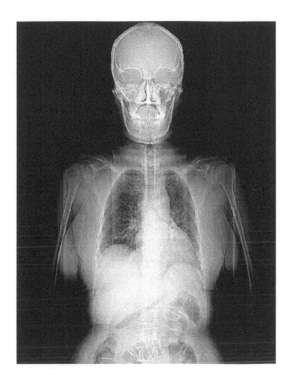

FIGURE 1.8
CT scout image attained when x-ray tube is at 0° position.

acquisition, which is made when the table is not moving, results in a set (or stack) of orthogonal 2-D cross-sectional (transverse or axial) images of discreet thickness equal to the scan slice thickness. Axial scanning was often the preferred sequence for high-quality CT imaging, as the table does not move during the image acquisition process, and image artifacts are reduced, but multislice CT (MSCT) scanner technology has allowed spiral acquisitions to attain axial images with similar or improved image quality.

1.2.3 Spiral Sequences

In spiral (or helical) acquisitions, the x-ray tube rotates around the patient, and the table moves continuously through the gantry at some predefined constant table speed throughout the entire scan. They are no interscan delays between scans as in axial acquisitions, and spiral scanning is often chosen when a large target volume needs to be scanned very quickly. The name of the acquisition is derived from the trajectory of the image data set relative to the table motion, which traces out in 3-D space a helical or spiral path along the scanner z-axis or long axis of the table, as seen

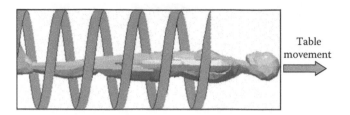

FIGURE 1.9
Illustration of spiral scan data set orientation with respect to table travel. The "articulated humanoid body" (Nancy) shown here has been programmed into MATLAB by Walterio Mayol-Cuevas from H-Anim working group, and can be obtained from the MATLAB Central\File Exchange.

in Figure 1.9. The spiral illustration in Figure 1.9 was generated with the following script using the nancy_body script to plot out the "articulated humanoid body" figure, which had been programmed into MATLAB by Walterio Mayol-Cuevas from the H-Anim working group, and can be obtained from the MATLAB Central\File Exchange online directory. The MATLAB figure can be manipulated by the script to view the entire 3-D plot from different angles. We used the part of the script to produce the helical function shown in Figure 1.10 to illustrate the z-interpolation.

```
% Draw Nancy Body
nancy_body;
hold on;
% Define a 3D helix whose parametric equation,
% [x(t),y(t),z(t)], is given as follows
t = 0:0.1:10*pi
```

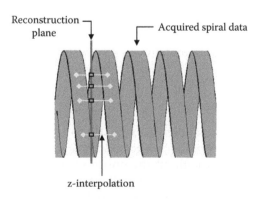

FIGURE 1.10
Calculation of an axial slice through z-interpolation in spiral CT. The acquired spiral data are demonstrated by a 3-D helix function.

```
X = cos(t);
Y = sin(t);
Z = t;
% Here we plot a number of helixes each being shifted
% a little bit in the z direction of the helix
% The z dimension of the helix made coincide with the
% superior-inferior direction of the humanoid.
for i=0:0.1:pi
   if i == 0 | i > pi - 0.1
      plot3(cos(t+i)/3.2,Z/25,sin(t+i)/3.2,'k','LineWidth',2);
   else
      plot3(cos(t+i)/3.2,Z/25,sin(t+i)/3.2,...
      'Color',[0.502,0.502,0.502],'LineWidth',2);
   end
end
axis off
set(gca,'Xlim',[-0.25 0.2]);
set(gca,'Zlim',[-0.32 0.32]);
```

The volume coverage that is attained during a helical scan acquisition is determined by a scan parameter called a *helical pitch* or simply *pitch,* and is defined (for single-slice CT scanners) as

$$\text{Helical Pitch} = \frac{\text{TF}}{\text{SC}} \tag{1.4}$$

where TF is the table feed per rotation (mm/rotation) and SC is the section collimation or slice thickness (mm). The choice of the helical pitch value, and hence the TF and SC values, is examination dependent, and it involves a trade-off between coverage and effective slice thickness accuracy. At a pitch value of 1.0, x-ray beam edges are continuous with no overlap with consecutive helical data loops; at pitch values > 1.0, a gap exists between x-ray beam edges and helical data loops (thus increasing coverage); and at pitch values < 1.0, x-ray beam edges of consecutive loops overlap, thus increasing irradiation of underlying tissues (improving image quality by reducing image noise).

Because the table is in constant motion throughout the acquisition, there is not enough projection data collected on any one helical data loop to reconstruct a 2-D axial slice as is the case in axial acquisitions; all the helical data for a given number of spiral turns are acquired, and then the 2-D axial images are reconstructed for any given z-axis position. Image reconstruction in a spiral CT is performed in the same way as for an axial CT, but before the image reconstruction, an interpolation is performed that utilizes data from adjacent helical loops (see Figure 1.10) to provide the additional projection data needed to complete the formation of the 2-D image. Interpolation is essentially a weighted average of the data from either side of the reconstruction plane, with slightly different weighting factors used for each projection plane. Reconstructing 2-D images from any one 360° spiral segment without interpolation would result in 2-D images corrupted by motion artifacts, which have the same appearance as those obtained at axial CT acquisitions when the patient moves.

A variety of interpolation algorithms is available to calculate planar data sets from spiral volume scans; the simplest approach is to use linear z-interpolation (LI) between successive spiral segments, measured at the same angular position θ and computed from data that is 360° apart (360° LI). Even though these algorithms are easy to implement, they tend to significantly broaden slice sensitivity profiles (because a data range of 2 × 360° is accessed), and 180° LI techniques are used instead of. Techniques 180° LI introduce fewer image misrepresentations and image artifacts because they use data points that are closer together and only 180° apart.

1.2.4   CT Fluoroscopy

Real-time CT fluoroscopy can be achieved by continuous dynamic scanning, as is the case in spiral CT, but the scanner is modified to allow for real-time table-side image viewing, table control positioning via joystick, and foot-pedal-controlled acquisitions. Images are continuously acquired for a fixed z-axis position and are updated several times per second (typically 6 frames/s) by continually adding new data to the reconstruction data set and dropping off oldest data. CT fluoroscopy is often used to guide biopsy and aspiration procedures, but poses the risk of significant x-ray radiation to the patient. To minimize patient exposure, the recent trend has been to replace continuous acquisition with a series of discrete rapid acquisitions. The temporal resolution gained in this acquisition is considerably better than expected owing to the modern CT scanner's faster x-ray tube rotation speeds.

1.2.5   Multislice CT Scanners

MSCT scanners are similar in concept to single-slice CT (SSCT) scanners, with the exception that the detector array comprises more than one row of detectors, each of which when exposed to transmitted x-ray radiation can generate a single image upon one complete rotation of the x-ray tube. Depending on the manufacturer, MSCT scanners can generate anywhere between 64 and 256 images (announced in 2007, RSNA annual meeting) per x-ray tube rotation. MSCT detector arrays can be of the matrix (see Figure 1.11) or adaptive structured types, where each detector element on the row is of the same (isotropic) or of different widths with respect to the row center along the scanner z-axis. The major benefits MSCT has over conventional single-slice CT are substantially shorter acquisition times, retrospective creation of thinner or thicker sections from the same raw data, increased speed of volume coverage (which has a major impact on CT angiography and cardiology procedures that rely heavily on precise

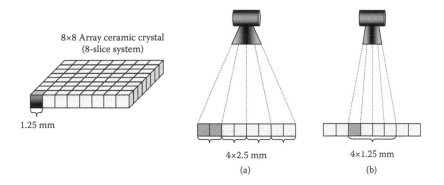

FIGURE 1.11
Multislice matrix array detector design for spiral CT. Four image acquisition detector configurations for 2.50 mm (a) and 1.25 mm (b) slice thickness. The indicated detector rows are parallel to the scanner z-axis or table long axis.

timing to ensure good temporal resolution), and the ability to achieve isotropic voxel resolution even on routine studies (which means that maximum image quality is not restricted to images in the axial plane; and, therefore, studies can be freely viewed in any desired plane with the same resolution and with diminished helical artifacts). The added image slice data that are now available provide a means of attaining even larger and more accurate volume data sets, which can improve 3-D reconstruction and rendering techniques. Some vendors even introduced a 64-slice dual x-ray tube and detector array CT scanner design to increase temporal resolution by reducing the rotation angle required to reconstruct a complete image, thus permitting cardiac studies without the use of heart-rate–lowering medication, as well as permitting imaging of the heart in systole. The dual x-ray tube design makes possible the use of dual energy imaging as well, which improves estimations of voxel total attenuation and atomic number, thus permitting automatic differentiation of calcium (in bone or diseased arteries) from iodine (contrast media) or titanium (in stents) and improved tumor differentiation arising from better tissue characterization.

In SSCT, the slice thickness is determined by mechanical adjustment of a predetector collimator whose width is always smaller than the detector width. In MSCT scanners, slice thickness is determined by electronically binning together different numbers of detector elements and physically moving the collimator to the two outermost edge elements.

The volume coverage that can be acquired during an MSCT procedure, as is the case in spiral CT, depends on the selection of slice thickness and the helical pitch value, which has been defined as follows:

$$\text{MSCT Helical Pitch} = \frac{\text{TF}}{n \cdot \text{SC}} \qquad (1.5)$$

where TF is the table feed per rotation (mm/rotation), n is the number of active detector rows, and SC is the width (in mm) of a single-section collimation.

Image reconstruction for spiral MSCT is similar to that in spiral SSCT, with the exception that cone-beam projections are used instead of fan-beam projections, and more complex MSCT linear z-interpolation (180° MLI) algorithms are used instead of the standard 180° LI techniques. In 180° MLI techniques, the planar image data are not interpolated between two measured data points 180° apart on the same helical loop, but instead, data obtained by rebinning all of the available helical loops are used, and the two closest points to the desired planar image z-axis position are used for the interpolation.

The high sampling density of the data along the z-axis in MSCT offers many suitable points for measurements in the vicinity of the reconstruction plane, and thus has provided the means during interpolation to select an effective slice thickness by weighting all suitable points with some filter function (180° MFI). An advantage of this interpolation technique is that the width of the filter function, and thus the effective slice thickness, can be user selectable depending on clinical needs; thus, the width of the reconstructed images is not dependent on the slice collimation or the reconstruction process as is the case for spiral SSCT. Even though this filtering technique is possible for spiral SSCT scanners as well, it is with MSCT scanners that it has become truly realized, as acquisitions are routinely carried out with thin slices even for very large volumes. It should be mentioned, though, that the effective slice thickness can only be increased, but never decreased below the value of the original slice collimation (SC) or thickness.

A comprehensive discussion of the topics pertaining to SSCT or MSCT spiral CT can be found in Kalender [3].

1.2.6 Image Quality

In this section, we will discuss some of the fundamental factors affecting image quality in CT, such as noise, resolution, and the helical pitch.

Noise in CT images is usually measured by calculating the standard deviation of a region of interest in a homogeneous water phantom. The predominant factor affecting noise is the fluctuation in the number of x-ray quanta. This in turn is affected by the attenuation of the object of scan, the tube current, and the size of the detector. The standard deviation of the CT value in an image can be given by Kalender [3]

$$\sigma = C_R \sqrt{\frac{I_0/I}{\varepsilon QS}} \tag{1.6}$$

where C_R is due to the reconstruction algorithm (mainly the reconstruction filter), ε is the efficiency of the overall system, Q is the current-scan time product (mAs), and S is the slice thickness. For the mathematical derivation of the noise in CT, the reader can refer to Macovski [4]. The ratio I_0/I refers to the attenuation of the object. A higher ratio indicates higher attenuation, which in turn gives rise to higher noise. Because the attenuation in large patients is larger, the CT image of large patients will be noisier unless it is scanned with a larger tube current to compensate for this factor. Note that the factors are not linearly related to the noise; to reduce the noise by a factor of 2, the slice thickness needs to be increased by a factor of 4. It should be also noted that the noise significantly impacts the low-contrast delectability of a system. The noise level in single-slice or multislice spiral CT systems is different from that of sequential CT (see Problems).

In-plane (i.e., transaxial plane) spatial resolution in CT is a function of several factors. These are focus size, detector size (or detector aperture), and the movement of the focus as the x-ray source moves continuously during the scan. The type of filter used in image reconstruction and its parameters also influence in-plane resolution. In-plane resolution can be measured quantitatively using wire phantoms that provide us with a line-spread function, whose Fourier transform will give us the modulation transfer function (MTF) of the system. The reader can refer to Application 2 for a discussion of the calculation of MTF from a line spread function. Comprehensive discussion of the axial resolution can be found in Kalender [3].

The spiral CT image quality on single-slice CT continuously decreases with increasing helical pitch value primarily for two reasons: nominal slice thickness (or slice sensitivity profile) broadening occurs with increasing table speed, and the z-interpolation errors increase during image reconstruction, which results from increases in the z-axis interpolation distances between adjacent measured data (stretching of the helical data loops).

1.3 Magnetic Resonance Imaging

Magnetic resonance imaging (MRI or MR) can be simply defined as imaging the macrolevel behavior of atomic nuclei that possess magnetic property, under a strong magnetic field. The term *magnetic property* will be explained later in the section. For clarification purposes we should mention that hydrogen (H) is the most commonly used atom in MRI. Before moving forward, it is worthwhile to mention several unique advantages of MRI over other imaging modalities. Unlike computer tomography (CT), single photon emission computed tomography (SPECT), and positron emission tomography (PET), MRI operates at radio-frequency (RF) range; thus, there is no ionizing radiation involved.

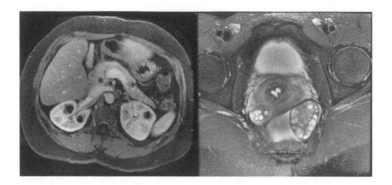

FIGURE 1.12
Body MR images demonstrating the exquisite soft tissue contrast that can be obtained using MR imaging.

Furthermore, MRI can generate excellent soft tissue contrast, as shown in Figure 1.12.

MR is also capable of producing three-dimensional (3-D) volumetric images, and has the capability of producing images at any orientation, while CT is limited to axial slices, other orientations being reconstructed through postprocessing interpolation. Moreover, the information content of MR images is extremely rich compared to other imaging modalities.

Image pixel values depend on various intrinsic properties of the tissue; hence, exquisite images can be obtained by simply enhancing or suppressing the effects of the desired parameters in terms of anatomical, functional, and molecular imaging. Figure 1.13 demonstrates three different images acquired with three different contrasts from the same subject.

Similar to all imaging systems, MRI can be divided into three steps: signal generation, detection, and reconstruction.

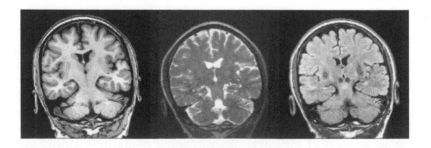

FIGURE 1.13
Different contrasts, hence information content, can be acquired with MR by manipulating intrinsic magnetic properties of spins such as T1 and T2.

1.3.1 Signal Generation

A fundamental property of nuclei is that those with odd atomic weights or atomic numbers possess angular momentum, often called *spin*. A nucleus with a nonzero spin rotates around its own axis. If there is a net electrical charge associated with that nucleus, it creates a magnetic field around the nucleus, according to Faraday's law of induction. For example, H has one proton and therefore has a net angular momentum. Due to its abundance in the human body such as in water (H_2O), it is usually the element of interest in MR imaging. However, under normal conditions, the direction of the field is random because of thermal random motion resulting in zero net magnetization. For imaging purposes, a strong external magnetic field, B_0, is needed to create coherence or bulk magnetization, M, among the spins and to eliminate the effect of thermal random motion. This coherence alone is not sufficient to generate a detectable signal, as static magnetic fields do not generate any signal. Once coherence is achieved, an input signal (RF excitation), denoted by $B_1(t)$, is applied to the system to change the direction of M, which induces a change in the magnetic field and generates a response to be recorded as the output signal. The purpose of RF excitation is twofold:

1. Disturb the equilibrium (static) condition generated by the magnetic field B_0.
2. Establish phase coherence in the transverse plane, and generate a response or output signal to be measured.

$B_1(t)$ is applied perpendicular to B_0 for a short duration that falls into the RF range, and hence is generally called *RF pulse*. A typical RF pulse takes the following form:

$$B_1(t) = B_{e1}(t)e^{-i(w_0 t + \phi)} \tag{1.7}$$

where $B_{e1}(t)$ is the envelope of the pulse, w_0 is the excitation carrier frequency, and ϕ is the initial phase, generally assumed to be zero. As mentioned in the beginning of this section, spins with magnetic properties rotate around their own axis at a frequency w, which is expressed as

$$w = \gamma B_0 \tag{1.8}$$

where γ is the gyromagnetic ratio constant **and** is characteristic of a particular nuclide. w_0 needs to be in resonance with w to provide coherent transition of spins from the equilibrium state to another:

$$w_0 = \gamma B_0 \tag{1.9}$$

This so-called **Larmor frequency** lies within the radio frequency range, which is why there is no ionizing radiation involved in MR.

1.3.2 Signal Detection: Relaxation

After a magnetized spin system is perturbed from its equilibrium condition by an RF pulse, it will return to the equilibrium state after a sufficient time once the perturbation is removed. This process is known as *free induction* decay or relaxation, which was first discovered by Bloch in his seminal work [5]. The recovery of the longitudinal component $\mathbf{M}_z$ is called *longitudinal* or T_1 relaxation, whereas the decay of the transverse magnetization $\mathbf{M}_{xy}$ is called *transverse* or T_2 relaxation. The underlying mechanism is quite complicated; hence, only the dominant mechanism will be mentioned without going into further details. Accounting for the T_1 and T_2 relaxations, the Bloch equation describes the magnetization process as follows:

$$\frac{d\mathbf{M}}{dt} = \mathbf{M} \times \gamma \mathbf{B} - \frac{\mathbf{M}_x \mathbf{i} + \mathbf{M}_y \mathbf{j}}{T_2} - \frac{(\mathbf{M}_z \mathbf{i} + \mathbf{M}_0)\mathbf{k}}{T_1} \tag{1.10}$$

$\mathbf{M}$ and $\mathbf{B}$ are the vector forms of magnetization and the magnetic field, respectively, and $\mathbf{i}$, $\mathbf{j}$, and $\mathbf{k}$ are unit vectors along x, y, and z, respectively. In the Bloch equation, the cross product term, which is the first term on the right-hand side, describes the rotational (precessional) behavior, whereas the relaxation terms describe the exponential behavior of the transverse and longitudinal magnetization components. Although the precession does not alter the magnitude of the magnetization vector, the relaxation processes do.

1.3.3 Longitudinal Relaxation

The longitudinal relaxation process is governed by

$$\frac{dM_z}{dt} = \frac{(M_z - M_0)}{T_1} \tag{1.11}$$

where T_1 is the spin-lattice time constant, and characterizes the return to equilibrium along the direction of the B_0 field. The solution of this equation is given by

$$M_z = M_0 + (M_z(0) - M_0)e^{\frac{-t}{T_1}} \tag{1.12}$$

Following a 90° excitation, $\mathbf{M}_z(0) = 0$; simplifying the preceding equation,

$$M_z = M_0(1 - e^{\frac{-t}{T_1}}) \tag{1.13}$$

where T_1 is a field-strength-dependent parameter and is a measure of the amount of energy exchanged between the nuclei and the surrounding lattice. Randomly fluctuating magnetic dipoles between the different energy states shortens the T_1 and helps longitudinal relaxation. Greater energy exchange is required at higher frequencies to switch between states; hence, T_1 increases with increasing B_0.

1.3.4 Transverse Relaxation

The transverse component of magnetization behaves according to [5]

$$\frac{dM_{xy}}{dt} = -\frac{M_{xy}}{T_2} \tag{1.14}$$

where T_2 is the spin–spin time constant and describes the decay of the transverse magnetization. After a 90° excitation, that is, $M_{xy}(0) = M_0$, Equation (1.14) simplifies to

$$\frac{dM_{xy}}{dt} = -\frac{M_{xy}}{T_2} \tag{1.15}$$

In longitudinal relaxation, fluctuating magnetic dipoles with an xy-component at the spin resonant frequency are responsible for T_1 relaxation. In transverse relaxation, in addition to the xy-component fluctuations, z-component fluctuations also account for T_2 relaxation. Therefore, T_2 is greater than T_1. Furthermore, z-component fluctuations often dominate T_2 relaxation; hence, T_2 is largely independent of field strength.

1.3.5 Selective Excitation

In the presence of B_0, all spins possess the same resonant frequency, w_0. A transverse RF magnetic field, B_1, tuned to the Larmor frequency of spins, tips all spins; thus, the excitation is nonselective. In this case, the entire volume contributes to the signal recorded by the receiver. The 3-D imaging task can be reduced to 2-D by selectively exciting a plane, as shown in Figure 1.14.

Selective excitation is achieved by applying B_1 in the presence of B_0 and the linear gradient field G_z. Linear gradients are used to linearly change

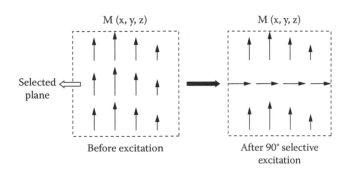

FIGURE 1.14
Selective excitation on a spin system. Arrows represent spin magnetization. After a 90° selective excitation, only the spins in the selected plane are excited.

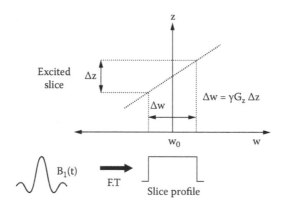

FIGURE 1.15

Selective excitation using gradient G_z. Resonant frequency of spins varies linearly with z. A sinc-shaped RF pulse ($\mathrm{sinc}(x) = \sin(\pi x)/(\pi x)$) creates a rectangular slice profile exciting the desired plane of thickness Δz.

the magnetic field strength, and thus the resonant frequency of spins, along the axis to which they are applied. By turning on G_z, the resonant frequency of the spin is varied with z-position. To excite a plane perpendicular to z-axis of thickness Δz, B_1 must possess a frequency bandwidth of $[yG_z \, \Delta z]$ in order to match the resonant frequencies of interest. Exciting a slice of thickness of Δz requires a rectangular slice profile, which demands a B_1 with a rectangular frequency content. Such frequency content can be achieved by a sinc-shaped $B_1(t)$. Figure 1.15 demonstrates the selective excitation process.

1.3.6 Spatial Encoding

According to Faraday's law of induction, the changing magnetic field induces an electromotive force, EMF. The RF coil that generates the RF excitation field can be used to detect this signal, commonly known as *free induction decay* (FID). Sets of these FIDs are used to reconstruct the image, and the method is explained in the next section.

Selective excitation only reduces the imaging task to 2-D. Within the selected slice, all the spins have the same resonant frequency and behave similar to oscillators, inducing signals at that frequency. It is impossible to differentiate contributions of spins at different locations, as the total signal generated by all the oscillators of the excited region is recorded in a single time waveform. Similar to selective excitation, magnetic field gradients G_x and G_y can be applied to produce spatial variation in the strength of magnetization. For example, if a gradient G_x is applied in the x direction, as in Figure 1.16, then the applied field is $B_0 + xG_x$.

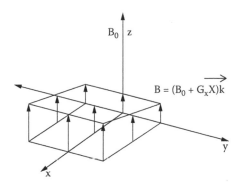

FIGURE 1.16
Spatial encoding using magnetic field gradients. A spin at a higher x position experiences a stronger field than a spin at a lower x position and therefore generates a signal at a higher frequency, enabling the spatial resolvability of its location.

The most important point in Figure 1.16 is that the gradient only changes the strength of the magnetization vector, not its direction; hence, the spins are still pointing in the z direction (hence, the use of unit vector $\mathbf{k}$). As a result of this linear variation in field strength, spins at different locations precess at different frequencies. Thus, the spatial position of a spin along the x-axis or y-axis can be encoded in the frequency of spins, which can be decoded during the reconstruction process. This is known as frequency encoding. In our example, the frequency of spins becomes

$$w(x) = \gamma(B_0 + G_x x) = w_0 + \gamma G_x x \tag{1.16}$$

The position along the frequency-encoding axis is resolved using the spatial dependence on precession frequency. Spatial location along the remaining axis, that is, the y-axis, can be encoded by phase. A spin at position y will accumulate a phase shift that is equal to the time integral of the precession frequency:

$$\phi(t) = 2\pi\gamma y \int_0^t G(\tau)d\tau \tag{1.17}$$

By applying a gradient pulse G_y for a duration of T_y, the spatial position along the y-axis can be resolved. Incorporating the frequency-encoding and phase-encoding gradients, the transverse magnetization becomes

$$m(x,y,t) = M_{xy}e^{-iw_0 t}e^{-i\gamma G_x xt}e^{-i\gamma G_y yT_y} \tag{1.18}$$

1.3.7   Image Reconstruction

The excited spins, acting as RF sources, have a distribution $m(x, y)$, which we wish to image. As spins induce EMF in the receiver coil through precession, gradients G_x and G_y are applied to encode the spatial information in the FID signal. As the receiver coil encompasses the entire region of interest, the received signal $S_R(t)$ will be

$$S_R(t) = \int_x \int_y M_{xy} e^{-iw_0 t} e^{-i\gamma G_x x t} e^{-i\gamma G_y y T_y} dxdy \qquad (1.19)$$

where T_y is the duration that G_y is turned on. We are actually interested in the baseband signal $S(t)$, which can be extracted by ignoring the high-frequency factor $e^{-iw_0 t}$:

$$S_R(t) = \int_x \int_y M_{xy} e^{-i\gamma G_x x t} e^{-i\gamma G_y y T_y} dxdy \qquad (1.20)$$

At this point, two new terms, $k_x(t)$ and $k_y(t)$, are introduced as the time integrals of $G_x(t)$ and $G_y(t)$. They are given by

$$k_x(t) = \frac{\gamma}{2\pi} \int_0^t G_x(s)ds \qquad (1.21)$$

$$k_y(t) = \frac{\gamma}{2\pi} \int_0^t G_y(s)ds \qquad (1.22)$$

Intuitively, $k_x(t)$ and $k_y(t)$ represent the coordinates of the path followed by the spatial encoding gradients G_x and G_y. In most situations, G_x and G_y are constant; hence

$$k_x = \frac{\gamma}{2\pi} G_x t \qquad (1.23)$$

$$k_y = \frac{\gamma}{2\pi} G_y T_y \qquad (1.24)$$

and the recorded signal becomes the 2-D Fourier transform of M_{xy}:

$$S(t) = \int_x \int_y M_{xy} e^{-i2\pi k_x x} e^{-i2\pi k_y y} dxdy \qquad (1.25)$$

Once the signal is recorded, the inverse Fourier transform gives the image or spin distribution, $m(x, y)$. Figure 1.17a, b shows the timing diagram for pulse sequence and the corresponding Fourier domain or k-space coverage to collect the data. Because the timing diagram corresponds to the k-space coverage of a single line, this sequence must be repeated to cover the entire k space. Each time the value of G_y is changed to cover a different line. To extend the 2-D acquisition to 3-D, just add another phase-encode gradient similar to the one applied along G_y in the slice direction.

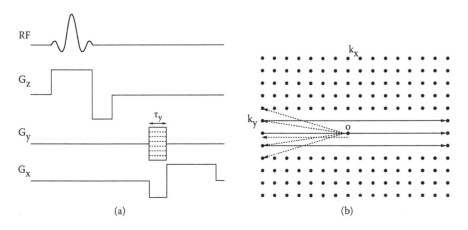

FIGURE 1.17

Timing diagram for a simple pulse sequence and the corresponding k-space coverage. A G_z gradient is applied together with an RF pulse for selective excitation. G_x and G_y are applied simultaneously in reception. The origin in k-space is denoted by O. Each time G_y is changed, as shown with the dotted lines, another line in k-space is acquired. The negative lobe at the beginning of G_x is needed to move from the center of k-space to the beginning of each k-space line, as indicated by the dotted arrows.

There exist several acquisition techniques that allow traveling multiple lines per sequence to speed up the acquisition. One approach to speeding up acquisition, known as *parallel imaging*, utilizes multiple receivers to simultaneously acquire data. Multiple receivers allow skipping k-space lines during acquisition, which can be synthesized using the relationships between the acquired signals from different receivers.

1.4 Gamma Cameras and Single Photon Emission Tomography

Single photon emission computer tomography (SPECT), similar to the other tomographic modalities discussed in this chapter, provides a volumetric image of the human body. It has been known to be a functional imaging modality as it images the functional activities, such as blood flow in the heart. However, imaging modalities in nuclear medicine have been undergoing a paradigm shift. They are evolving from functional imaging toward molecular imaging as technology and science advance.

In emission tomography, the source lies within the structure of interest; hence the name *emission tomography*. In SPECT imaging, the radiopharmaceutical or the tracer, which is a compound labeled with a radioisotope, is injected or inhaled into the body. The radioisotope decays by emitting a single or multiple γrays; hence the name *single photon emission computed tomography*.

TABLE 1.1

Common SPECT isotopes

Isotope	Half-life (h)	γ Energy (keV)	Examples of applications
Technetium-99m	6.01	140.5	To image the skeleton, heart muscle, brain, thyroid, lungs (perfusion and ventilation), liver, spleen, and kidney (structure and filtration rate)
Thallium-201	73	69–80,167	Coronary artery disease and other heart conditions
Iodine-123	13.2	159	Diagnosis of thyroid function
Gallium-67	78	93,184,296	Tumor imaging, localization of inflammation

The gamma camera detector detects these gamma rays that emanate from within the body, and localizes them. Table 1.1 enlists the most commonly used isotopes, of which Technetium-99m is the most widely used one in nuclear medicine.

Figures 1.18 and 1.19 show the hardware components of a gamma camera system and a top view of the detector illustrating the arrangement of the photomultiplier tubes, respectively. The main component, the detector, consists of the crystal and the photomultiplier tubes. The detector or the camera head is mounted on a rotating gantry to enable it to acquire the SPECT data. The collimator, made of tungsten or lead, mounted on the

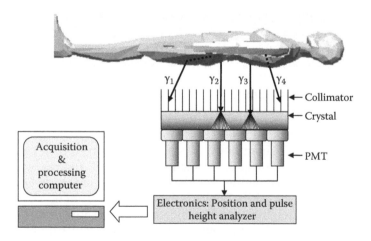

FIGURE 1.18
Schematic picture of a gamma camera system. The articulated humanoid body (Nancy) shown here has been programmed into MATLAB by Walterio Mayol-Cuevas from H-Anim working group and can be obtained from the MATLAB Central\File Exchange.

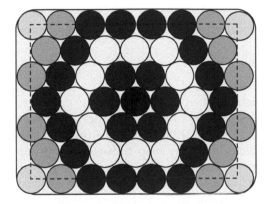

FIGURE 1.19
Top view of the gamma camera shown in Figure 1.18 in which the individual PMTs, which are coupled to the crystal, are closely packed in a hexagonal pattern.

detector with thousands of holes, allows only the γ rays that are at right angle to the detector (e.g., γ_2 and γ_3 in Figure 1.18) and stops the other rays from reaching it.

Gamma camera systems can operate in two modes. In planar imaging, the gamma camera captures the projection image of the body or organ. In SPECT mode, however, it acquires a number of 2-D projections at equally spaced angular distances around the body (see Figure 1.22). Volumetric images are reconstructed from the projections using an iterative tomographic image reconstruction method or the well-known filtered back-projection (FBP) technique.

Gamma cameras may have one or multiple detectors to increase the sensitivity and to reduce the acquisition time. Dual-head gamma camera systems are the most common ones used in clinics today. Further, gamma cameras are capable of imaging multiple isotopes simultaneously. In the last decade, there has been a lot of effort to combine different imaging modalities to improve disease diagnosis. Recently, SPECT/CT systems have been introduced into the clinical service, combining the SPECT and CT modalities to better localize disease and for more accurate attenuation correction. Today, major vendors provide SPECT/CT systems with diagnostic-quality CTs. In the following sections, we will discuss gamma cameras (see Figure 1.18) along with their performance characteristics and SPECT. The coverage of the topic is in a way limited here. We advise the readers interested in further detail to look up the books and articles referred to at the end of this chapter. In the following sections, we will briefly discuss the essential aspects of the gamma camera systems. It may sound as if the gamma camera and SPECT are two different hardware systems. In fact, gamma camera is the name of the imaging equipment that operates in both planar and SPECT modes. By the term *gamma camera system*, we refer to the entire system, including the detectors and collimators. In the subsequent sections, we will discuss the characteristics of gamma cameras.

1.4.1   Collimator

Collimators are made of lead or tungsten, with holes of round or hexagonal shape, which may be parallel, diverging, or converging. The septa between the holes stop γ rays that are not perpendicular to the collimator (e.g., γ_1 and γ_4 in Figure 1.18). Hence, collimators, which are directly placed on the detectors, mainly help reduce the amount of scattering γ photons. However, they significantly reduce the overall detection efficiency of gamma camera systems. Normally, 1 out of every 5000 γ photons is transmitted to the crystal; so their efficiency is around 0.02%.

Collimators are important factors that limit image resolution, as well. The intrinsic (without the collimator in place) resolution of a gamma camera is around 3.5 mm at full-width-at-half-maximum (FWHM), whereas the extrinsic resolution varies between 7 and 12 mm at FWHM. The spatial resolution for parallel-hole collimators is expressed in terms of the effective length of the collimator holes, L_{eff}, the diameter of the hole, d, and the distance from the source to the collimator, b as Cherry, Sorensen, and Phelps [6]

$$R_{coll} \approx d(1 + b/L_{eff}) \tag{1.26}$$

where the effective length is given by $L_{eff} = L - 2\mu^{-1}$, L being the depth of the collimator and μ, the attenuation coefficient of the collimator material. This relation clearly shows that a smaller b and d result in better (smaller) resolution, and the collimator length L_{eff} is inversely related to the resolution. To demonstrate how the length L_{eff} affects the collimator resolution, the following script calculates and plots the resolution values for the specified range of length and fixed values of b and d. Figure 1.20 shows the graph generated by the following MATLAB script.

```
leff = 0.05:0.05:2.5; % cm
d = 0.25; % cm
b = 10; % cm
R = d*(leff + b)./leff;
plot(leff, R);
ylabel('R_{coll} (cm)');
xlabel('L_{eff} (cm)');
```

The overall detector resolution can be expressed in terms of the intrinsic, and the collimator resolutions as

$$R_{det} = \sqrt{R_{coll}^2 + R_{in}^2} \tag{1.27}$$

Manufacturers provide a variety of collimators with different performance characteristics. Low-energy high-resolution collimators (LEHR) have good

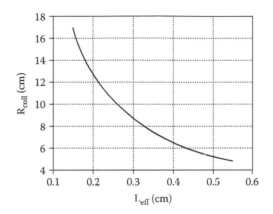

FIGURE 1.20
Collimator resolution as a function of effective length for fixed b and d.

resolution characteristics and are used with low-energy isotopes. There is always a trade-off between resolution and efficiency in collimators. The relationship between the collimator efficiency and the collimator resolution is approximately given by Cherry, Sorensen, and Phelps [6]

$$g_{coll} \approx R_{coll}^2 \tag{1.28}$$

Therefore, while designing a collimator, one needs to optimize these two conflicting factors. This trade-off is also the reason why there exist different types of collimators for different applications.

1.4.2 Crystals

Crystals (see Figure 1.18), which are usually made of NaI(Tl) and typically are 9.5–15.6 mm thick, convert the γphotons to light photons. A little impurity of Tl is added to enable the doped crystals to scintillate much more efficiently at room temperature. Single slabs of NaI(Tl) crystals may be manufactured in different sizes of up to 60 × 40 cm. Light photons reach the photomultiplier (PM) tubes that are normally arranged in a hexagonal pattern (see Figure 1.19) and are coupled to the crystal. The thickness of the crystal is an important factor defining the detection efficiency and the resolution of the gamma camera system. Thicker crystals result in higher detection efficiency but lower resolution.

1.4.3 Photomultiplier Tubes and Other Components

Light photons are converted to photoelectrons at the photocathode of the PM tubes. The conversion efficiency is around 1–3 photoelectrons per 10 visible light photons [6]. Then, the photoelectrons are amplified by the dynodes of the PM tube, which are positively charged metal plates. The multiplication factor is ×3 to ×6 per dynode. Total multiplication is typically around 10^6 for a 10-stage PM tube [6]. At the output of the PM tubes, the electrons are converted to electrical current or a voltage pulse. The amplitude of the pulse is related to the amount of energy deposited by the gamma rays in the crystal.

The pulses are sent to a pulse height analyzer, by which the energies of the detected events are determined based on the amplitude of each pulse. Signals from the PM tubes are used to obtain the x and y locations of the scintillation event, using the analog-positioning circuit. The located events are finally saved as a 2-D image.

1.4.4 Image Acquisition Modes

1.4.4.1 Planar Imaging

In gamma camera systems, images are acquired in two modes: (1) 2-D planar and (2) SPECT volumetric. The planar is the simplest method. Planar imaging includes static, dynamic, or whole-body imaging; the image of a particular projection of the body is acquired according to the time, total counts, number of heart beats, or by a specified length of the patient. Planar images are the projection of a 3-D distribution of the activity inside the body into the gamma camera field of view (FOV). The detected signal at a location represents the sum of the activity along the line traversing the body perpendicular to the gamma camera. The detected signal is not linearly dependent on the sum of the activity along this line of response because of the attenuation in tissue. Unlike that of PET, attenuation in SPECT is a function of the distance that the gamma ray travels within the tissue before it reaches the detector. In planar imaging, tissue attenuation is not an issue; but in SPECT imaging, to accurately estimate the amount of activity inside the tissue volume, attenuation correction has to be performed. In clinical SPECT systems, attenuation correction is done either by using external radionuclide sources as in SPECT-only systems, or by using the CT image as in SPECT/CT systems.

Planar imaging is also performed in a continuous mode to scan the entire body from head to toe. In this mode, the patient or patient bed moves under the gamma camera, whereas the gamma camera itself remains in a fixed position. This scan is widely known as a whole-body scan. Bone scans, such as those shown in Figure 1.21, in nuclear medicine are typical examples.

1.4.4.2 SPECT Imaging

Figure 1.22 shows the SPECT image acquisition process. As seen in the figure, a single or multiple detectors rotate around the patient at certain angular steps. At each step, normally a 64×64 or 128×128 2-D projection image is acquired for a specified time period. The acquired projections

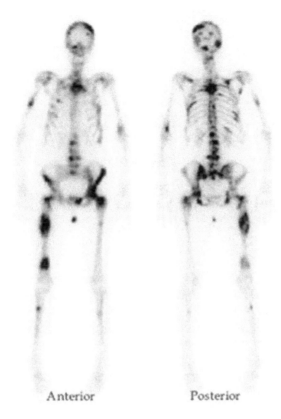

Anterior   Posterior

FIGURE 1.21
Whole-body bone scan of a female patient with history of breast cancer acquired using
99Tc-MDP. The planar images were acquired by a dual-head gamma camera. Both anterior
(left) and posterior (right) views were acquired simultaneously. The regions with darker
intensities in the images indicate widespread bone metastasis.

are finally reconstructed into $64 \times 64 \times 64$ or $128 \times 128 \times 128$ tomographic
volumes using either the FBP or an iterative method such as the ordered
subset expectation-maximization (OSEM) method. Recently, venders have
developed improved versions of their iterative reconstruction methods
that incorporate system characteristics and image formation processes to
recover some of the lost resolution and to improve contrast [7].

In a gamma camera system, the extrinsic (with collimators in place)
resolution is a function of the distance between the activity source and
the collimator, as we discussed earlier. Thus, their resolution is normally
specified at a certain distance (usually 10 cm) from the collimator. The
image resolution is also a function of the characteristics of the collimator,
such as septal thickness, the thickness of the wall between holes, and the
lengths and diameters of the holes. Further, the characteristics of the reconstruction filter (windowing functions in the FBP and postreconstruction

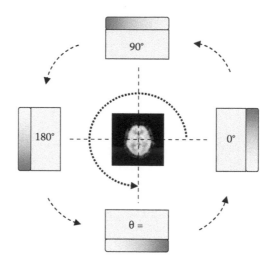

FIGURE 1.22
A diagram showing the image acquisition process in SPECT mode.

filtering in the OSEM) and the angular sampling around the body will also influence the SPECT resolution.

In Chapter 10, in one of the applications, we discuss in detail how to measure and calculate some of the performance characteristics of gamma camera systems. In addition to Cherry, Sorensen, and Phelps [6], an in-depth discussion of these topics can also be found in Wernick and Aarsvold [8].

1.5   Positron Emission Tomography

Positron emission tomography (PET) is a functional imaging modality that has also been evolving into a molecular imaging modality. Clinically, PET has been used in disease diagnosis, staging of various cancer types, and

TABLE 1.2

Common PET isotopes and their emission characteristics

Isotope	Half-life (minimum)	Maximum positron energy (MeV)	Positron range in water (mm) (maximum, mean)
F-18	109.7	0.635	(2.4, 0.6)
C-11	20.4	0.96	(4.1, 1.1)
N-13	9.96	1.19	(5.1, 1.5)
O-15	2.07	1.72	(7.3, 2.5)
Rb-82	1.25	3.35	(14.1, 5.9)

Source: D. L. Bailey, D. W. Townsend, P. E. Valk, and M. N. Maisey, *Positron Emission Tomography: Basic Sciences*, London: Springer-Verlag London Limited, 2004.

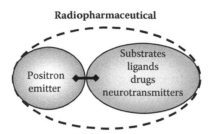

FIGURE 1.23
PET radiopharmaceutical is a compound labeled with a positron emitter.

assessing response to therapy. PET is becoming an almost indispensable tool in preclinical and clinical drug studies to study drug delivery and efficiency.

In PET imaging, similar to SPECT imaging, compounds labeled with radioisotopes are injected into the human body, which is scanned after a certain uptake period. Unlike SPECT, PET uses naturally occurring radioisotopes such as oxygen, carbon, nitrogen, and fluorine with shorter half-lives than those of the SPECT; so PET requires an on-site cyclotron to produce its isotopes. Table 1.2 shows the most common positron-emitting isotopes used in PET. The half-lives and the maximum energy of the emitted positron are also given in the table. PET measures the distribution of the positron-emitting isotope inside the tissue. As Figure 1.23 shows, a number of compounds such as drugs, ligands, neurotransmitters, or genes and gene products can be labeled with a positron-emitting isotope to image their distribution in living tissue. Therefore, PET measures the functional/biochemical or molecular activity within the tissue.

For instance, the most commonly performed ^{18}F-labeled fluoro-deoxy-glucose (abbreviated as ^{18}F-FDG) imaging reveals glucose metabolism in the tissue. Because cancerous tissue in the body is metabolically much more active, a high uptake relative to the surrounding tissue may be an indication of abnormal activity. The major advantages of PET over SPECT include higher sensitivity (approximately 20 times), electronic collimation, a better resolution than that of clinical SPECT, and the use of naturally occurring isotopes.

1.5.1 Positron Emission and Annihilation

The positron was first postulated by Paul Dirac around 1928 and was later discovered by Carl D. Anderson in 1932. It ($\beta+$ particle) is the antimatter of an electron. It has the same mass as electron but with a positive charge. The radioisotopes used in PET are proton-rich isotopes that decay through the emission of positrons.

After emission, the positron travels inside the tissue for a short while, interacting with electrons inside the tissue. It loses its energy and momentum after each interaction. Before it comes to a complete halt, it meets with an electron, and both are annihilated together. From this annihilation, two gamma photons, each with an energy of 511 keV, are produced. The energy of each photon can be calculated by Einstien's well-known equation:

$$E = mc^2 \qquad (1.29)$$

where m is the mass of the electron or positron and c is the speed of light.

These two photons travel almost in opposite directions at about 180° from each other. PET detectors detect these two photons—supposedly produced by the same annihilation event—in coincidence, and register it as an event.

Figure 1.24 shows the positron emission and annihilation process schematically. The distance that the positron travels inside the tissue before annihilation is called the positron range (PR). This distance is a function of the energy of the positron immediately after emission. As Table 1.2 shows, each isotope emits positrons with different maximum energies, and the PR is directly related to its maximum energy. It is not easy to estimate the PR, as the positron travels in a very zigzag path through tissue. The values given in Table 1.2 are empirically determined average mean distances. We should note that the PR is our uncertainty about the point of annihilation when we try to locate the radioisotope distribution. The PR is also a function of the density of the matter.

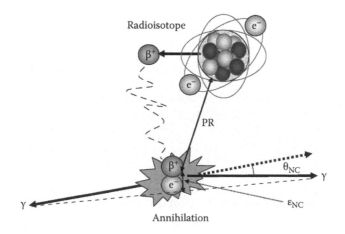

FIGURE 1.24
Positron emission and annihilation process. (Modified from S. R. Cherry, J. A. Sorenson, and M. E. Phelps, *Physics in Nuclear Medicine*, third edition, Philadelphia, Pennsylvania: Saunders, 2003. With permission.)

The two photons resulting from the annihilation event are not always at 180° to each other. The residual energy the positron may have before annihilation results in a deviation in the angle from 180°. This is called photon noncolinearity (NC). In Figure 1.24, this deviation is denoted by θ_{NC}. When the angle is different from 180°, the line of response (LOR), which is the line along which the two photons travel, is wrongly estimated— as the dotted line shown in Figure 1.24—because the detection process always assumes that the angle is 180°. The error committed due to the NC in estimating the actual location of annihilation is denoted by ε_{NC} in Figure 1.24. The NC ultimately influences the image resolution, as we will discuss later.

1.5.2 Coincidence Detection

As mentioned, PET detects the two photons traveling in opposite directions in coincidence. If two opposing detectors (A and B in Figure 1.25, for instance) detect photons within a short time window (e.g., ~12 ns), then an event is registered for those two particular detectors. The LOR in this case is a line—or rather a rectangular prism whose base is equal to the surface

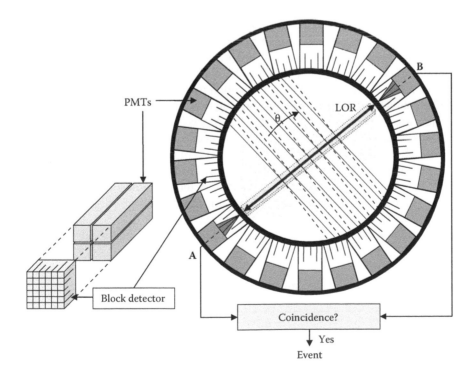

FIGURE 1.25
A block detector and a single ring of block detectors. In conventional PET systems, the blocks of detectors are arranged in a ring shape.

of the detector—between the two opposing detectors. If we keep registering events for a time period, which is called the *scan time*, the resultant number of events will be the sum of the distribution of the activity or the line integral along the LOR.

1.5.3   Photon Detection and Event Registration

The photon detection process in PET is very similar to that of gamma cameras. However, different types of crystals are used as we are dealing with higher-energy gamma photons. There are four different types of crystals used in today's commercial PET scanners. These are bismuth germinate (BGO), gadolinium oxyorthosilicate (GSO), lutetium oxyorthosilicate (LSO), and yttrium oxyorthosilicate (YSO). Each has its own characteristics that make it superior or inferior depending on the application in which it is used. Here, we will mention only four important properties. More in-depth information can be obtained from [9]. These properties are density, decay constant, light output, and energy resolution.

Table 1.3 shows these properties of the crystals used in today's commercial PET scanners. The shaded figures are the best ones among their counterparts. Ideally, it is desired to have a higher density, higher light yield or output, lower decay constant, and smaller energy resolution. The first increases the stopping power, the second improves the energy resolution, the third reduces the dead time and randoms, and the last one enables better rejection of the scattered photons. Among the ones given in Table 1.3, LSO crystals seem to have the best properties needed in an ideal scintillator, whereas GSO crystals have the advantage of having the best energy resolution.

There are three types of events in PET. A *true* event results when the two photons come from the same annihilation event. A *scatter* results when one or both photons, having undergone scattering in the tissue, are detected as though they have originated from the same annihilation event. A *random* event is registered by an opposing pair of detectors when two unrelated photons are detected within the same coincidence timing window.

Figure 1.25 shows block detectors and a ring of detectors. Crystals are normally cut in blocks (typically 6 × 6 or 8 × 8 elements) and attached to the PM

TABLE 1.3

Properties of the crystals commonly used in PET (the shaded figures are the best properties)

Crystal types	BGO	GSO	LSO	YSO
Density (g/cm³)	7.13	6.71	7.4	4.53
Light yield (photons/KeV)	6	10	29	46
Decay constant (ns)	300	60	40	70
Energy resolution, $\Delta E/E$ (%)	10.2	8.5	10	12.5

Source: D. L. Bailey, D. W. Townsend, P. E. Valk, and M. N. Maisey, *Positron Emission Tomography: Basic Sciences*, Springer-Verlag London Limited, 2004.

tubes. In current clinical PET systems, it is very common to have at least three crystal rings. In some systems, the rings are separated by movable septa made usually of tungsten. When the septa are extended, only certain rings are in coincidence with each other. This mode of acquisition is called 2-D. When the septa are retracted, however, almost every ring of the detector is in coincidence with the others. The mode of operation in this case is called 3-D. The major difference between these two modes of operation is in the proportion of the scattered photons and the overall sensitivity of the system. The sensitivity in 3-D mode is higher (approximately fivefold), but so also is the scatter fraction. The scatter fraction in 2-D mode is approximately 15%, whereas in 3-D mode, it is 45%. However, some of the current commercial systems do not have any septa, and therefore always operate in 3-D mode.

As we have mentioned earlier, the registered events represent the summation of activity within the tissue along the LORs. Thus, at the end, parallel LORs rearranged into a sinogram are reconstructed by a reconstruction algorithm into a volumetric image that represents the distribution of the activity in the tissue volume. We will not discuss the reconstruction algorithms here, but they can be found in many relevant textbooks. However, it is probably worth mentioning that the statistical iterative methods have almost become the standard method, mainly for two reasons, as computer technology and algorithms have advanced. First, it is possible to reconstruct images within a reasonable time. Second, these techniques have the advantage of being able to model the noise and imaging systems and incorporate them into the reconstruction process to improve the signal-to-noise ratio and resolution.

1.5.4 Axial Sampling in PET

A clinical PET camera typically consists of three blocks of rings. Each block may have 6×6 or 8×8 detector elements. If the latter is the case, we have a total of 24 rings of detectors spanning the entire axial FOV. A PET system with these characteristics will produce a volume image with 47 planes or slices. Where do the extra 23 slices come from? The 24 image planes are formed from the LORs between the detectors within each individual detector ring (see Figure 1.26). These are called *direct planes*. The remaining planes are formed by the LORs between the detectors of the adjacent rings (see again Figure 1.26). These planes are called *cross planes*, which fall halfway between the direct planes. Thus, a system with n detector rings will generate an image of $2n - 1$ planes. This is how the axial sampling is improved in PET. Figure 1.26 illustrates the direct and cross planes of a hypothetical six-ring system.

1.5.5 Spatial Resolution in PET

The resolution in transaxial FOV or in-plane resolution is not shift invariant. That is, the resolution varies in a transaxial slice depending on the

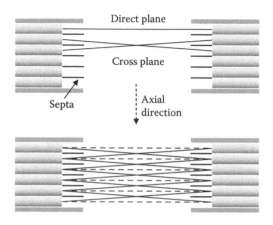

FIGURE 1.26

Top: Cross section of a detector with six rings. Axial sampling in 2-D mode (septa extended). The direct planes are due to the LORs between the detectors within a ring. The cross planes are formed by the LORs between adjacent rings The straight line at the top denotes the first plane (slice), whereas the two crossed lines denote the fourth plane. Bottom: Dashed lines denote the six direct planes, whereas solid lines denote the five cross planes.

location. It is different at different radial locations within the transaxial FOV. Resolution has two components, the transaxial (in-plane) and axial. The in-plane resolution has two components, namely, radial and tangential (see Figure 1.27). There are a number of factors determining the resolution of a PET system. The resolution of PET is normally measured with a small (≤1 mm in diameter) point source of activity in terms of FWHM. The resolution in PET will also differ depending on the mode of operation—2-D or 3-D.

Here, we will briefly discuss the important factors affecting PET resolution. The first factor is the size of the individual detector crystal, which may vary in the range (4–6) × (4–6) × (30) mm. The contribution of this

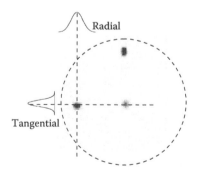

FIGURE 1.27

Images of three point sources showing the components of the transaxial resolution.

factor is about $d/2$, where d is the face size of the crystal. The second factor is the internal coupling within the block detector and the anger logic, which is the method used to position the signal within the block. The third factor is photon noncolinearity, which was discussed earlier. This is a function of both the ring diameter and the radioisotope (see Table 1.2). The θ_{NC} (see Figure 1.24) is about $\pm 0.5°$, and its contribution to overall resolution, in terms of FWHM, is given by [1]

$$R_{NC} = 0.0022D \qquad (1.30)$$

where D is the detector ring diameter. For example, for a PET scanner with a 80 cm ring diameter, R_{NC} would be 0.176 mm (0.0022*800). The fourth important factor influencing the resolution is the positron range. Let us remember that we can determine the position of the annihilation but not the actual location of the radiopharmaceutical. The difference between the two positions is the positron range, which also contributes to the overall blurring (resolution) in the image. Remember also that the positron range is a function of the energy of the emitted positron. It is, for instance, about 0.2 mm for ^{18}F and 2.6 mm for ^{82}Rb [1]. The last critical factor affecting the resolution is the reconstruction filter. The overall image resolution in PET can therefore be given by

$$R_{image} = \sqrt{R_{det}^2 + R_{PR}^2 + R_{NC}^2 + R_{recon}^2} \qquad (1.31)$$

There are also other factors affecting the resolution such as the stopping power of the crystal, incident angle of the photon on the detector, and the distance between the individual detectors [9]. Given all these factors, the current commercial systems have an overall in-plane resolution of 4–7 mm at 10 cm from the center.

Due to undersampling in the axial direction, it is difficult to measure the axial resolution from a point source. For instance, in a 47-slice clinical PET with an axial field of view (FOV) of approximately 150–160 mm, the slice thickness is around 3.27 mm (156/47). This is equivalent to sampling the point spread function once, because such a system would have an axial resolution of about 5 mm. Moving the source in small steps and recording the peak count, as suggested in Bailey et al. [9], may provide a solution to the undersampling problem in the axial direction.

1.5.6 Quantization in PET

PET is an innately quantitative imaging modality. However, to obtain an accurate measurement of the radiopharmaceutical concentration, the PET data have to be corrected for a number of degrading factors. These are attenuation, scatter, and randoms. The scanner also has to be calibrated for detector efficiency differences and geometric factors due to the curvature of the rings. The latter calibrations are all done as part of the quarterly tests/calibration procedures known as normalization.

Here, we will discuss the corrections for the attenuation and normalization for detection efficiency differences, as they are more relevant to the subject of image processing. The discussions about the corrections for scatter and randoms can be found in Bailey et al. [9].

1.5.7　Normalization

The physical properties of the individual detectors vary; so do the detector efficiencies. The correction for this problem is fairly straightforward. A uniform source of activity is used to uniformly irradiate all the detectors. Therefore, if the detector efficiencies were the same, the counts for all the LORs would be the same. The detectors are calibrated for differences in their efficiencies using an external positron source. If a uniform source irradiates the detectors, all lines of response (LORs) will approximately have the same coincident photon flux. A long (~12 h) scan is acquired with a uniform source. The correction factors are calculated as

$$F_{i,j}^{norm} = \frac{N_{i,j}}{\frac{1}{n}\sum_{k=1}^{n} N_{i,j}} \tag{1.32}$$

where $N_{i,j}$ are the counts of the LOR for the pair of detectors i and j, and n is the number of detector pairs. Then each acquired clinical image $C_{i,j}$ is corrected as follows:

$$C_{i,j} = \frac{C_{i,j}}{F_{i,j}^{norm}} \tag{1.33}$$

Note that this correction is performed on the raw or sinogram data before the reconstruction is carried out.

Let us demonstrate this process on a hypothetical image generated by the MATLAB function randn (see Figure 1.28, left image). Let us suppose that this image shows the acquired image using an external source during calibrations. The normalization factors are then calculated by computing the average of the counts for all LORs and dividing the individual count of every detector pair by the average. The following MATLAB script creates the acquired image, computes the normalization factors, and lastly normalizes the acquired image:

```
nimg = round(10*randn(8) + 50);
fimg = img/mean2(nimg);
cimg = nimg./fimg;
```

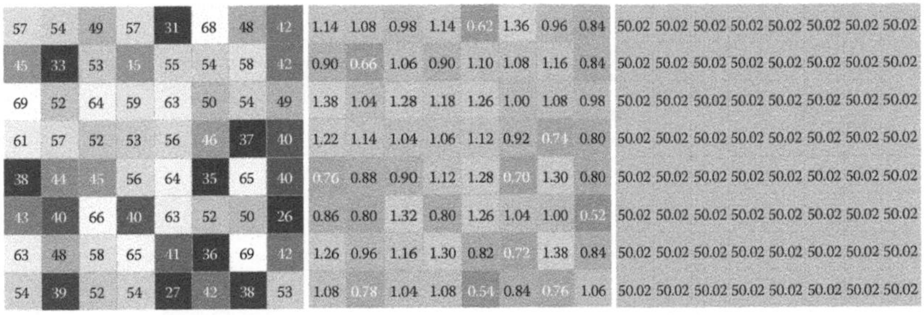

57	54	49	57	31	68	48	42	1.14	1.08	0.98	1.14	0.62	1.36	0.96	0.84	50.02	50.02	50.02	50.02	50.02	50.02	50.02	50.02
45	33	53	45	55	54	58	42	0.90	0.66	1.06	0.90	1.10	1.08	1.16	0.84	50.02	50.02	50.02	50.02	50.02	50.02	50.02	50.02
69	52	64	59	63	50	54	49	1.38	1.04	1.28	1.18	1.26	1.00	1.08	0.98	50.02	50.02	50.02	50.02	50.02	50.02	50.02	50.02
61	57	52	53	56	46	37	40	1.22	1.14	1.04	1.06	1.12	0.92	0.74	0.80	50.02	50.02	50.02	50.02	50.02	50.02	50.02	50.02
38	44	45	56	64	35	65	40	0.76	0.88	0.90	1.12	1.28	0.70	1.30	0.80	50.02	50.02	50.02	50.02	50.02	50.02	50.02	50.02
43	40	66	40	63	52	50	26	0.86	0.80	1.32	0.80	1.26	1.04	1.00	0.52	50.02	50.02	50.02	50.02	50.02	50.02	50.02	50.02
63	48	58	65	41	36	69	42	1.26	0.96	1.16	1.30	0.82	0.72	1.38	0.84	50.02	50.02	50.02	50.02	50.02	50.02	50.02	50.02
54	39	52	54	27	42	38	53	1.08	0.78	1.04	1.08	0.54	0.84	0.76	1.06	50.02	50.02	50.02	50.02	50.02	50.02	50.02	50.02

FIGURE 1.28
Illustration of the correction for the differences in detector efficiencies. Left: Image supposedly acquired during a quarterly calibration. Middle: Calculated during quarterly calibrations. Right: Factors applied to the image on the left.

The middle image in Figure 1.28 shows the normalization factors. The right image, however, is the corrected image. All the intensities are the same in the calibrated since we calibrated the image from which we calculated the factors. Note that here we normalized the image supposedly acquired during calibrations to show the process, but normally the acquired image is used only once to calculate the factors, and then the factors are applied to routine clinical images.

1.5.8 Attenuation Correction

Photoelectric absorption and Compton scattering may result in the total absorption (or attenuation) of gamma photons. The degree of absorption depends on the electron density of the tissue and the total length traveled by the two photons that emanate from the positron annihilation. At 511 keV, the photoelectric absorption is almost negligible. Most interactions occur in the form of a Compton interaction, in which the photon interacts with a loosely bound electron and gets deflected, and as a result, loses some of its energy. The deflected photons may get out of the FOV and escape detection. The absorption of photons within the tissue affects the accurate measurement of the in vivo concentration of radiopharmaceuticals labeled with positron emitters. Attenuation correction (AC) in PET is therefore required to accurately quantify the distribution of radiopharmaceuticals in the tissue.

If the survival probability of γ_1 photon, shown in Figure 1.29, is $p_1 = e^{-\mu a}$, where μ is the attenuation coefficient of the tissue and the survival probability of γ_2 is $p_2 = e^{-\mu b}$, then the survival probability of both photons is

$$p_{12} = e^{-\mu a}e^{-\mu b} = e^{-\mu(a+b)} = e^{-\mu D} \tag{1.34}$$

as they are two independent events.

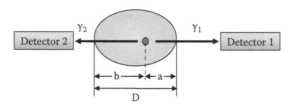

FIGURE 1.29
Attenuation of gamma photons.

The attenuation in PET, thus, is a function of the total body length D. Therefore, attenuation correction factors (ACFs) can easily be calculated if we acquire a transmission reference scan. ACFs are computed by taking the ratio (pixel-by-pixel) of the blank reference scan, normalized for the scan duration, to the transmission scan. We will refer to this ratio as the measured attenuation correction (MAC) factor. A high-count blank reference scan is normally acquired at the beginning of the day without a subject in the gantry, and transmission scans are acquired after positioning subjects in the scanner. In both scans, external radioactive sources are used. The MAC is then performed simply by multiplying (pixel-by-pixel) every emission sinogram with the ACFs. This method of correction has become obsolete with the introduction of PET/CT scanners. Now, in PET/CT scanners, the CT scan is used to obtain ACFs at 511 keV. We know that CT scans are normally acquired at a different energy than that of 511 keV; therefore, they represent the attenuation at this lower energy. The CT values represented in Hounsfield units are mapped to the attenuation factors at 511 keV using methods such as bilinear mapping [10].

1.5.9   Absolute Quantification

Absolute quantification (AQ) is expressing activity in terms of the activity per unit volume. To do this, a calibration factor that maps counts per second (cps) into activity per unit volume (mCi/cc or MBq/cc) is generated. This process, which is illustrated in Figure 1.30, is fairly straightforward. A known amount of activity is injected into a water phantom, whose volume is also known, and scanned with the PET scanner. From the volume image, this factor is calculated and used later to quantify patient images. Note that this factor is applied to voxels of the reconstructed tomographic image, whereas the other corrections discussed previously are applied to the sinogram data.

[18]F-labeled flourodeoxyglucose (FDG) PET has been proved effective in characterizing the nature of tumor lesions by measuring glucose metabolism. The standard uptake value (SUV), a semiquantitative determination of tissue activity, represents the amount of uptake in a given volume of

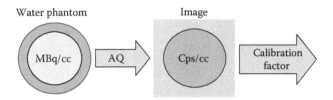

FIGURE 1.30
Absolute quantification process.

interest (VOI) normalized by the injected dose and the body weight. It is given by

$$SUV = \frac{\text{Tissue activity } (\mu Ci/cc)}{\text{Injected Dose}(\mu Ci)/\text{Body Weight (g)}} \qquad (1.35)$$

Although there are a number of factors affecting the SUV, such as blood glucose, partial volume effect, body composition and habitus (e.g., fat has a lower uptake), and uptake period (elapsed time from tracer injection to the time of PET scan), nowadays it is common practice to report the activity values in terms of SUV. The SUV may be helpful to distinguish benign tissue from malignant, and to assess the response to therapy.

1.5.10 Scan modes in PET

There are two scan modes in PET: static and dynamic. These modes should not be mixed with the 2-D and 3-D data acquisition modes that we discussed earlier. In the subsequent sections, we will briefly discuss these two scan modes.

1.5.11 Static Scan

Clinical scans are usually static scans in which patients are scanned after an uptake period of approximately 1 h. As the axial FOVs for most clinical scans are typically around 16 cm, it takes several axial FOVs, which is also called bed positions, to scan a whole body. In a PET/CT scanner, the CT scan of the whole body is usually performed in a helical mode. Then the PET scan is performed in a step-and-shoot mode, acquiring for about 2–4 min at each bed position. Hence, a whole-body PET scan takes about 20–25 min, depending on the number of bed positions needed to cover the length of the patient and the preferred scan time per bed position. Figure 1.31 shows transaxial slices at the thorax level from a whole-body PET/CT image acquired by a GE Discovery ST PET/CT scanner.

Static brain imaging has found widespread applications in areas such as oncology, in which accurate detection of recurrent brain tumors after

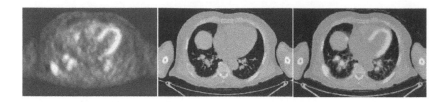

FIGURE 1.31
Transaxial PET/CT images at the thorax level acquired by a GE Discovery ST scanner. Left: FDG PET image. Middle: CT image. Right: Fused PET and CT images.

treatment is needed, and epilepsy. Current image registration algorithms, of which the mutual-information-based one is the most popular, allow accurate registration of PET and MR volume images. This significantly improves the detection and/or localization of the tumor uptake in PET. Figure 1.32 shows transaxial slices from the brain images of a patient with a brain tumor. The images were registered using a commercial software package. The PET, MR, and fused images are shown from left to right, respectively. The uptake denoted by the arrow indicates that the tumor, which is discernible in the MR image, is metabolically active only in its center.

MR images, in which the tumor boundary is usually better discernable than in PET, can help us to identify the tumor lesion and to quantify the uptake in PET. Image segmentation methods, which are discussed in Chapters 6 and 7, can be used to identify the tumor tissue. The registration of the two modalities also can be helpful in guiding tumor biopsy to the most active part of the tumor, as tumor uptake is often heterogeneous.

1.5.12 Dynamic Scan

FDG is an analog of glucose. It is chemically similar to glucose, and is transported through the blood–brain barrier by a facilitated transfer. The

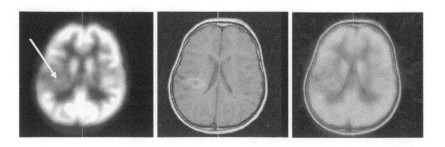

FIGURE 1.32
PET and MRI images of a patient with a brain tumor. Images are registered using registration software and then fused. From left to right are PET, MR, and fused images, respectively. PET image indicates a higher activity in the center of the tumor, pointed by arrow.

glucose is phosphorylated by hexokinase to glucose-6-PO_4, which is further metabolized in the glycolytic pathway. FDG, similar to glucose, is also phosphorylated to FDG—6-PO_4; therefore, it is a competitive substrate with glucose in this phosphorylation step. FDG—6-PO_4, however, is not a substrate for further metabolism, and it also does not diffuse across cell membranes; therefore, it is metabolically trapped inside the cell. This characteristic of FDG makes it an ideal tracer for imaging metabolic activity in the tissue. Thus, the rate of the phosphorylation of the FDG—6-PO_4 will reflect the rate of glycolysis in the tissue.

In static FDG PET, images show the accumulation of FDG—6-PO_4 within the tissue, and FDG in the tissue and plasma. As we have mentioned previously, there are a number of factors affecting the amount of activity measured via static imaging. For this reason, the tracer distribution measured from a static image is regarded as a semiquantitative measure. The term *quantitative measure* refers to the metabolic rate of FDG obtained via dynamic imaging by means of kinetic modeling. The dynamic scan is the imaging of the time course of the activity distribution in the tissue. It involves capturing the volume distribution of the activity at certain time intervals for certain time durations. Because of the normally longer scan time and their cumbersomeness, dynamic scans are not preferred in routine clinical studies. Moreover, kinetic modeling requires sampling of an arterial input curve. This is a process that may further complicate the imaging procedure. The two major advantages of quantification via a dynamic scan, however, are the ability to quantify the actual glucose metabolism (μmole/g/min) and avoidance of most factors affecting the activity measured by a static scan. Despite their difficulties, dynamic scans are often preferred and carried out in clinical trials or research studies.

We will not discuss the details of kinetic modeling in PET here, but interested readers may refer to Hobbie and Roth [1] and Macovski [4] for further knowledge. Readers interested in learning more about PET instrumentation may refer to the articles in references [11–13]. For a comprehensive review of PET/CT scanners, the reader can also refer to David, Thomas, and Todd [14].

Problems

1. Calculate the energy of one of the γ photons produced from the annihilation of a positron and an electron in terms of keV.

2. Show that the FWHM of two cascade imaging systems is equal to $FWHM_{cascaded} = \sqrt{FWHM_1^2 + FWHM_2^2}$, where $FWHM_i$ ($i = 1, 2$) is the FWHM of the ith system. Assume that the transfer function of the two subsystems are approximated by the Gaussian function of σ.

3. The measured line integral for each ray in an x-ray projection is given by $P = \ln\left(\frac{N_0}{N}\right) = \int \mu dx$, where N_0 and N are the average number of x-ray photons entering the tissue, and transmitted to the detector, respectively. Calculate the mean and the variance of the line integral, assuming that the line integral P is a function of the random variable X: $P = \ln\left(\frac{N_0}{X}\right)$, where X is Poisson distributed.

4. In spiral CT, the simple z-interpolation (see Figure 1.10) known as 360 LI is given by Kalender [3] $P_z(i,\theta) = (1-w) \cdot P_j(i,\theta) + w \cdot P_{j+1}(i,\theta)$ where $w = (z_R - z)/d$ and $P_j(i,\theta)$ is the projection in the jth rotation at position $z_j < z_R \cdot z_j$ is the closest distance to z_R, d is the table feed distance in mm/rotation, and z_R is the location of the calculated projection. For a 360° spiral rotation, the weights w and $1 - w$ vary between 0 and 1 but are the same for all the rays (i s). Compute the variance of the calculated projection P_z if the variances of the individual projections are equal to σ.

5. Calculate the resolution (FWHM) of a low-energy collimator with a depth of 2.4 cm and hole diameter of 0.25 cm at source distances $b = 0$ cm and $b = 10$ cm.

6. Calculate the collimator resolution (FWHM) of a gamma camera system with an intrinsic resolution of 3.5 mm at 10 cm from the detector and an extrinsic resolution of 12 mm at 10 cm from the detector.

7. Figure 1.26 shows the axial sampling for direct and cross planes, when the ring difference is 0 and ±1, respectively. Draw the axial sampling for direct and cross planes for ring differences of 0 and ±1 for direct planes and ±1 and ±3 for cross planes.

References

1. R. K. Hobbie and B. J. Roth, *Intermediate Physics for Medicine and Biology*, 3rd ed., New York: Springer-Verlag, 1997.
2. A. C. Kak and M. Slaney, *Principles of Computerized Tomographic Imaging*, New York: IEEE Press, 1988.
3. W. A. Kalender, *Computed Tomography: Fundamentals, System Technology, Image Quality, Applications* Publicis MCD. Munich, Germany: Verlag, 2000.
4. A. Macovski, *Medical Imaging Systems*. Englewood Cliffs, NJ: Prentice-Hall, 1983.
5. F. Bloch, Nuclear induction, *Physical Review*, 70: 460–474, 1946.
6. S. R. Cherry, J. A. Sorenson, and M. E. Phelps, *Physics in Nuclear Medicine*, 3rd ed. Philadelphia, PA: Saunders, 2003.

7. M. T. Madsen, Recent advances in SPECT imaging. *J Nucl Med* 48: 661–673, 2007.
8. M. N. Wernick and J. N. Aarsvold, *Emission Tomography: The Engineering and Physics of PET and SPECT*. San Diego, CA: Academic Press, 2004.
9. D. L. Bailey, D. W. Townsend, P. E. Valk, and M. N. Maisey, *Positron Emission Tomography: Basic Sciences*, London: Springer-Verlag London Limited, 2004.
10. P. E. Kinahan, B. Hasegawa, and T. Beyer, x-ray-based attenuation correction for positron emission tomography/Computed tomography scanners. *Semin. Nucl. Med* XXXIII: 166–179, 2003.
11. F. H. Fahey, Data Acquisition in PET Imaging. *J Nucl Med Technol* 30: 39–49, 2002.
12. G. Tarantola, F. Zito, and P. Gerundini, PET Instrumentation and Reconstruction Algorithms in Whole-Body Applications. *J Nucl Med* 44: 756–769, 2003.
13. T. G. Turkington, Introduction to PET instrumentation. *J Nucl Med Technol* 29: 4–11, 2001.
14. W. T. David, B. Thomas, and M. B. Todd, PET/CT scanners: A hardware approach to image fusion. *Semin Nucl Med* 33: 193–204, 2003.

2

Fundamental Tools for Image
Processing and Analysis

CONTENTS

2.1   Introduction

In this chapter, we introduce and discuss some fundamental image processing and analysis techniques using MATLAB®. The techniques presented here are utilized throughout the book. We also present some advanced techniques for the efficient processing and analysis of two-dimensional (2-D) and three-dimensional (3-D) images.

The MATLAB Image Processing Toolbox includes many basic functions that are used in typical image processing applications. The MATLAB documentation contains plenty of information about these functions and examples about their use. The concepts introduced and functions provided in this chapter in general differ from those available in the Image Processing Toolbox. Some topics available in MATLAB are included only for completeness.

We intend to introduce image processing tools that can be used to help build applications for solving general image processing and analysis problems. As our experience is primarily with medical and biological images, these will dominate the examples provided throughout the book.

We will demonstrate the use of these techniques and functions on 2-D or 3-D images, the latter being emphasized more when deemed necessary. Although MATLAB has been improving its library of functions applicable directly to 3-D volumetric images, to date there has generally been little emphasis on 3-D image processing and analysis. We will extend some of our 2-D analysis techniques to 3-D analysis, if not straightforward to do so. In order to follow this chapter, the readers should be familiar with the general matrix operations in MATLAB and have a basic level of programming experience and knowledge.

2.2 Definition of Digital Image

A digital image is a discrete function defined over a rectangular grid (lattice) representing the characteristics of the objects being imaged. In 2-D images, each grid element, or "pixel," is defined by a location and a value representing a characteristic of the object at that location (see Figure 2.1). Different names may be used to refer to the pixel value; for example, gray value, gray-level intensity, intensity, and brightness. Depending on the modality used to generate an image, intensity value may represent different characteristics of the object under investigation. Pixel intensity represents the attenuation of tissue to x-ray in computer tomography (CT), the amount of light in family pictures taken by a CCD camera, proton density in magnetic resonance imaging (MRI), tissue reflectivity at the boundaries in the case of ultrasound (US), radioactivity concentration within the body in positron emission tomography (PET) or single photon emission tomography (SPECT), and so on. Chapter 1 discussed major medical imaging modalities in more detail.

Images in which each pixel is assigned a single value, as in the above examples, are called *scalar-valued images*. Images in which each pixel is represented by a vector are called *vector-valued* or *multispectral images*. Typical examples of multispectral images in medicine and biology are red green blue (RGB) color images and magnetic resonance (MR) diffusion tensor images. Multispectral images such as color images will have pixels

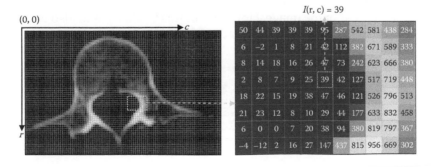

FIGURE 2.1
A 2-D image where *r* and *c* represent the row and column numbers respectively, of each pixel.

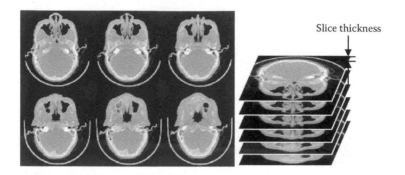

FIGURE 2.2
Transaxial slices from a 3-D CT image $I(x, y, z)$, where z refers to the slice number.

represented by vectors. Each pixel will therefore have more than one intensity value. In multispectral images, the third dimension is referred to as the spectrum, band, or channel.

Images can be 3-D, four-dimensional (4-D), or N-dimensional for that matter. Generally, 2-D images are represented by 2-D matrices, $I(x, y)$; 3-D (or volume) images are represented by a stack of 2-D images, $I(x, y, z)$ (see Figure 2.2). In a 3-D volumetric image of a body, obtained by a CT scan for example, although it may not be obvious, each slice has a thickness representing the characteristics of a slab of body tissue. 4-D images are generally sets of 3-D images taken over time, $I(x, y, z, t)$ (see Figure 2.3). The dynamic PET image data set is a typical example of a 4-D image. Such volumetric PET images represent tissue activity distribution acquired at specified intervals for the purpose of quantifying actual metabolic activity in tissue. Although most of the concepts and methods discussed here can be extended to 4-D images, for the remainder of this text we will limit our discussion to 2-D and 3-D images.

It should be noted that indexing in MATLAB is different from the conventional indexing, $I(x, y)$, in which x and y denote the column and row numbers, respectively. Using MATLAB indexing, the (1,1) point is the upper left corner of the image. However, in this book, we will also use the convention of $I(x, y)$ in the presentation of topics.

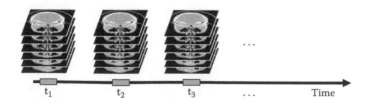

FIGURE 2.3
A 4-D image generally is a set of 3-D images acquired over time.

2.3 Image Types in MATLAB

In the MATLAB Image Processing Toolbox, there are four types of images:

- Indexed
- Intensity
- Binary
- RGB

An indexed image consists of a data matrix and a colormap matrix. The colormap matrix is an m-by-3 array of class double containing floating-point values in the range [0, 1] [Image Processing Toolbox User's Guide]. The data matrix value for each pixel in the indexed image is an index to the colormap matrix. The value 1 points to the first row of the map, the value 2 points to the second row, and so on.

An intensity image consists of a single data matrix, each element of which denotes the intensity of the corresponding pixel. As imaging scientists in the medical imaging field, the images we work with are mainly intensity images.

A binary image is stored as a logical array. Each element of the array takes one of two values (i.e., each pixel is turned on or off), and is represented by a byte. The following excerpt from the Image Processing Toolbox User's Guide describes the color images in MATLAB!

> "An RGB image, sometimes referred to as a truecolor image, is stored in MATLAB as an m-by-n-by-3 data array that defines red, green, and blue color components for each individual pixel. RGB images do not use a palette. The color of each pixel is determined by the combination of the red, green, and blue intensities stored in each color plane at the pixel's location. Graphics file formats store RGB images as 24-bit images, where the red, green, and blue components are 8 bits each. This yields a potential of 16 million colors. The precision with which a real-life image can be replicated has led to the commonly used term true color image."

The Toolbox includes various functions to convert between these different image types. For detailed information, the reader can again refer to the MATLAB help pages.

2.4 Image Display

The Image Processing Toolbox has several functions to display 2-D images. These are imshow, image, imagesc, subimage, and imview. The function imagesc is the same as the function image except that it automatically scales the image intensities before display. The function subimage is used together with subplot to display multiple images in a single figure window. The attributes of each subimage (e.g., colormap) can be set separately. The image functions mentioned return a handle to the image object that enables changing image attributes. The two functions iptgetpref, and iptsetpref can get and set the preferences of the Image Processing Toolbox. Volume images or multiple 2-D images can be displayed slice by slice or all together using the montage function in MATLAB. In Section 2.8.3, we present an image display tool, imlook3d, to display 3-D images. The imlook3d graphical user interface (GUI) includes some basic processing functions as well.

2.4.1   Superimposing a Binary Image on a Gray-Level Image

It is often necessary to display a gray-level image overlaid with its processed (e.g., segmented) version. Here, we present a simple function code that can accomplish this task. The function overlays a binary image, the second input argument, onto the gray-level image gimg, the first input argument with a color of choice

```
% function J = mipimoverlay (gimg,bimg,c)
% c = 1: red, 2:green, 3:blue, 4:white
function J= mipimoverlay(gimg,bimg,c)
Mx = max(gimg(:));
gimg(bimg==1) = 0;
J=cat(3,gimg,gimg,gimg);
if Mx < 255
    gimg(bimg==1) = 255;
else
    gimg(bimg==1) = 65535;
end
J(:,:,c) = gimg;
if c==4
    J = cat(3,gimg,gimg,gimg);
else
J(:,:,c) = gimg;
end
```

This function creates a color image in which one component (e.g., red if c = 1) is zero everywhere except for pixels that are 1 in the binary image. These pixels are assigned values 255 or 65535, depending on the maximum intensity in the intensity image. The other two components retain their original intensities.

Let us demonstrate how to overlay a binary image on an intensity image using the "rice" image available in MATLAB. First, we create a binary image using a threshold of 150, and then detect the boundary pixels using

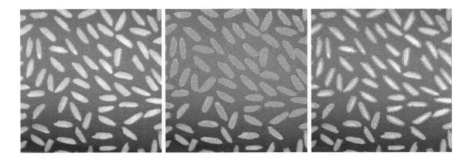

FIGURE 2.4
Left: Original rice image. Middle: Color image on which binary regions are overlaid. Right: Color image on which the boundaries are overlaid.

bwperim function. Lastly, we overlay the binary boundary image on the original rice image using our mipimoverlay function. The following code identifies the rice boundaries and overlays them on the intensity image:

```
I = imread('rice.png');
BW = I > 150;
BWP = bwperim(BW,8);
J = imoverlay(I,BWP,1);
imagesc(I); imagesc(J);
```

In Figure 2.4, the original rice image and the overlaid images are shown. In the middle image, binary rice regions are overlaid, whereas in the right image, boundaries are superimposed only.

2.4.2 Image Fusion

With the introduction of hybrid imaging modalities and robust image registration software programs, it has become routine to display images from different modalities that are superimposed or fused. In medical imaging, the term *image fusion* may be used to mean both image registration and superimposition of already registered images. When we use the term image fusion here, we mean the superimposition of two images from different modalities that are already registered into a common coordinate system. We will demonstrate how this can be done in MATLAB using the PET and CT images that are obtained by a PET/CT scanner. Such hybrid scanners acquire the PET and CT images registered (hardware registration) in the same coordinate system. PET images show functional biochemical activity, whereas CT images show anatomical structures. In the former, the boundaries of anatomical structures are not very clear due largely to the limited resolution. The CT image of the PET/CT scanner is used mainly to locate the functional activity identified in the PET image.

Let us suppose that `PETImg` and `CTImg` are names of arrays that each holds a single slice of a PET and a CT image, respectively. First, let us set the number of gray levels displayed to 255.

```
numGrayLevels = 255;
```

Because a CT image has a wide range of intensities, we like to limit our range by −600 and 1250; this range is very similar to the bone window used in radiology. We assign all pixels outside the range the value nan.

```
CTLower = -600;
CTUpper = 1250;
CTImg(CTImg < CTLower) = nan;
CTImg(CTImg >= CTUpper) = nan;
```

Similarly, let us also limit the range of PET values,

```
PETLower = 2;
PETUpper = 20;
PETimg(PETimg < PETLower) = nan;
PETimg(PETimg >= PETUpper) = nan;
```

As we know, PET values represent the distribution of a radiopharmaceutical in the tissue, whereas CT values represent tissue attenuation. In the next step, we normalize CT values between [0–numGrayLevels] and PET values between [numGrayLevels+1–2*numGrayLevels].

```
% Normalize CT image between 0 and numGrayLevels
normCTimg = CTimg - min(CTimg(:));
normCTimg = normCTimg/max(normCTimg(:));
normCTimg = numGrayLevels*normCTimg;

% Normalize PET image between numGrayLevels+1 and 2*numGrayLevel
normPETimg = PETimg - min(PETimg(:));
normPETimg = normPETimg/max(normPETimg(:));
normPETimg = numGrayLevels + 1 + numGrayLevels*normPETimg;
```

Then, we create a common colormap to display the values between 0 and 2*numGrayLevels.

```
% Create a common colormap
commonCMAP = [gray(numGrayLevels); hot(numGrayLevels)];
```

It should be noted that the CT values will be represented by the first 256 3-tuple elements of the common map, whereas PET values are represented by the colors from the popular colormap known as *hot*. One can use different colormaps for each intensity range depending on preference. Now we are ready to display the CT and PET images on the same axis.

```
figure (1);
hCTImage = image(CTImg);
hold on;
hPETImage = image(normCTimg);
colormap(commonCMAP);

opacityValue = 0.25;
opacityValues = opacityValue*ones(size(normPETimg));
set(hPETImage,'alphadata',opacityValues);
axis('image');
axis('off');
```

Figure 2.5 shows the separate PET and CT images acquired by a PET/CT scanner and the one fused using the script just mentioned. In our example, the *alphadata* property is manipulated to display the two images in the

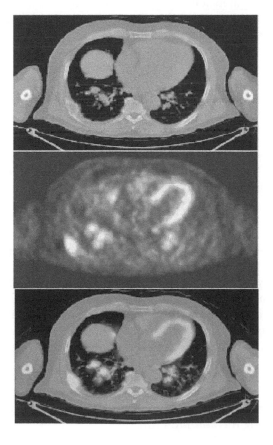

FIGURE 2.5
Images acquired by a PET/CT scanner. Top: CT image shown with bone window. Center: PET image. Bottom: Fused image.

same axis. We set opacity for the PET image to lower values of the whole range, making it partially transparent so the CT image will also be visible. This process is normally applied to the entire volume image rather than a single slice so the slices can be browsed through.

2.5   Image Manipulations

In this section, we will be discussing basic image manipulation techniques using MATLAB.

2.5.1   Row or Column Ordering

While doing matrix operations, it is often most efficient to perform the operation in one dimension. To convert an image matrix, which can be two, three, or multidimensional, to a one-dimensional (1-D) matrix (column vector) we simply use the statement

```
Img = Img(:);
```

For example, if `Img` is a 32×32 image matrix, `nImg = Img(:)` will be a 32*32×1 column vector. To try this out with MATLAB, first create a 32×32 matrix of random numbers using

```
Img = rand(32,32),
```

Then convert this to a column matrix by

```
nImg = Img(:).
```

You can see the sizes of the matrices by typing the command `whos` at the command line.

Before we convert the image matrix into a column vector, we need to be careful that we are using the same variable name to save the column vector, as with this conversion we lose the dimension information regarding our image matrix.

To retain the size information for later use, we must save it into a variable

```
sizeIMG = size(Img);
```

Now, the image matrix can be easily put back into its original multidimensional format using the `reshape` function.

```
Img = reshape(Img, sizeIMG);
```

By the way, the reshape function used here is a handy and most versatile function. Mastering this useful function is important for writing an efficient code. For instance, we can use it to extract a slice from a 3-D image. Let us assume that the image Img(x, y, z) consists of transverse slices (z). The entire image can easily be transformed into coronal views (or slices) using this simple code:

```
[r,c,z]=size(Img);
for i=1:c
 cImg(:,:,i)= reshape(Img(:,i,:),[r z]);
end
```

Similarly, the sagittal slices can be extracted with a little modification in the script:

```
for i=1:r
 sImg(:,:,i)= reshape(Img(i,:,:),[c z]);
end
```

However, this is not the most efficient way for generating orthogonal views. We will discuss codes that are more efficient later in the chapter.

2.5.2 Maximum Intensity Projection (MIP) Images

Maximum intensity projections (MIPs) are frequently used in medical imaging to generate movies in which each frame is the MIP projection of a volume at a different orientation. Let us find the MIP of a 3-D image along one of the orthogonal dimensions. To demonstrate this, we will be using the MR image available in the MATLAB image library. Let us load the image, find the size, and convert the 4-D image to 3-D.

```
% load image
load mri
[r,c,s,z]=size (D);
% convert 4-D image to 3D image here s is 1
Img = reshape(D,[r c z]);
```

Note that we can also use squeeze(D) function to remove singleton dimensions. Then, we find the maximum along the rows; as a result, the image reduces to [c 1 z], and finally remove the singleton dimension again to reduce it to [c z].

```
pimg = squeeze(max(Img,[],1));
```

This process can be generalized as seen in the following function for three orthogonal planes:

```
function pimg = miporthogonal(img,plane)
switch (plane)
    case 1
        pimg = max(img,[],3); % transverse
    case 2
        pimg = squeeze(max(img,[],2)); % coronal
    case 3
        pimg = squeeze(max(img,[],1)); % sagittal
end
```

Figure 2.6 shows the orthogonal MIP projections of a whole-body CT image.

2.5.3　Image Transformations

Image transformations and rotations can be performed using the trans-pose, flipdim, fliplr, flipud, permute, ipermute, and imrotate functions in MATLAB. For an image, transpose operation is equal to a flip and a 90-degree clockwise (CW) rotation. The permute function

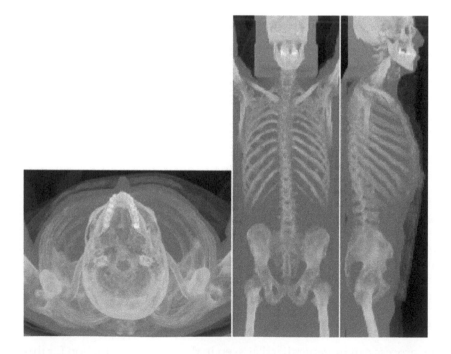

FIGURE 2.6
Orthogonal MIP projections of a whole-body CT image. Left: Transverse. Middle: Coronal. Right: Sagittal.

rearranges the dimension of arrays, and thus can be a useful tool to flip and rotate images faster. `permute` and `ipermute` are generalizations of the function `transpose`.

2.5.4 Changing Image Intensities

In MATLAB, this subject is generally discussed under the title of indexing. We will demonstrate through examples how image intensities can be changed using what is known as the logical indexing method.

We can change all zero intensities to one using

```
Img(Img==0) = 1;
```

This can also be carried out using a *for* loop, in which we visit every element sequentially, but this would be inefficient. Using the aforementioned technique, one can replace a range of numbers. For instance, instead of `Img == 0`, one can use `Img > 200` to change all the intensities greater than 200 in the image. We can change the numbers greater than 10 and less than and equal to 50 in an image by

```
Img (Img > 10 & Img <= 50) = 20;
```

An alternative method of changing the elements of an image matrix is the use of the `find` function. This function locates the intensities specified by an expression. The following script finds the intensities larger than `I1` and replaces them with `I2`:

```
INDX = find (Img > I1);
Img(INDX) = I2;
```

This function can accept any expression usually consisting of variables or smaller expressions joined by relational operators (e.g., lower limit < `Img` < upper limit). The image matrix can have two or more dimensions. `INDX` is a column vector including the location of those intensities specified by the expression.

2.5.5 Replacing `infs` and `nans`

As a result of an image division (element-by-element) operation in which the divisor image has zero elements, we may have nan and `inf`, at the end of the image arithmetic. The following function replaces the infs and nans in a matrix with zero.

```
function Img = mipremoveundefinedNums(X)
sizeX = size(X);
```

```
X = X(:);
X(isnan(X)) = 0;
X(isinf(X)) = 0;
Img = reshape (X, sizeX);
```

Here, we employ the same approach that was used to change the image intensities. Also note the column ordering done before the replacement operation. See also the MATLAB help pages for isnan and isinf.

2.5.6 Concatenating Images

It may be necessary to concatenate images, for instance, to display multiple images together horizontally in a row or vertically in a column format. Images can be concatenated horizontally:

```
ImgH = [Img1, Img2, Img3,…];
```

or vertically

```
ImgV = [Img1; Img2; Img3;…];
```

The image can be displayed using the code

```
Imagesc(ImgH); or Imagesc(ImgV);
```

The cat function can be used to concatenate images as well. To concatenate horizontally or along the second dimension, we use

```
ImgH = cat(2, Img1, Img2, Img3,…);
```

and vertically or along the rows

```
ImgV = cat(1, Img1, Img2, Img3,…);
```

The cat function can also be used to form 3-D volume images from 2-D slices:

```
Newimage = cat(3, Img1, Img2, Img3,…);
```

where Img1 through Img3 are 2-D images.

2.5.7 Plotting Intensity Values in a Row or Column

The following statement plots the intensity profile along the 20th row in a 2-D image:

```
plot(Img(20,:));
```

Similarly, to plot the intensity profile along the 20th column:

```
plot(Img(:, 20))
```

To plot profiles across row and column #20, respectively, in a certain slice of a 3-D image

```
plot(Img(20,:,sliceNum));
plot(Img(:,20,sliceNum));
```

To plot or extract any profile interactively or noninteractively from 2-D images, MATLAB offers the function improfile. When executed, this function allows one to choose the beginning and the end of a line segment along which the intensity values will be extracted or plotted. It can also be used to calculate the intensity profile along a line segment specified by a set of points (r_i, c_i). The reader can refer to the help pages in MATLAB for further explanation of the usage of this function.

2.5.8 Resizing Images

Resizing images (downsampling or upsampling) may be required for processing, analysis, or display purposes (e.g., zooming in or out). There are two functions, imresize and interp2, available in MATLAB for resizing 2-D images. To interpolate (or resize) 3-D images in the 3-D image space, the interp3 function can be used. Alternatively, 3-D images can be resized slice-by-slice if the slice thickness is to be retained. An interpolation method can be specified as an input argument. The nearest, bilinear and bicubic methods are the available one. In the following example script, we create an 11×11 image of a 2-D Gaussian function with $\sigma = 2$ using fspecial, and then upsample it with a ratio of 4:1.

```
Img = fspecial('gauss',[11 11],2);
[r,c]=size(Img);
Img1= imresize(Img,4,'bilinear');
```

Images can be resampled at some new x and y grid points using interp2 function as shown in the following code:

```
[xnew,ynew] = meshgrid(0.25:0.25:r-0.25,0.25:0.25:c-0.25);
[xold,yold] = meshgrid(0.5:r-0.5,0.5:c-0.5);
Img2 = interp2(xold,yold,Img,xnew,ynew);
```

The original and resampled images are shown in Figure 2.7. Note that one can resize or interpolate the entire image or a subregion (subvolume of 3-D image) of an image, which can be specified by meshgrid points, xnew and ynew. For further information about the usage of these functions, the reader can refer to the MATLAB help pages.

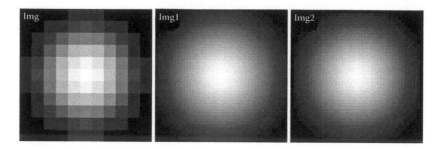

FIGURE 2.7
A 2-D Gaussian function before (left) and after resampling using `imresize` (middle) and `interp2` (right).

2.5.8.1   *Resizing by Pixel Binning*

In the previous section, we discussed image resizing using interpolation methods. Every now and then one may need to create an image at a desired pixel size. This can be done by binning the pixels (i.e., summing the intensities together). We will use the MATLAB function `blkproc` to bin image pixels. To bin (sum) n pixels per resulting pixel along the rows, we use the statement

```
bimg = blkproc(img,[n 1],'sum');
```

To bin n pixels along the columns, we change the second argument as follows:

```
bimg = blkproc(img,[1 n],'sum');
```

We can bin $n \times n$ pixels to obtain a smaller image using the script

```
timg = blkproc(img, [n 1],'sum');
bimg = blkproc(timg,[1 n],'sum');
clear tmpimg;
```

Note that the size of the final image is reduced by $n \times n$.

The Medical Image Processing Toolbox includes the function `mipimbin` that can be used to bin pixels along rows, columns, or both dimensions. For example, to calculate the uniformity of a gamma camera, the pixel size is required to be within a certain range. To fulfill this requirement, images are either acquired with a larger pixel size or the pixels are binned after the acquisition. The following statement executes our function and bins the original image by binning each 4×4 block into a single pixel. Note that binning will change the mean intensity of the image.

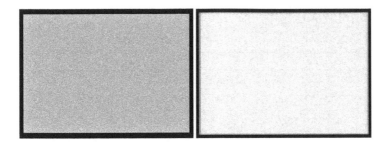

FIGURE 2.8
Uniformity image acquired by a gamma camera before (left) and after (right) binning.

```
Img = mipimbin(img,[4 4],3);
```

Figure 2.8 (left) shows the original 512×512 flood field uniformity image acquired by a gamma camera. The right part of the figure shows the original image after being binned to a size of 128×128.

2.5.9 Image Padding

Zero padding or, padding images with any number, may be necessary in spatial filtering operations to correctly handle edge pixels. While processing the border regions, extra rows and columns around an image must be added so that the sliding kernel neighborhood extends beyond the boundary of the image. The paddarray function has three modes: *circular, replicate,* and *symmetric.* The padding size can also be entered as an input argument. The symmetric mode is commonly used to pad a mirror image. The paddarray function can operate on two- or multidimensional images. The details about these modes can be found in the MATLAB help pages.

2.5.10 Finding Minimum or Maximum Intensity

If one requires just the minimum intensity of an image, then min(Img(:)) would do the job; but if one is interested in the location of the intensity value, then the following code can be used:

```
[r, c, z] = find(Img == min(Img(:)));
```

Similarly, the maximum intensity of an image and its location can be obtained by

```
maxInt = max(Img(:));
[r, c, z] = find(Img == maxInt);
```

TABLE 2.1

List of MATLAB functions for image arithmetic

Function	Description
imabsdiff	Absolute difference of two images
imadd	Add two images
imcomplement	Complement an image
imdivide	Divide two images
imlincomb	Compute linear combination of two images
immultiply	Multiply two images
imsubtract	Subtract two images

Note that there may be more than one pixel with the value of maxInt in the image.

2.5.11 Image Arithmetic

Although image arithmetic can be performed using normal matrix operations, the Image Processing Toolbox includes special functions for it. Table 2.1 lists some such functions. Their main advantages, as mentioned in the MATLAB help pages, are

- No conversion to double data type is necessary. It should be noted that the operations are executed in double precision internally.
- Overflow is handled automatically

On Intel architecture processors, such functions can take advantage of the Intel Performance Primitives Library (IPPL), thus accelerating their execution time. The IPPL is a collection of basic functions used in signal and image processing.

2.5.12 Block Processing of Images

At times, block processing may be required when images exhibit some type of inhomogeneity, such as spatially varying noise characteristics, or when it is necessary to perform processing locally inside the image. In block processing, the image is divided into small distinct or overlapping blocks, and each block is processed separately. A nonuniform background or illumination is one of the best examples in which block processing may be helpful. Recall also that in Section 2.5.8.1, we performed pixel binning by using the block processing function. There are several functions in MATLAB that allow us to perform block processing: blkproc, im2col, col2im, nrfilter, and colfilt.

`blkproc`	Implement distinct block processing
`im2col`	Rearranges image blocks into columns
`col2im`	Reverses the operation of `im2col`, rearranges the columns into blocks
`nrfilter`	Perform general sliding-neighborhood operations
`colfilt`	Perform neighborhood operations using columnwise functions

For the usage of these functions, the reader can refer to the MATLAB help pages.

2.6   Image Histogram

An intensity histogram represents the frequency of occurrence of intensities in an image. It is the approximation of the probability distribution function that intensities follow. Image histograms can be computed in several ways. For instance, the following statement

```
[h,cbins] = hist(Img(:),nbins);
```

creates an image histogram in which `nbins` is the desired number of bins, and `cbins` denotes their centers. Figure 2.9 shows a synthetic image consisting of two normally distributed regions with means 10 and 20 and a standard deviation 2. Then the following code computes the histogram using 64 bins. The computed histogram is shown on the left of the Figure 2.9 using a bar plot.

 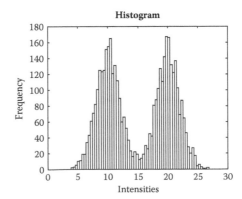

FIGURE 2.9

A gray-level image consisting of two normally distributed regions and its histogram on the right.

```
Img = [normrnd(10,2,64,32), normrnd(20,2,64,32)];
[h,cbins]=hist(Img(:),64);
bar(cbins,h,1);
```

The functions `imhist` and `histc` are the other alternatives in computing image histograms. For the usage of these functions, the reader can refer to MATLAB help pages.

2.6.1   2-D Histogram

The 2-D histogram, also known as cooccurrence matrix, was first suggested by Haralick [1] to classify/identify regions in an image on the basis of its textural characteristics. A cooccurrence matrix shows the frequency of cooccurrence of image intensities. It is a function of distance and angle. For instance, $h(i, j; \theta, D)$ indicates the frequency of occurrence of the intensities i and j at an angle θ (e.g., 0, 90, 45, 135) and a distance D. In other words, a cooccurrence matrix is the number of times a pair of intensities occurs at a certain distance and orientation. The following MATLAB code can be used to calculate the cooccurrence matrix of an image for a distance of 1 unit and an angle between 0 and 180 (see Figure 2.10):

```
function H = histo2d(Img)
maxI = max(Img(:));
levels = maxI+1;
H = zeros (levels, levels);
[r c] = size(Img);
Img = padarray(Img,[1 1],'replicate','both');
for I = 2:r
 for j = 2:c
        m = Img(i,j)+1;
        n = Img(i,j-1)+1;
        (m,n) = H(m,n)+1;
        n = Img(i,j+1)+1;
        H(m,n) = H(m,n)+1;
  end
end
```

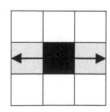

FIGURE 2.10
Dark center pixel and its neighbors at a distance of 1 and angle of 0 and 180.

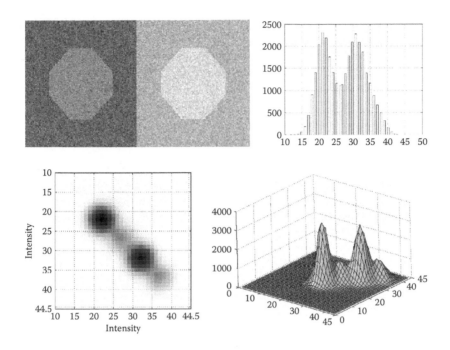

FIGURE 2.11
The image on the top left is the image of two hexagons with normally distributed regions. The graph on the top right shows the histogram of the image. The image on the bottom left shows the cooccurrence matrix. The mesh plot on the bottom right is the graph of the cooccurrence matrix.

Let us demonstrate the use of our function `miphisto2d` on a simulated hexagon image as shown in Figure 2.11 (top left part). The following script generates the image and computes the cooccurrence matrix. The graphs of the matrix are illustrated in Figure 2.11 (bottom).

```
himg1 = round(hexagon(20,25,128) + imgauss([128 128 1],1,5));
himg2 = round(hexagon(30,35,128) + imgauss([128 128 1],1,5));
himg = [himg1 himg2];
H = miphisto2d(himg,0) +...
    miphisto2d(himg,90) +...
    miphisto2d(himg,45) +...
    miphisto2d(himg,135);
surfl(H);
imagesc(H);
imagesc(himg);
```

The 2-D histogram in Figure 2.11 exhibits four peaks, corresponding to the two regions in the hexagon image. The diagonal elements of the histogram correspond to the cooccurrence of the elements within the nearly uniform regions, whereas off-diagonal elements are the cooccurrence of the intensities around the edges. As seen in Figure 2.11 (top right), the normal histogram of the image exhibits two peaks only. The regions of the hexagons are hidden in these two peaks. A 2-D histogram with four obvious peaks reflects more faithfully the number of regions that may be available in the image.

2.6.2 Computing a Joint Histogram

The joint histogram has found an important application in image registration. The mutual information based on the joint histogram is a widely used similarity measure in this area. A joint histogram represents the frequency of a pair of intensities given two images. Let $f(x, y)$ be gray-level intensity of the first image at location (x, y), and $g(x, y)$ the intensity of the second image at the same location. Then the joint histogram is $P(f(x, y) = m$ and $g(x, y) = n)$, where $m \in \{1, 2, \dots, M\}$ *and* $n \in \{1, 2, \dots, N\}$. The joint distribution function can also be used in image segmentation by thresholding. The following MATLAB code computes such a histogram given two images of the same size. This definition of the joint distribution function can be extended to 3-D.

```
% Histogram of joint distribution
% FUNTION h2d = mipjhist (im1,im2,mn1,mn2,mx1,mx2,b1,b2)
% Form the 2 dimensional histogram of two arrays.
% Result(i,j) = density of value i in im1,
% and value j in im2.
% Input images must be, of course, the same size....
% im1 & im2 are input arrays
% mn1 and mn2 are desired minimums for the histogram
% (defaults are image mins)
% Similarly, mx1 and mx2 are desired maximums
% (defaults are image maximums)
% b1 and b2 are bin sizes for im1 and im2 respecively;
% defaults
% are 1
%

function h2d = mipjhist (im1,im2,mn1,mn2,mx1,mx2,b1,b2)
%Find extents of arrays
MX1 = max(im1(:));
MX2 = max(im2(:));
MI1 = min(im1(:));
MI2 = min(im2(:));
if nargin < 8, b1=1; end
if nargin < 7, b2=1; end
if nargin < 6, mx2=MX2; end
if nargin < 5, mx1=MX1; end
if nargin < 4, mn2=MI1; end;
if nargin < 3, mn1=MI2; end;
```

```
m1 = floor((mx1-mn1)/b1)+1; % Get # of bins for each
m2 = floor((mx2-mn2)/b2)+1;
if (m1 <=0 | m2<=0), disp('Illegal bin size'); end;
if ((mn1==0 & mn2==0) & (b1==1 & b2==1) & (mx1<= m1 & ...
  mx2<=m2)& (mn1>=0 & mn2>=0))
  h = m1 * im2 + im1;
elseif (b1==1 & b2==1)
  h = m1*((im2 < mx2) - mn2 > 0)+ ((im1 < mx1) - mn1 > 0);
else
  h = m1*(((im2 < mx2) - mn2 > 0)/b2) + (((im1 < mx1) ...
  - mn1 > 0)/b1)
end;
h = h+1; % to handle the intensity level zero h(1) = ...
  p(0), probability of zero;
h1d = hist(double(h(:)),1:m1*m2); %Get the 1D histogram
% reform the histogram to produce 2D histogram
h2d = reshape(h1d,m1,m2);
% h2d = h2d';
% h2d = h2d/sum(sum(h2d));
```

2.7 Image Simulation

The MATLAB Statistical Toolbox has many functions that would allow us to draw random numbers from many distributions. These functions generate a single number or an array of random numbers, depending on the input argument one specifies during the function call. The functions in Table 2.2 are probably the most relevant ones for image simulations.

Using these functions, we can simulate images with different noise distributions. For detailed descriptions of these distributions and their input arguments, the readers can refer to the MATLAB help pages. We know that the variance of the Poisson noise is equal to its mean. The poissrnd function accepts a lambda value and the size of the output matrix as input arguments. If we specify an array of lambdas instead of a single lambda value, the output image will have a nonuniform noise distribution; in other words, the variance of the noise at each pixel will vary depending on the lambda value. This situation occurs in the projections in x-ray computer tomography. The x-rays traverse through thick or thin tissue paths. Because photon counting statistics obey Poisson's law, the noise at every projection point varies depending on the thickness of the path.

Rayleigh distribution is used to model noise in ultrasound (US) images, whereas a Weibull distribution can be used to model pulsetile or long-tailed noise distributions. Normal distribution, perhaps the most common distribution in medical imaging, could be used to model noise in various imaging modalities.

TABLE 2.2

Some of the MATLAB functions for generating random numbers

Function	unifrnd	poissrnd	normrnd	weibrnd	raylrnd
Distribution	Uniform	Poisson	Normal	Weibull	Rayleigh

There are two pseudorandom number generators available in MATLAB, rand and randn. It is possible to generate the same set of random numbers by setting the generator to the same state. For instance,

```
rand('state',1);
a = rand(1,5);
```

The repeated execution of this command generates the same set of numbers. To avoid it, one can use the following script that sets the random generator's state to a different number each time it is executed:

```
rand('state', sum(100*clock));
```

The following script generates a phantom image with a circle and ellipse using the MATLAB function phantom. Then, normally distributed noise is added to the phantom image. Figure 2.12 shows the resultant image.

```
E = [1 0.4 0.4 0.5 0 0;1 0.5 0.3 -0.4 0.5 0];
Img = phantom (E,64);
imagesc (10*Img+normrnd(0,1,64,64)));
```

2.7.1 Generating Images with Correlated Pixels

So far, we have discussed how to simulate images with pixels having independent identical distributions. What if we wanted to generate images with correlated pixels? It is more realistic to model pixels in an image with some degree or type of correlation, because due to the point

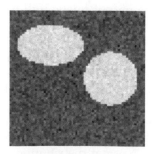

FIGURE 2.12

Image of a circle and an ellipse with normally distributed noise added.

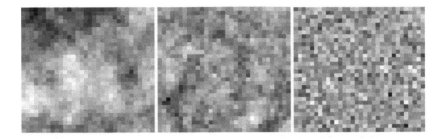

FIGURE 2.13
Images with correlated pixels. The parameter ρ, from left to right, was set to 0.95, 0.5, and 0.01, respectively.

spread function, the intensity of a pixel may contain information from its neighboring pixels.

Let us assume that an image is a random field in which each pixel is a random variable. We will also assume that these pixels are correlated with each other according to a correlation function. Different correlation functions can be used to model this random field. As an example, we will assume that the correlation is a function of the Euclidean distance between pixels. The following description is based on the treatment of Jain [2]. In general, isotropic and separable correlation functions commonly used in image processing are given by

$$c(x,y) = \sigma^2 \rho_1^{|x|} \rho_2^{|y|} \qquad \rho_1 \le 1 \qquad \rho_2 \le 1 \tag{2.1}$$

where σ^2 is the variance of the random field. An example of a nonseparable covariance function can be given by

$$c(x,y) = \sigma^2 \exp(-\sqrt{\alpha_1 x^2 + \alpha_2 y^2}) \tag{2.2}$$

When $\alpha_1 + \alpha_1 = \alpha$, then the covariance becomes a function of the Euclidean distance $d = \sqrt{x^2 + y^2}$, that is,

$$c(x,y) = \sigma^2 \rho \tag{2.3}$$

where $\rho = \exp(-\sqrt{\alpha})$. Such types of functions are called *isotropic* or *circularly symmetric*. The following MATLAB function `mipcorrimage` creates images with correlated pixels:

```
function [nImg,uImg] = mipcorrimage (ImSize,rho,sigma,muImg)
% IMSIZE : [row col]
% RHO : A number between 0 and 1.0
%        0 no correlation and 1 maximum correlation
% The covariance function is defined as
```

```
% covmatrix = sigma*rho.^(d) where d
% is the euclidean distance between pixels
% SIGMA : sigma of the normal distribution
% MUIMG : matix specifying the mean value for each pixel
% Output:
% NIMG,UIMG: Output images

if prod(size(muImg)) ~= prod(ImSize)
    error('Mean image (muImg) has to have the same ...
      dimensions');
end;
[r,c]   = find(ones(ImSize));
d       = squareform(pdist([r c],'euclidean'));
muvec   = muImg(:);
covmat  = sigma*rho.^(d/2);
nImg    = reshape(mvnrnd(muvec,covmat,1),ImSize);
uImg    = normcdf(nImg);
```

And then use inverse cumulative distribution function (CDF) to transform from uniform to other desired distributions. We can, for instance, transform to a Poisson distribution as follows:

```
posImg = poissinv(U, 10);
```

2.7.2   Creating Circular Disk and Sphere Images

Images of circles and ellipses can be created using phantom function. P = phantom(E,N) generates a user-defined phantom, where each row of the matrix E specifies an ellipse in the image. E has six columns, with each column containing a different parameter for the ellipse:

Column 1: A the additive intensity value of the ellipse

Column 2: a the length of the horizontal semiaxis of the ellipse

Column 3: b the length of the vertical semiaxis of the ellipse

Column 4: x0 the x-coordinate of the center of the ellipse

Column 5: y0 the y-coordinate of the center of the ellipse

Column 6: phi the angle (in degrees) between the horizontal semiaxis
           of the ellipse and the x-axis of the image.

Using the following code, one can create a 64×64 image of a circle and an ellipse:

```
E = [1 0.4 0.4 0.5 0 0; 1 0.5 0.3 -0.4 0.5 0];
Img = phantom(E,64);
imagesc (Img)
```

The image of the circle and the ellipse is shown in Figure 2.14 (left). The phantom function is very useful for creating multiple circles and ellipses in a single image. But we can also create circle images using the following approach. First, let us create a 100×100 meshgrid

```
[x,y] = meshgrid(1:100);
```

Then, using this meshgrid we can create a circle image, whose center is at (50, 50), as follows:

```
imCircle = sqrt((x-50).^2 + (y-50).^2);
```

By thresholding this image, imCircle, we can create a binary disk image of any size less than 100. For example, a disk of 30 can be created simply by

```
ImDisk = imCircle <= 30;
```

Here is a function that can accomplish a generalized task of creating a disk image:

```
function imDisk = mipdiskimage(imSize,Radius,Center);
[x, y] = meshgrid(1:imSize(1), 1:imSize(2));
imCircle = sqrt((x-Center(1)).^2 + (y-Center(2)).^2);
imDisk = imCircle<=Radius;
```

If required, one can further add noise to the binary disk image, using the methods just mentioned. Usually, noisy images are further smoothed to mimic a real image acquisition system, in which smoothing simulates the effect of point-spread function of an imaging system. Note that the smoothing process will also result in some type of correlation among pixels.

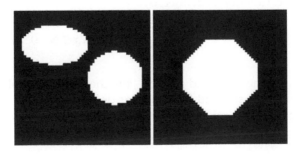

FIGURE 2.14
Left: Image of a circle and an ellipse created with the phantom function. Right: Image of a hexagon.

The `mipdiskimage` function can easily be expanded to 3-D to create spheres as seen in the following the function `mipsphereimage`:

```
function imSphere = mipsphereimage(imSize,Radius,Center,...
    delta);
[x, y,z] = meshgrid(1:imSize(1), 1:imSize(2),1:imSize(3));
imSphere = sqrt((x-Center(1)).^2 + (y-Center(2)).^2 + ...
    (z Center(3)).^2);
imSphere = imSphere<=Radius;
```

2.7.3   Creating Hexagon Image

The MATLAB code given here can be used to generate a binary image of a hexagon. An example of such an image is shown in Figure 2.14 (right). This function uses the MATLAB function `roipoly` to draw the hexagon. The input arguments of `roipoly` are an image and the vertex coordinates of the polygon forming the shape, in this case a hexagon. Note that the vertices of the hexagon are scaled according to the desired image size I1 and I2 are the background and foreground intensity values. To learn more about the function `roipoly`, the reader can refer to the MATLAB help pages.

```
% function im = hexagon(I1,I2, imSize);
% I1 and I2 are the background and foreground levels,
% respectively.
function im = hexagon(I1,I2, imSize)
tmp = zeros(imSize)
r =[14 26 38 50 50 38 26 14]/(64/imSize)
c =[26 14 14 26 38 50 50 38]/(64/imSize)
hx = double(roipoly(tmp,c,r))
im = (hx+I1).*(hx ==0)+(hx+I2-1).*(hx~=0)
```

2.7.4   Sigmoid Image

The 2-D sigmoid function is defined by

$$S(x,y) = \frac{A}{((1+e^{[-m*(x-c_x)]}))((1+e^{[-m*(y-c_y)]}))} \quad 0 \leq x \leq N,\ 0 \leq y \leq M \quad (2.4)$$

where $0 \leq m \leq 1$ is the slope and c_x and c_y are the amounts of shifts in the x and y directions. The sigmoid function S is defined over the $N \times M$ grid. The following MATLAB code implements the 2-D sigmoid function:

```
% function simg = mipsigmoid2d (A,m,M,N)
% This generates a 2D sigmoid image
% for a given amplitude A and a matrix size of MxN
% where the slope m varies between 0 and 1
function S = mipsigmoid2d(A, m, M,N)
```

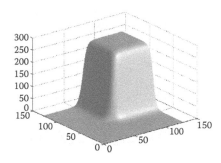
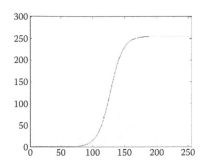

FIGURE 2.15
Left: `mipsigmoid2d` (255, 0.3, 128, 128). Right: `mipsigmoidoned` (255, 0.1, 255).

```
cx = M/2; cy = N/2;
[x,y] = meshgrid(0:M,0:N);
S = A./((1+exp(-m*(x-cx))).*(1+exp(-m*(y-cx)))));
```

The following function code implements a 1-D version of the sigmoid function:

```
% function [S,sx] = mipsigmoidoned(A,m,W)
% This generates a 1D sigmoid function of width W
% The slope m varies between 0 and 1
function S = mipsigmoidoned (A,m,W)
cx=W/2; x=linspace(0,W,W+1);
S = A./(1+exp(-m*(x-cx)));
```

On the left of Figure 2.15 is shown the graph of a 2-D sigmoid function viewed as a surface in $\mathbb{R}^3$, and on the right, the graph of a 1-D sigmoid function is given.

2.7.5 Creating Hollow Spheres

Hollow spheres filled with radioactivity are often used in nuclear medicine to study the image quality and resolution in SPECT and PET. Thus, we thought it would be helpful to show how one can create a synthetic hollow sphere in MATLAB. We have included the function `sh = mipshereshell(pixel size,slice thickness,R1,R2)` in our library. The last two variables are the inner and outer radiuses of the spherical shell (see Figure 2.16, top right), that is, R2 > R1. The interested reader can study the code for further details. The images shown in Figure 2.16 are generated with `sh = mipshereshell(1,1,10,15)`. On the lower left is the binary image sh displayed using `montage(sh)`, whereas on the lower right is the same image corrupted by uniform noise using the command `sh + rand(size(sh))`. On the top left is the surface-rendered image of the hollow sphere, and on the top right, the drawing of the cross section of the sphere is shown.

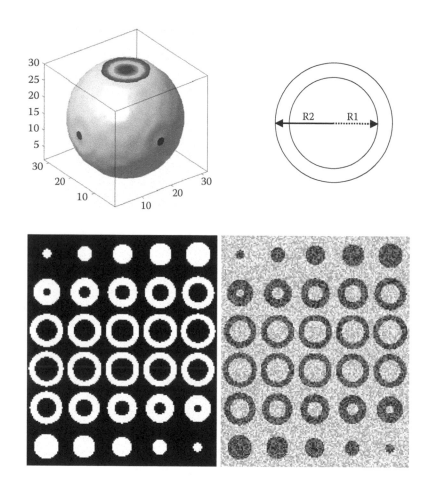

FIGURE 2.16
Top left: Volume-rendered image of the spherical shell. Top right: Cross section of the spherical shell. Bottom left: Slices of the spherical shell. Bottom right: After adding uniform noise.

2.8 Examples of 3-D Processing

2.8.1 Slicing Orthogonal Views

In medical imaging, reslicing a volume image is often required to visualize the three orthogonal views: transverse, coronal, and sagittal. In fact, it is routine to display all the orthogonal views simultaneously on a dual monitor workstation. In MATLAB, there are a number of ways to reslice a volume image. We have already discussed one approach in Section 2.5.1 while introducing the function reshape. However, that approach involves a *for* loop and is therefore computationally inefficient. The alternative

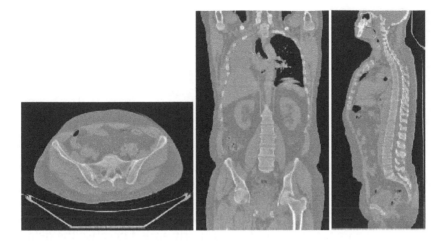

FIGURE 2.17
Transverse (left), coronal (middle), and sagittal views of a whole-body CT image.

function is `permute` that can be used for the same purpose. The following statement converts transverse slices to coronal views:

```
cviewImage = permute(Img, [2 1 3])
```

Similarly, to convert transverse slices to sagittal views

```
SviewImage = permute(Img,[1 3 2])
```

To generate an individual slice of one of the orthogonal views, we can extract the slice as shown in the following code and use the `squeeze` function to remove the singleton dimension. Slice 32 of the coronal view can be extracted by

```
I = squeeze(Img(:,32,:))
```

or similarly, that of the sagittal view by

```
I = squeeze(Img(32,:,:))
```

Figure 2.17 shows the three orthogonal views of a whole-body CT image.

2.8.2 Setting Data Aspect Ratio for Volume Images

When medical images are displayed in sagittal or coronal views, pixels become anisotropic; that is, the x and y dimensions of the pixel in the new view are not equal. In these views, the y dimension is the slice thickness, whereas the x dimension is either x (coronal) or y (sagittal)

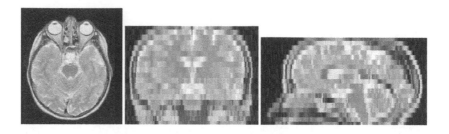

FIGURE 2.18
The three orthogonal views of a MRI brain image: transverse (left), coronal (middle), and sagittal (right).

dimension of the pixel in the transverse slice. Therefore when displayed in a figure, the images may not look properly scaled because the default assumption is that the voxel dimensions are equal. Therefore, we need to set the DataAspectRatio property of the axis to properly scale pixels. The DataAspectRatio, as described in MATLAB help pages, is "a three-element vector controlling the relative scaling of data units in the x, y, and z directions. For example, setting this property to [1 2 1] causes the length of one unit of data in the x direction to be the same length as two units of data in the y direction and one unit of data in the z direction."

We will show how to set the aspect ratio of an MRI volume image of a brain (see Figure 2.18). This volume has 19 slices with a voxel dimension of 0.4883×0.4883×6 mm^3. Obviously, the voxel dimensions are severely aniso-tropic. Hence, using a data aspect ratio of [1 1 1] would incorrectly scale the pixel dimensions in coronal and sagittal views.

After reading the image data, we can display the axial slices using a data aspect ratio of [1 1 1] as pixel dimensions are equal in the axial plane. Because this is the default setting, we do not need to do anything.

To display the coronal or sagittal view properly scaled, however, the DataAspectRatio property of the axis should be set correctly. The pixel dimension in coronal and sagittal views is 0.4883×6 mm^2. Therefore, we need to set DataAspectRatio property by

```
set(gca,'DataAspectRatio',[1 0.4883/6 1]);
```

This statement indicates that one unit of data in the x direction is the same as 0.4883/6 units of data in the y direction.

2.8.3   The Function `Imlook3d`

Here, we present an image display GUI, which we named `imlook3d` to display primarily 3-D images. The screenshot of the GUI is shown in Figure 2.19. `imlook3d` can read images of the main modalities such as MRI, CT, PET, and SPECT.

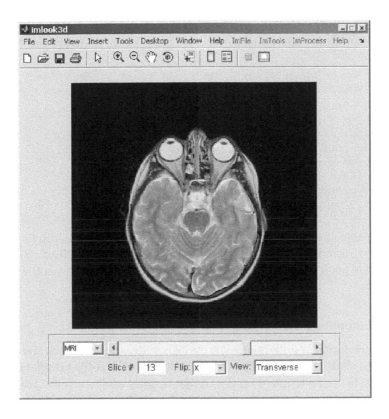

FIGURE 2.19
Screenshot of the Imlook3d image display GUI showing the transverse view of an MRI brain image.

A number of colormaps (jet, hot, gray, and inverse gray) have been included on a context menu. Some basic functions (pixval, improfile, and histogram) are included on a pull-down menu.

One can also convert the image from transverse to other orthogonal views: coronal and sagittal. The most current version of this GUI can be downloaded from the MATLAB File Exchange Web site. Because we share the source code of the GUI, even a novice reader can learn more about DICOM images of different modalities by examining the source code. Appendix D also discusses extensively the DICOM image file format.

2.8.4 Removing Small Structures from an Image

This may be necessary after an image segmentation operation. In a segmented binary image, in addition to the structures of interest, there may be small undesired structures due to noise or fragmentation. If such undesired structures are smaller than a certain size, then the following function code can be used to remove them from the binary image:

```
% MIPRMDEBRISN removes the objects with size less than
% excSize
% oimg = miprmdebrisn(image,excSize)
% image: input image should be a binary image
% oimg : output, a binary image
function oimg = miprmdebrisn(image,excSize)
L = bwlabeln(image,4);
S = regionprops(L,'Area');
oimg = ismember(L,find([S.Area] >= excSize));
```

First the objects in the binary image are labeled, and then, using the function `regionprops`, areas are computed. In the last step, the `ismember` function is used to exclude the structures that are smaller than the exclusion size.

2.8.5   Computing 3-D Normalized Cross-Correlation

Cross-correlation is widely used in pattern matching, in which the aim is to locate a structure with a known shape and size. First the template of the structure is created, and then the image is correlated with the template. The cross-correlation operation is simply a convolution operation except that the kernel (i.e., template) is not flipped. The normalized correlation coefficient in 2-D can be written as

$$r_2(X,Y) = \frac{\sum_{i=1}^{n}\sum_{j=1}^{m} X_{ij}Y_{ij} - nm\overline{X}\,\overline{Y}}{\left(\sum_{i=1}^{n}\sum_{j=1}^{m} X_{ij}^2 - nm\overline{X}^2\right)\left(\sum_{i=1}^{n}\sum_{j=1}^{m} Y_{ij}^2 - nm\overline{Y}^2\right)} \tag{2.5}$$

The original image is searched using the template of the known structure. The normalized correlation coefficient in 3-D is given by

$$r_3(X,Y) = \frac{\sum_{i=1}^{n}\sum_{j=1}^{m}\sum_{k=1}^{l} X_{ijk}Y_{ijk} - nml\overline{X}\,\overline{Y}}{\left(\sum_{i=1}^{n}\sum_{j=1}^{m}\sum_{k=1}^{l} X_{ijk}^2 - nml\overline{X}^2\right)\left(\sum_{i=1}^{n}\sum_{j=1}^{m}\sum_{k=1}^{l} Y_{ijk}^2 - nml\overline{Y}^2\right)} \tag{2.6}$$

where X is the reference image and Y is a subimage (of the same size as the template image) from the original image, and n, m, and l are the dimensions of the images. The following MATLAB code computes the normalized correlation coefficient of an input image given the kernel h:

```
% This function calculates the correlation coefficient in 3D
% function ccf = mipcorrcoef3d(img,h)
% img : input image
% h : kernel
% ccf : output-correlation coefficient
function ccf= mipcorrcoef3d(img,h)
[hr,hc,hz] = size(h);
Ksize = hr*hc*hz;
h1 = ones(hr,hc,hz);
th = h(:);
th = th-mean(th);
hh = sum(sum(th.*th));
avgimg = imfilter(img,h1/ksize);
imgsq = img.*img;
imgsq = imfilter(imgsq,h1);
imgsq = imgsq-ksize*avgimg;
cor = imfilter(img,h);
cor = cor - ksize*avgimg*mean(th);
ccf = cor./sqrt(imgsq*hh);
```

The resultant image ccf has a bright spot where the object in the image matches the kernel. The aforementioned code can be frustratingly slow when working on large images; in such cases, one needs a more efficient code. Figure 2.20 illustrates the cross-correlation. The CT image of small hollow spheres shown in the left of the figure was cross-correlated with the synthetically created template hollow sphere shown in the middle. The image on the right is the cross-correlation of the two.

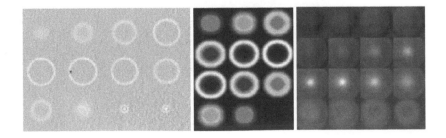

FIGURE 2.20
Left: CT images of a spherical shell phantom. Sphere diameters R1=12.5, R2=16, and the slice thickness = 3.2. Middle: Smoothed images of a spherical shell. Right: Normalized cross-correlation image.

2.8.6   Computing a Bounding Box in 3-D

A bounding box in 3-D is the smallest rectangular prism (see Figure 2.21) containing the 3-D object. In image analysis, it is often needed to extract an object from a larger image. To define the sub-volume to extract, we need to know the extensions, in other words, the bounding box of the object in 3-D. This is straightforward in 2-D, as the MATLAB Image Processing Toolbox already has a function called regionprops that computes the bounding box of an object in a 2-D image.

   The following function computes the bounding box of an object in 3-D whose pixel list is given by Ldata, the input argument. The output can directly be used as an input argument to the function subvolume to extract the object from the volumetric image.

```
function Ldatao = mipboundingboxe3d(Ldata,ImSize)
aborder = [1 ImSize(2) 1 ImSize(1) 1 ImSize(3)];
ido = [1,3,5];
ide = [2,4,6];
constant = 1;
bbox = zeros(1,6);
nObjects = length(Ldata);
Ldatao = Ldata;
for i=1:nObjects
   p = Ldata(i).PixelList;
   minp = min(p,[],1);
   maxp = max(p,[],1);
   bbx = [minp(1)-constant, maxp(1)+constant,...
     minp(2)-constant,maxp(2)+ constant,...
     minp(3)-constant maxp(3)+constant];
   % checks for the borders of the image since
```

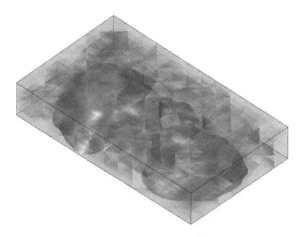

FIGURE 2.21
Rendered image of an object and its bounding box in 3-D.

```
% we add and subtract 1 from the minima and maxima,
% respectively.
bbox(1,ido)  = max(bbx(1,ido),aborder(1,ido));
bbox(1,ide)  = min(bbx(1,ide),aborder(1,ide));
Ldatao(i).BoundBox = bbox;
end
```

2.8.7 Defining Region or Volume of Interests Using Isolines

2.8.7.1 Region of Interest

Defining a region of interest (ROI) in anatomical modalities such as CT and MR requires the segmentation of the organ or object and its boundaries that are generally well defined. In functional modalities such as SPECT and PET, the organ boundaries are not very clear due to severe limitations in resolution. In functional modalities researchers are usually interested in regions of high uptake, which may refer to abnormal functional activities in the tissue. A high-uptake region may not necessarily constitute the entire organ in which it lies; it may rather be the portion of an organ. The boundaries of such regions are usually fuzzy due again to the limited resolution and partial volume effect. Hence, segmentation methods are not directly applicable to these cases.

We will discuss and demonstrate a widely used method of defining ROIs in functional modalities. It does not require the segmentation of a region. The method will be demonstrated on PET images, but it can be applied to SPECT images as well. We will accomplish this using the *isoline* method applied to 2-D transaxial slices or 3-D volume images consisting of multiple slices.

Isoline is the contour along which the intensity values are greater than or equal to a constant value. In this case, we will define our ROI as the isoline that is equal to some percentage of the maximum intensity value within the ROI. It is common to take 50% of the maximum intensity within the ROI. Figure 2.22 (left) shows the isoline that is equal to 50% of the maximum intensity of 11.96. In the figure, the gray-level image taken from a PET image shows a region of high uptake. On the right is the binary image in which the pixels within the ROI are assigned value 1 whereas the ones outside are assigned 0. Now the binary image can be used as a mask to calculate the intensity statistics such as the average, minimum, maximum, or standard deviation within the ROI.

The following script extracts the isolines for a given image gimg and the percentage value P:

```
maxIntensity = max(gimg(:));
P = 0.5;
C = contourc(gimg, maxIntensity*[P,P]);
CC = mipdecomposeContourCurves (C);
tempimg = roipoly(gimg,[CC.x],[CC.y]);
```

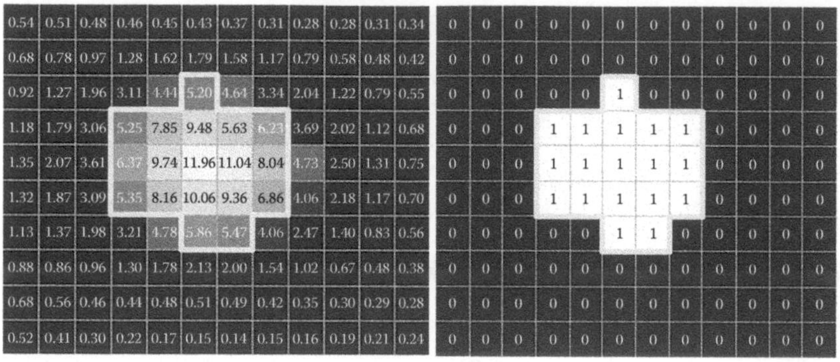

0.54	0.51	0.48	0.46	0.45	0.43	0.37	0.31	0.28	0.28	0.31	0.34
0.68	0.78	0.97	1.28	1.62	1.79	1.58	1.17	0.79	0.58	0.48	0.42
0.92	1.27	1.96	3.11	4.44	5.20	4.64	3.34	2.04	1.22	0.79	0.55
1.18	1.79	3.06	5.25	7.85	9.48	5.63	6.23	3.69	2.02	1.12	0.68
1.35	2.07	3.61	6.37	9.74	11.96	11.04	8.04	4.73	2.50	1.31	0.75
1.32	1.87	3.09	5.35	8.16	10.06	9.36	6.86	4.06	2.18	1.17	0.70
1.13	1.37	1.98	3.21	4.78	5.86	5.47	4.06	2.47	1.40	0.83	0.56
0.88	0.86	0.96	1.30	1.78	2.13	2.00	1.54	1.02	0.67	0.48	0.38
0.68	0.56	0.46	0.44	0.48	0.51	0.49	0.42	0.35	0.30	0.29	0.28
0.52	0.41	0.30	0.22	0.17	0.15	0.14	0.15	0.16	0.19	0.21	0.24

0	0	0	0	0	0	0	0	0	0	0	0
0	0	0	0	0	0	0	0	0	0	0	0
0	0	0	0	0	1	0	0	0	0	0	0
0	0	0	1	1	1	1	1	0	0	0	0
0	0	0	1	1	1	1	1	0	0	0	0
0	0	0	1	1	1	1	1	0	0	0	0
0	0	0	0	0	1	1	0	0	0	0	0
0	0	0	0	0	0	0	0	0	0	0	0
0	0	0	0	0	0	0	0	0	0	0	0
0	0	0	0	0	0	0	0	0	0	0	0

FIGURE 2.22
Left: The isoline is overlaid on the gray-level image. Right: The ROI defined by the isocontour on the left image.

The script uses the MATLAB function contourc, rearranges the boundary points into new format using our function mipdecompose-ContourCurves, and finally creates the binary mask image using the MATLAB function roipoly. Note that to extract a single isoline, the second argument of the function should be a two-element vector whose elements are equal as in [Ig,Ig]. Note that the percentage will affect the ROI size. A larger percentage will result in a smaller ROI and vise versa. Our function mipdecomposeContourCurves decomposes the contour curves produced by contourc and also finds out if the contour is a closed one. The contour has to be a closed one to be able to use it as an ROI. To learn more about our function, the reader can examine the code further. The reader should also go through the help pages of the function contourc to learn about its output format.

2.8.7.2 Volume of Interest

Volumes of interest (VOIs) can be determined using the same approach mentioned in the previous section as applied to each individual slice of a volume image. The resulting isoline contours of all slices will specify the VOI defined in 3-D. To accomplish this, the script mentioned earlier has to be run for each slice separately.

Let us demonstrate this on the PET image of a phantom consisting of small spheres filled with activity of higher concentration compared to its background region. These small spheres are meant to simulate small lesions in a human body. The following script computes the VOI for one such small sphere cropped from the original image:

```
for i=1:size(oimg,3)
    Img(:,:,i) = imresize(oimg(:,:,i),2,'bilinear');
end
```

```
P = 0.4;
maxIntensity = max(Img(:));
simg = zeros(size(Img));

for i=1:size(Img,3)
    C = contourc(Img(:,:,i), maxIntensity*[P,P]);
    tt = mipdecomposeContourCurves (C);
    if ~isempty(tt)
        simg(:,:,i) = roipoly(Img(:,:,i),[tt.x],[tt.y]);
        imshow(Img(:,:,i),[]);hold on;
        plot([tt.x],[tt.y],'b','linewidth',2);
    end
    clear C
end
```

As seen in the script, we first upsample each slice 2:1 to improve the definition of the ROIs. The script plots the contour lines on the gray-level image for display purposes. Figure 2.23 shows the slices and the overlaid isolines. The image saved into simg variable is the binary VOI or mask image. It also shows the surface-rendered image of the binary VOI image. Note that in the script, we used 40% of the maximum intensity for all slices.

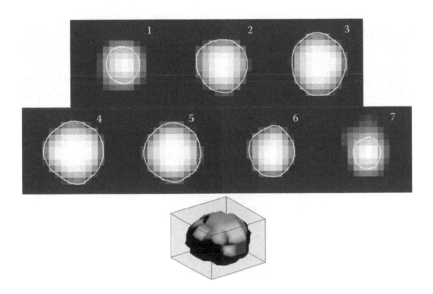

FIGURE 2.23
Consecutive slices of a volume image (top). The computed isoline contours, which constitute the VOI, are overlaid on each slice. The bottom plot shows the surface-rendered image of the binary image of the VOI.

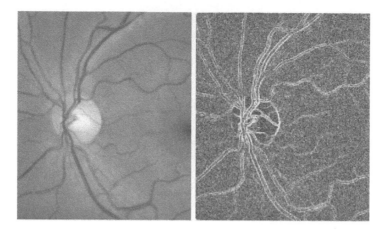

FIGURE 2.24
The green channel of the image of the retina (left) and local standard deviation (right).

2.9   Vectorized Neighborhood Calculations

In image processing, neighborhood processing is often costly. It requires visiting every pixel within two *for* loops in a 2-D image. This operation can be vectorized to substantially speed up the process, at the expense of more memory. As computer memories are affordable nowadays, one may want to use the following approach for neighborhood processing to substantially reduce the processing time. We will demonstrate how one can vectorize a neighborhood operation with a min–max filter example. In other words, we will filter an image by taking the minimum or maximum intensity in a 3×3 neighborhood. We can perform this by going to every pixel and finding the minimum or maximum intensity in the neighborhood, then replacing the central pixel intensity with it. We assume that the reader is familiar with neighborhood systems in a 2-D or 3-D image. We discuss such systems in chapter 7. For an 8-neighborhood, we need to create 8 images each representing one of the 8 neighbors of all the pixels in the image. The size of the combined neighborhood image is the size of the original image times the number of pixels in the designated neighborhood. For a 4-neighborhood, it is 4*prod(size(image)), whereas for an 8-neighborhood it is 8*prod(size(image)). It is important to note that such systems do not include the center pixel. It is straightforward to extend the following functions to include center pixels:

```
% function Nimg = mipneighborhood2d(img,nhood)
% output image will have the size r*c*nhood
```

```
% where r and c are the number of rows and columns of
% input image
% nhood can be either 4 or 8
function Nimg = mipneighborhood2d(img,nhood)
[R,C]=size(img);
Nimg = zeros(R,C,nhood);
r0=2:R-1;
c0=2:C-1;
switch nhood
    case 4
        Nimg(r0,c0,1) = img(r0-1,c0);
        Nimg(r0,c0,2) = img(r0,c0+1);
        Nimg(r0,c0,3) = img(r0+1,c0);
        Nimg(r0,c0,4) = img(r0,c0-1);
    case 8
        % from upper-left corner in clock-wise direction
        Nimg(r0,c0,1) = img(r0-1,c0-1);
        Nimg(r0,c0,2) = img(r0-1,c0);
        Nimg(r0,c0,3) = img(r0-1,c0+1);
        Nimg(r0,c0,4) = img(r0,c0+1);
        Nimg(r0,c0,5) = img(r0+1,c0+1);
        Nimg(r0,c0,6) = img(r0+1,c0);
        Nimg(r0,c0,7) = img(r0+1,c0-1);
        Nimg(r0,c0,8) = img(r0,c0-1);
    otherwise
        errorgdlg('Neighborhood is unknown');
end
```

Let us first create an 8-neighborhood image.

```
Nimg = mipneighborhood2d(Img,8)
```

Then we can perform a minimum filtering by

```
Fimg = min(Nimg,[],3)
```

Doing this in two-nested *for* loops would be computationally expensive. As we have said, the only disadvantage of this approach is the memory needed. Working with 3-D images can be worse when we have larger numbers of neighbors: 6-, 18-, and 26-neighborhoods. The code for the 3-D neighborhood is

```
% function Nimg = mipneighborhood3d(img,nhood)
% output image Nimg will have the size r*c*nhood
% where r and c are the number of rows and columns of
% input image
% nhood can be 6,18, or 26
% This is a memory demanding approach
```

```
function Nimg = mipneighborhood3d(img,nhood)
[R,C,Z]=size(img);
Nimg = single(ones(R,C,Z,nhood));
r0=2:R-1;
c0=2:C-1;
z0=2:Z-1;
switch nhood
    case 6 % six faces
        % 4 neighboors on the middle plane
        Nimg(r0,c0,z0,1) = img(r0-1,c0,z0);
        Nimg(r0,c0,z0,2) = img(r0,c0+1,z0);
        Nimg(r0,c0,z0,3) = img(r0+1,c0,z0);
        Nimg(r0,c0,z0,4) = img(r0,c0-1,z0);
        % top voxel
        Nimg(r0,c0,z0,5) = img(r0,c0,z0-1);
        % bottom voxel
        Nimg(r0,c0,z0,6) = img(r0,c0,z0+1);
    case 18 % six faces and 12 edges
        Nimg = neighborhood18(Nimg);
    case 26 % six faces, 12 edges and 8 corners
        Nimg = neighborhood18(Nimg);
        % four corners-top
        Nimg(r0,c0,z0,19) = img(r0-1,c0-1,z0-1);
        Nimg(r0,c0,z0,20) = img(r0-1,c0+1,z0-1);
        Nimg(r0,c0,z0,21) = img(r0+1,c0+1,z0-1);
        Nimg(r0,c0,z0,22) = img(r0+1,c0-1,z0-1);
        % four corners bottom
        Nimg(r0,c0,z0,23) = img(r0-1,c0-1,z0+1);
        Nimg(r0,c0,z0,24) = img(r0-1,c0+1,z0+1);
        Nimg(r0,c0,z0,25) = img(r0+1,c0+1,z0+1);
        Nimg(r0,c0,z0,26) = img(r0+1,c0-1,z0+1);
    otherwise
        errorgdlg('Neighborhood is unknown');
end

function Nimg = neighborhood18(Nimg)
        % 8 neighbors on middle plane
        % from upper-left corner in clock-wise direction
        Nimg(r0,c0,z0,1) = img(r0-1,c0-1,z0);
        Nimg(r0,c0,z0,2) = img(r0-1,c0,z0);
        Nimg(r0,c0,z0,3) = img(r0-1,c0+1,z0);
        Nimg(r0,c0,z0,4) = img(r0,c0+1,z0);
        Nimg(r0,c0,z0,5) = img(r0+1,c0+1,z0);
        Nimg(r0,c0,z0,6) = img(r0+1,c0,z0);
        Nimg(r0,c0,z0,7) = img(r0+1,c0-1,z0);
        Nimg(r0,c0,z0,8) = img(r0,c0-1,z0);
        % five voxels on top plane
        Nimg(r0,c0,z0,9) = img(r0,c0,z0-1); % center
        % 4-neighbors
        Nimg(r0,c0,z0,10)= img(r0-1,c0,z0-1);
```

```
Nimg(r0,c0,z0,11) = img(r0,c0+1,z0-1);
Nimg(r0,c0,z0,12) = img(r0+1,c0,z0-1);
Nimg(r0,c0,z0,13) = img(r0,c0-1,z0-1);
% five voxels on bottom plane
Nimg(r0,c0,z0,14) = img(r0,c0,z0+1); % center
% 4-neighbors
Nimg(r0,c0,z0,15) = img(r0-1,c0,z0+1);
Nimg(r0,c0,z0,16) = img(r0,c0+1,z0+1);
Nimg(r0,c0,z0,17) = img(r0+1,c0,z0+1);
Nimg(r0,c0,z0,18) = img(r0,c0-1,z0+1);
    end
end
```

Another example in which we can use this function is to calculate local standard deviation. In the following statements, the neighborhood function is run on the green channel of the image of the retina saved in array R, and the local standard deviation is computed. The retina image and the local standard deviation image (Istd) are shown in Figure 2.24

```
N = mipneighborhood2d(R,8);
Istd = std(N,0,3);
```

2.10 Numerical Derivative in Image Space

We are often interested in the change of intensity in an image defined in x–y space with the change in the x or y direction. We know from basic calculus that the derivative of an analog function $f(x)$ is defined as

$$f'(x) = \lim_{h \to 0} \frac{f(x+h) - f(x)}{h} \tag{2.7}$$

The discrete analog of this is given by the finite difference equation (see Figure 2.25)

$$\frac{\partial I}{\partial x} = I_x = \frac{I(x+h) - I(x)}{h} \tag{2.8}$$

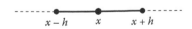

$$x - h \qquad x \qquad x + h$$

FIGURE 2.25
Three adjacent discrete locations along x direction separated by a distance h.

This is known as *forward differencing* for the spacing h between pixel centers. It can be shown by using Taylor's series expansion that this has an error of the order $O(h)$. One could also estimate the derivative using the backward difference equation

$$I_x = \frac{I(x)-I(x-h)}{h} \tag{2.9}$$

Again Taylor series expansion of $f(x \pm h)$ near x is given by

$$
\begin{aligned}
f(x+h) &= f(x)+hf'(x)+O(h^2) \\
f(x-h) &= f(x)-hf'(x)+O(h^2)
\end{aligned}
\tag{2.10}
$$

Multiplying the second equation by minus one and adding both sides of the two equations gives us the following relation for the first derivative:

$$f'(x) = \frac{f(x+h)-f(x-h)}{2h} \tag{2.11}$$

The discrete analog of this equation is the well-known central differencing equation:

$$I_x = \frac{I(x+h)-I(x-h)}{2h} \tag{2.12}$$

Note that the error in this case is of the order $O(h^2)$. Note also that the central difference is equal to (forward difference + backward difference)/2, that is, the average of the forward and backward differences.

On the other hand, the second derivative of function f by definition is

$$f''(x) = \lim_{h \to 0} \frac{f'(x+h)-f'(x)}{h} \tag{2.13}$$

If we substitute the first derivative into the second derivative, we get the following relation for the second derivative:

$$f''(x) = \frac{f(x+h)-2f(x)+f(x-h)}{h^2} \tag{2.14}$$

The discrete analog of this function is given by

$$I_{xx} = \frac{I(x+h)-2I(x)+I(x-h)}{h^2} \tag{2.15}$$

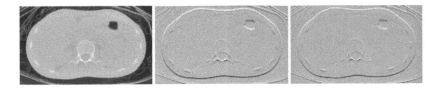

FIGURE 2.26
Original CT image (left) of a patient at the chest level. Forward (middle) and central (right) differences in the y direction.

Note that the second derivative may also be computed by repeated application of the first derivative. To compute the derivative of an image in the x or y direction, we will use the finite difference equations discussed here. In an image the change in intensity can be computed using forward, backward, or central differences. Figure 2.26 shows an axial slice from a CT image (left) and its forward (middle) and central (right) differences in the y direction. The pixel spacing is assumed to be 1.

In calculating the forward difference, the following script pads the array using the "symmetric" option only on one side, computes the forward difference in x direction, and then reduces the image size back to the original:

```
Img = padarray(Img,[0 1],'symmetric','post');
[row,col]=size(Img);
Fdx = zeros(row,col);
Fdx(:,1:col-1) = Img(:,2:col)-Img(:,1:col-1);
Fdx = dimg(:,1:end-1);
```

These difference functions are implemented in `mipforwarddiff`, `mipbackwarddiff`, and `mipcentraldiff`, and are included in the Medical Image Processing Toolbox.

As mentioned earlier, the higher-order derivatives can always be computed by recursively applying the difference operators.

2.10.1 Image Gradient

The gradient of an image I is defined by the vector

$$\nabla(I(x,y)) = \left[I_x = \frac{\partial I}{\partial x}, \quad I_y = \frac{\partial I}{\partial y} \right] \tag{2.16}$$

The elements of the vector are the partial derivatives of the image. This vector points in the direction along which the rate of change of I is maximum. The magnitude of the gradient, which is the quantity most frequently needed, is given by

$$\| \nabla I \| = \left(I_x^2 + I_y^2 \right)^{1/2} \tag{2.17}$$

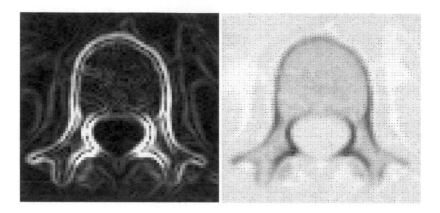

FIGURE 2.27
Left: The magnitude of the gradient. Right: The direction of the gradient plotted with the quiver function.

But it is also common to approximate it by $\|\nabla I\| \approx |I_x| + |I_y|$ due to the computational cost of the former one. The gradient function in MATLAB computes the gradient using the finite difference approach discussed earlier.

MATLAB has another convenient function, called quiver, which plots the gradient magnitude and direction. To demonstrate the computation of the gradient and the use of the quiver function, we cropped the lumbar disk from the CT slice shown in Figure 2.26 and computed its gradient using gradient. The following code computes the gradient and displays it using the quiver function. The array I in the script holds the cropped image.

```
[dx,dy] = gradient(I);
magnitudeI = sqrt(dx.^2+dy.^2);
imagesc(magnitudeI);
hold on; quiver(dx,dy);
```

Figure 2.27 shows the magnitude of the gradient (to the left), and the magnitude and direction of the gradient plotted with the quiver function. The lengths of the arrows are proportional to the magnitude of the gradient.

2.10.2 Directional Derivatives

The first directional derivative of an image in the direction of the unit vector $\mathbf{v} = [v_1, \ldots, v_p] \in \mathbb{R}^p$, where p is the dimension of the image, is given by

$$I_\mathbf{v} = \frac{\partial I}{\partial v} = \nabla I \cdot \mathbf{v} \qquad (2.18)$$

This is the dot product of the image gradient computed along the orthogonal directions and our unit direction vector **v**. It is easier to illustrate the concept in 1-D. Figure 2.28 shows the unit vector **v** (dotted) and the gradient I_x that are separated by angle θ. The first directional derivative can be viewed as the projection of the gradient vector onto the line running in the direction of the unit vector. We can express the dot product as $I_v = \| \nabla I \| \cdot \| \mathbf{v} \| \cos \theta$. Thus, we can see that the magnitude of the first directional derivative is maximum when the angle between the two vectors is zero. This reaffirms the fact that the derivative of a function at a given point will be maximum only in the gradient direction.

The first directional derivative for 2-D images is written as

$$\mathbf{v} = [v_1 \quad v_2], \quad I_v = v_1 I_x + v_2 I_y \tag{2.19}$$

Note that the directional derivative of image I in the direction of $\mathbf{v} = \begin{bmatrix} 1 & 0 \end{bmatrix}$ is equal to the gradient in the x direction. Similarly, for 3-D volume images

$$\mathbf{v} = [v_1 \quad v_2 \quad v_3], \quad I_v = v_1 I_x + v_2 I_y + v_3 I_z \tag{2.20}$$

The second directional derivative in the direction of $\mathbf{v} = [v_1, \ldots, v_p] \in \mathbb{R}^p$ can be expressed using the relation

$$I_{vv} = \frac{\partial^2 I}{\partial v^2} = \nabla(\nabla I.\mathbf{v}).\mathbf{v} \tag{2.21}$$

It can be shown that for 2-D images

$$I_{vv} = v_1^2 I_{xx} + 2v_1 v_2 I_{xy} + v_2^2 I_{yy} \tag{2.22}$$

And for 3-D images, it can be written as

$$I_{vv} = v_1^2 I_{xx} + 2v_1 v_2 I_{xy} + 2v_1 v_3 I_{xz} + 2v_2 v_3 I_{yz} + v_2^2 I_{yy} + v_3^2 I_{zz} \tag{2.23}$$

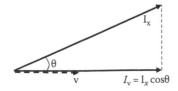

FIGURE 2.28
First directional derivative in the direction of the unit vector **v** in 1-D.

We will discuss later in this chapter how second directional derivatives can be expressed in terms of the Hessian matrix.

2.10.3 Gaussian Function and Its Derivatives

The *Gaussian function,* also known as the *Gaussian kernel,* is one of the most frequently used functions in image processing owing to its unique features. Its first and second derivatives and Laplacian are ubiquitously utilized in image processing applications such as filtering and edge detection. In this section, we will discuss how Gaussian functions in 1-D and 2-D and their derivates can be discretized in MATLAB, as we will frequently refer to them in the remainder of the book.

The continuous Gaussian function in 1-D and its first and second derivatives are given by

$$G = \frac{1}{(2\pi\sigma^2)^{1/2}} \exp\left(-\frac{x^2}{2\sigma^2}\right)$$

$$\frac{\partial G}{\partial x} = \frac{-x}{\sqrt{2\pi\sigma^3}} \exp\left(-\frac{x^2}{2\sigma^2}\right) \tag{2.24}$$

$$\frac{\partial^2 G}{\partial x^2} = \frac{1}{\sqrt{2\pi\sigma^5}}(-\sigma^2 + x^2)\exp\left(-\frac{x^2}{2\sigma^2}\right)$$

where σ is the standard deviation of the Gaussian function.

The total width of a Gaussian function is around $2*3\sqrt{2}\sigma$; therefore, when we discretize this function, the values of x should include the range $x \in [\mu - 3\sqrt{2}\sigma, \mu + 3\sqrt{2}\sigma]$ (see problem 6 as to why this is so). The discrete Gaussian kernels are normalized so that the area under the kernel adds up to unity to preserve the mean value after a convolution operation. Note that in the following script the kernel size is coerced to be odd. It is always desirable in a convolution operation to have a symmetric kernel.

```
ksize = ceil(sigma*8.5);
sqrt2pi = sqrt(2*pi);
if mod(ksize,2) == 0
     N = ksize-1;
else
     N = ksize;
end
x = -(N-1)/2:1:(N-1)/2;
g = ( 1./ ( sigma* sqrt2pi ) )*exp( -(x.*x)/(2*sigma^2) );
g = h/sum(g(:));
```

The derivative of a Gaussian (DoG) can be calculated using the following script:

```
dog = -x./( sigma^3*sqrt(2*pi)).*exp(-( x.*x )/
    ( 2*sigma^2));
```

The second derivative of a Gaussian (SDoG) can be computed by

```
sdog = (-sigma^2 + x^2)./(sigma^5*sqrt(2*pi)).*exp(-(
    x.*x )/( 2*sigma^2));
```

The Medical Image Processing Toolbox includes the function `mipgauss` that computes the Gaussian kernel up to 3-D, and the functions `mipdog` and `mipsdog` that compute the first and second derivatives of a 1-D Gaussian kernel, respectively, for a given σ or kernel size. The following script generates the kernels for $\sigma = 4$ and plots them on the same axis. The graphs of these functions are shown in Figure 2.29.

```
h = mipgauss(4);
dog = mipdog(4);
sdog = mipsdog(4);
% h is scaled for display purposes
plot(h/4); hold on;plot(dog);plot(sdog)
```

The extension of these functions to 2-D is fairly straightforward and will not be discussed here. The 2-D Gaussian function is a separable function, that is, it can be expressed in the form $G_x(\sigma, x)G_y(\sigma, y)$. Thus, one can perform 2-D convolution by convolving the image first in x using a 1-D Gaussian kernel, and then in y using its transpose. Similarly, the gradient and the second derivative of an image in the x and y directions can be computed using the 1-D kernels DoG and SDoG.

The MATLAB function `fspecial` can also generate Gaussian kernels of 1-D or 2-D form for a given σ and kernel size. Note that the `fspecial` function does not force the kernel size to be odd.

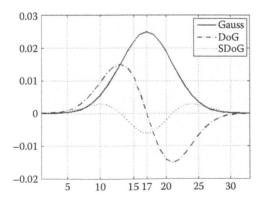

FIGURE 2.29
Gaussian function and its first and second derivatives, DoG and SDoG, respectively.

The Laplacian of a Gaussian is also widely used in image processing. The zero-crossing edge detectors proposed by Marr and Hildreth [3] are based on the zero crossing of the Laplacian of the image. One can compute the Laplacian of an image by convolving the image with the Laplacian of a 2-D Gaussian (LoG) kernel as the convolution is an associative and commutative operation. A 2-D Gaussian function with equal variance in both dimensions, that is, $\sigma_x = \sigma_y = \sigma$, is writen as

$$G = \frac{1}{\left(2\pi\sigma^2\right)^{1/2}} \exp\left[-\left(\frac{x^2}{2\sigma^2} + \frac{y^2}{2\sigma^2}\right)\right] \tag{2.25}$$

Taking advantage of the separability feature, the Laplacian of a Gaussian can be derived as

$$\nabla^2 G = \frac{\partial^2 G}{\partial x^2} + \frac{\partial^2 G}{\partial y^2} = \frac{1}{\sqrt{2\pi}\sigma^5}[-2\sigma^2 + x^2 + y^2]\exp\left(-\frac{x^2 + y^2}{2\sigma^2}\right) \tag{2.26}$$

In addition to helping the computation of the Laplacian of an image, the LoG kernel provides smoother images.

Note that when we discretize the Gaussian or its derivatives, we truncate the signal because the support region of a Gaussian function is theoretically unbounded. In the case of such a function, we normalize the area under the Gaussian curve so as not to introduce a bias to the final convolved signal, in other words, to preserve the mean signal or mean gray-level intensity. In the case of the Laplacian, however, the truncation of the signal at the tails may introduce a bias in the resultant image if the sum of the positive elements of the LoG is not equal to the sum of absolute values of the negative elements of the kernel. Hence, the effect of truncation will be worse as the size of the kernel becomes smaller for a given σ. Figure 2.30 shows the plots of the 2-D Gaussian (left) with $\sigma = 2.5$ and the Laplacian of the Gaussian (right) functions.

2.10.4 Gradient of Multispectral Images

A scalar image is defined as a mapping $I : \mathbb{R}^m \rightarrow \mathbb{R}$, whereas a multispectral image $\mathbf{I}$ can be defined as the mapping $\mathbf{I} : \mathbb{R}^n \rightarrow \mathbb{R}^m$. A color image, where m = 3, is a typical example of a multiple spectral image in which each pixel or voxel is a vector consisting of three intensities, known as Red (R), Green (G), and Blue (B) values, if the image is acquired in RGB format. We can consider a multispectral image as a vector $\mathbf{I} = (I_1, \dots I_m)$ and denote the ith component, which we will call *channel*, by I_i. We dropped the spatial variables x and y for brevity. In this section, we will discuss the computation of the gradient of multispectral images. We will use the

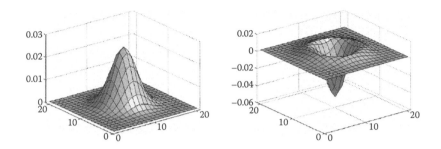

FIGURE 2.30

Plots of 2-D Gaussian (left) and Laplacian of Gaussian (right).

example of color images but the formulas that we present here can be expanded to the cases where $m > 3$.

There is more than one method, as there is more than one channel, to compute the gradient of a multispectral image. In the case of a color image, one approach is to convert the color image to a gray-level image using rgb2gray, and then compute the gradient of the converted image using the methods discussed earlier.

The second approach is to convert the image to the L*a*b color space and compute the gradient of the luminosity (L) channel only. We need to be aware of the fact that the L channel may not always capture all the local geometry information existing in the image. Figure 2.31 shows the individual channels of a color image converted to the L*a*b color space. As seen in the figure, the L image on the left does not reflect faithfully the local geometry information that is more pronounced on the color channels (see middle and right images).

The third approach is to compute the gradient of every pixel separately for each channel and combine the gradients using one of the vector norms. Note that the first and second approaches are for color images only and cannot be applied to multispectral images where $m > 3$ in general. The

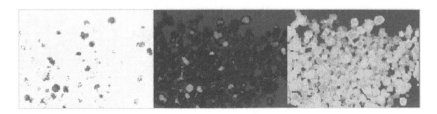

FIGURE 2.31

The individual channels of a L*a*b color image. The L (left), *a* (middle), and *b* (right) channels.

last approach, which we will discuss now, is applicable to the entire class of multispectral images.

Let us suppose that the gradient at a pixel in the ith channel is denoted by the vector $\nabla I_i = (I_{xi}, I_{yi})\, i = 1, \ldots m$, where $I_{xi} = \partial I_i / \partial x$ and $I_{yi} = \partial I_i / \partial y$. For 3-D volumetric images, the gradient vector is given by $\nabla I_i = (I_{xi}, I_{yi}, I_{zi})\, i = 1, \ldots m$.

Then, the resultant gradient magnitude at each pixel of a 2-D multispectral image can be computed using one of the following vector norms:

1. L-infinity (L_∞) norm

$$\| \nabla I \|_\infty = \max (|\nabla I|_i) \tag{2.27}$$

where $|\nabla I|_i = \sqrt{I_{xi}^2 + I_{yi}^2}$

2. L-1 (L_1) norm

$$\| \nabla I \|_1 = \sum_{i=1}^{m} |\nabla I|_i \tag{2.28}$$

L_1 norm is also known as the *city-block* or *Manhattan distance*, as one would travel the same distance to get from one point to another in a city.

3. L-P (L_p) norm

$$\| \nabla I \|_p = \left(\sum_{i=1}^{m} \left(|\nabla I|_i \right)^p \right)^{1/p} \tag{2.29}$$

Note that when $p = 2$, the above norm is the Euclidian norm.

The following script computes the gradients of a color image I using different methods and saves them into the variable `fgrad`:

```
% Convert color image to gray level image
% Then compute the gradient
Igray = rgb2gray(I);
[Ix,Iy] = gradient(single(Igray));
fgrad = sqrt(Ix.*Ix + Iy.*Iy);

% Transform RGB image to Lab space
cform = makecform('srgb2lab');
Lab = applycform(I,cform);
% Compute the gradient of the L band
L = Lab(:,:,1);
```

```
[Ix,Iy] = gradient(single(L));
fgrad = sqrt(Ix.*Ix + Iy.*Iy);

% Compute each band separately and combine them
[r, c, nChannels] = size(I);
for i=1: nChannels
    [Ix,Iy] = gradient(I(:,:,i));
    grad(:,:,i) = sqrt(Ix.*Ix + Iy.*Iy);
end

% L-infinity norm
fgrad = max(grad,[],3);
%L-1 norm
fgrad = sum(grad,3);
%L-p norm
p = 2;
ngrad = zeros(r,c);
for i=1:nChannels
    ngrad = ngrad + grad(:,:,i).^p;
end
fgrad = ngrad.^(1/p);
```

Figure 2.32 shows the gradients of a color image (image of islet cells, see Chapter 12: Application B) computed using different norms as shown in the just-mentioned script. The gray-level image shown on the top left of the figure was obtained using the function rgb2gray. It appears that different methods provide different results.

The gradients computed from the gray-level image and the L channels appear similar. There are minor differences among the gradients computed using the three norms. In the previous script, image gradients are computed using the function gradient.

They can be also computed using Gaussian kernels to smooth the image simultaneously during the gradient computation. The following script shows how this can be performed:

```
DoG = mipdog(1);
Ix = conv2(single(I),DoG,'same');
Iy = conv2(single(I),DoG','same');
gimg = mipgauss(1,2);
Ix = conv2(Ix,gimg,'same');
Iy = conv2(Iy,gimg,'same');
fgrad = sqrt(Ix.*Ix + Iy.*Iy);
```

This script uses a 1-D derivative of Gaussian to compute the image gradient in the x and y directions. The gradients in both directions are then smoothed again using a 2-D Gaussian kernel. The last line in the script computes the magnitude of the gradient. This method provides smoother gradient images.

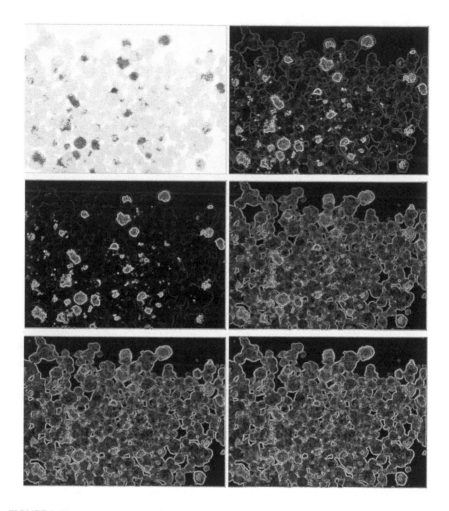

FIGURE 2.32
Top row: Gray-level image converted from an RGB color image. The gradient magnitude of the gray-level image on the left. Middle row: The gradient of the L band of the L*a*b image (left) and the L_1 norm (right) of the RGB image. Bottom row: The L_2 (left) and L_∞ (right) norms of the RGB image.

2.10.5 Hessian Matrix

The Hessian of a smooth image $I(x, y)$ at (x, y) is given by the matrix

$$\mathbf{H}(I(x,y)) = \begin{bmatrix} I_{xx} = \dfrac{\partial^2 I(x,y)}{\partial x^2} & I_{xy} = \dfrac{\partial^2 I(x,y)}{\partial x \partial y} \\[2ex] I_{yx} = \dfrac{\partial^2 I(x,y)}{\partial y \partial x} & I_{yy} = \dfrac{\partial^2 I(x,y)}{\partial y^2} \end{bmatrix} \tag{2.30}$$

where the elements of the matrix are the second-order partial derivatives of the image. Note that the Hessian matrix is computed at every pixel location. For a 3-D image, the matrix becomes

$$\mathbf{H}(I(x,y,z)) = \begin{bmatrix} I_{xx} & I_{xy} & I_{xz} \\ I_{yx} & I_{yy} & I_{yz} \\ I_{zx} & I_{zy} & I_{zz} \end{bmatrix} \tag{2.31}$$

If we consider our image surface as a function in 3-D, that is, $z = f(x,y)$, the Hessian matrix helps to determine whether a point on the surface is a local minimum or maximum. A maximum or a minimum of an image or any multidimensional function depends on the determinant of the Hessian matrix. For a 2-D image, for instance, the determinant of Hessian is given by

$$\det(\mathbf{H}) = |\mathbf{H}| = I_{xx}I_{yy} - (I_{xy})^2 \tag{2.32}$$

Indeed, $|\mathbf{H}|$ can be used as a discriminant measure to test for local extrema as follows:

If $|\mathbf{H}| > 0$ and $I_{xx} > 0$, then $I(x,y)$ has a local minimum.

If $|\mathbf{H}| > 0$ and $I_{xx} < 0$, then $I(x,y)$ has a local maximum.

If $|\mathbf{H}| < 0$, then $I(x,y)$ has a saddle point.

An important characteristic of the Hessian of an image is that the eigenvalues of the Hessian matrix gives the directions of the derivative and the relative magnitude of the second derivative. Let us suppose the eigenvalues of $\mathbf{H}$ and their corresponding eigenvectors are represented by λ_i (where $i = 1, 2$ and $\lambda_1 \geq \lambda_2$) and $\mathbf{e}_i$, respectively. The eigenvector ($\mathbf{e}_1$) corresponding to the largest eigenvalue represents the direction along which the second derivative is maximum. The two eigenvectors are orthogonal to each other.

Now, we will demonstrate the computation of the Hessian matrix of an image. Because MATLAB has a function, eig, that computes the eigenvalues of a matrix, we just need to fill our Hessian matrix by computing second-order derivatives at every pixel location.

```
[r,c] = size(I)
H = zeros(r,c,4);
dx = central_diff(I,'dx');
dy = central_diff(I,'dy');
H(:,:,1) = central_diff(dx,'dx');
H(:,:,2) = central_diff(dx,'dy');
H(:,:,3) = central_diff(dy,'dx');
H(:,:,4) = central_diff(dy,'dy');
E=zeros(size(I));
```

```
for i=1:r
    for j=1:c
        E(i,j,1:2) = eig([H(i,j,1) H(i,j,2);...
            H(i,j,3) H(i,j,4)]);
    end
end
MaxE = max(E,[],3);
```

This script computes the partial derivatives, fills the Hessian matrix **H**, computes the eigenvalues, and finally finds the maximum eigenvalue MaxE. Figure 2.33 shows a CT image of a lumbar disk and the maximum-eigenvalue image.

Recall that we previously discussed the second directional derivate in the direction of the unit vector v. We can also write the second directional derivate in terms of the Hessian matrix as

$$I_{vv} = \mathbf{vHv}^T \tag{2.33}$$

The directional derivate along the eigenvectors of the Hessian matrix can be computed using Equation (2.18). Then the local geometry information that includes the partial derivatives and first and second directional derivatives along the eigenvectors can be used to carry out the division of the image intensity surface into different categories such as peak, ridge, and saddle. This is known as the *topographic classification of intensity surface patches* [1].

2.10.6 Laplacian Operator

The Laplacian operator is one of the differential calculus operators used frequently in many image processing applications. Spatial filtering and edge detection are the prime examples of its use. The Laplacian operator in 2-D is defined by

$$\nabla^2 = \frac{\partial^2}{\partial x^2} + \frac{\partial^2}{\partial y^2} \tag{2.34}$$

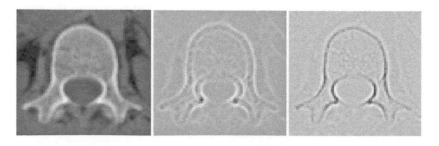

FIGURE 2.33
Left: CT image of a lumbar disk. Middle: Maximum-eigenvalue image. Right: Laplacian image.

We already know how to compute the second partial derivative of an image in 1-D. For a 2-D image, the Laplacian operator, which is the summation of the second partial derivatives in x and y directions, is then given by

$$\nabla^2 I = \frac{I(x+h_1,y)-2I(x,y)+I(x-h_1,y)}{h_1^2} +$$

$$\frac{I(x,y+h_2)-2I(x,y)+I(x,y-h_2)}{h_2^2} \tag{2.35}$$

If we assume that $h_1 = h_2 = 1$, the operator becomes

$$\nabla^2 I = I(x+1,y)+I(x-1,y)+I(x,y+1)+I(x,y-1)-4I(x,y) \tag{2.36}$$

This is also known as *five-point Laplacian* because it involves the five pixels in a 3×3 neighborhood: north, south, east, and west neighbors and the center pixel. The Laplacian operator, denoted by ∇^2, can be represented in matrix form as an averaging kernel or stencil as

$$\nabla^2 = \begin{bmatrix} 0 & 1 & 0 \\ 1 & -4 & 1 \\ 0 & 1 & 0 \end{bmatrix} \tag{2.37}$$

Therefore, the Laplacian of an image can be computed by convolving the image with the above stencil.

The function `del2` implements the Laplacian operation. The output of the `del2` function is $l = \frac{\nabla^2 I}{4} = \frac{1}{4}\left(\frac{\partial^2 I}{\partial x^2} + \frac{\partial^2 I}{\partial y^2}\right)$ when I is a 2-D array. If I is a multivariable function, then the output is

$$\frac{\nabla^2 I}{2N} \tag{2.38}$$

where N is the number of dimensions of I. This function also accepts pixel dimensions as input arguments. Figure 2.33 shows the Laplacian (right) of the lumbar image shown in the left of the figure computed with `del2`. Observe the differences between the Laplacian and the eigenvalue images. It can be shown that the Laplacian can also be written as

$$\nabla^2 I = trace(\mathbf{H}) \tag{2.39}$$

2.10.7 Example Applications: Gradient-Based Corner Detectors

Edges have large gradients only in one of the orthogonal directions, whereas object or region corners have gradients that are large in both directions. In this section, we will discuss a gradient-based corner detector widely known as the *Harris corner detector* [4] that is robust and simple to implement. This corner detector takes advantage of the aforementioned feature of corners.

Harris and Stephens defined the autocorrelation* function as

$$C_{x,y} = \sum_{dx,dy} w_{dx,dy} [I_{x,y} - I_{x+dx,y+dy}]^2 \qquad (2.40)$$

where $w_{dx,dy}$ are the weights. Note that this is the sum of the squared differences in a neighborhood between the center pixel and the neighboring pixels. They suggest using a Gaussian window for noisy images to enhance the robustness with respect to noise, that is,

$$w_{x,y} = \exp[-(x^2 + y^2)/2\sigma^2] \qquad (2.41)$$

Let us ignore the weights for a moment (which can always be incorporated later on). If we approximate the second term inside the square brackets in Equation (2.40) using Taylor's expansion, we obtain

$$C = \sum_{dx,dy} \left[I - I - [I_x + I_y] \begin{bmatrix} dx \\ dy \end{bmatrix} \right]^2 \qquad (2.42)$$

$$C = \sum_{dx,dy} \left[-[I_x + I_y] \begin{bmatrix} dx \\ dy \end{bmatrix} \right]^2 \qquad (2.43)$$

$$C = \sum_{dx,dy} [dxI_x + dyI_y]^2 = \sum_{dx,dy} I_x^2(dx)^2 + 2I_xI_ydxdy + I_y^2(dy)^2 \qquad (2.44)$$

Any 2-D quadratic function of the form $F(x, y) = Ax^2 + 2Bxy + Cy^2$ can be expressed in matrix form as $F = \mathbf{v}\mathbf{M}\mathbf{v}^T$, where $\mathbf{v} = [x\ y]$ and $\mathbf{M}$ is a 2×2 matrix written as $\mathbf{M} = \begin{pmatrix} A & B \\ B & C \end{pmatrix}$.

Thus, the functions of the form given in Equation 2.44 can be written in a matrix form as

$$\mathbf{C} = [dx \quad dy]\mathbf{M}[dx \quad dy]^T \qquad (2.45)$$

where dx and dy are the small shifts and $\mathbf{M}$, which is widely known as the structure tensor, is a 2×2 symmetric matrix written as

$$\mathbf{M} = \begin{pmatrix} I_x^2 & I_x \cdot I_y \\ I_x \cdot I_y & I_y^2 \end{pmatrix} \qquad (2.46)$$

---

* This term was used by Harris and Stephens in their original paper.

For every pixel in an image, Equation (2.40) is computed within a 3×3 window. The eigenvalues of **M** will indicate the gradient magnitude, whereas eigenvectors will denote the direction of the gradients. Harris and Stephens [4] defined the corner response function R as

$$R = \det(\mathbf{M}) - kTrace(\mathbf{M})^2 \qquad (2.47)$$

Note that the corner response function can be computed without the computation of eigenvalues, which requires extra computational effort. The factor k in Equation (2.47) is defined empirically. In the Problems section, the reader is asked to find the range of values that k may take on. It can be shown that the determinant and the trace of **M** are $(I_x I_y)^2 - \left(I_x^2 I_y^2\right)$ and $(I_x)^2 - (I_y)^2$, respectively. Note that the determinant and the trace of an $n \times n$ matrix **A** can be expressed in term of its eigenvalues λ_i as

$$\det(\mathbf{A}) = \prod_{i=1}^{n} \lambda_i$$

$$trace(\mathbf{A}) = \sum_{i=1}^{n} \lambda_i \qquad (2.48)$$

For our 2×2 matrix **M**, the determinant and the trace are $\lambda_1 \lambda_2$ and $\lambda_1 + \lambda_2$, respectively. So the corner response can also be written as

$$R = \lambda_1 \lambda_2 - k\left(\lambda_1 + \lambda_2\right)^2 \qquad (2.49)$$

The eigenvalues of the matrix **M**, λ_1 and λ_2, reveal information about the differential structures such as edges and corners in an image. Given the eigenvalues, there may be three cases:

1. Both λ_1 and λ_2 are too small so the autocorrelation function (given by Equation [2.40]) is flat; there is no change in the local neighborhood.
2. One of the eigenvalues is large whereas the other is small. This is an indication of an edge. There is little or no change along the edge but significant change along the orthogonal direction.
3. Both λ_1 and λ_2 are large, indicating the existence of a corner. That is, changes in both directions are large.

Images can be smoothed with a Gaussian kernel before computation of their gradients and also afterward using the Gaussian window as suggested earlier in Section 2.10.4.

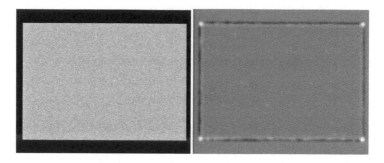

FIGURE 2.34
Left: The uniformity image of a gamma camera. Right: Harris and Stephens corner response.

We will leave it to the reader as an exercise to write a script or function code that implements a Harris and Stephens' corner detector, as it is reasonably straightforward.

Figure 2.34 shows the uniformity image of a gamma camera and the corner reponse of Harris and Stephens [4]. The value of k was set to 0.04 and a Gaussian window ($\sigma = 3$) was used. The bright spots at the corners of the field of view of the camera indicate the maximum response of the corner detector at the corners of a region.

We know Gaussian smoothing displaces image features. And this effect becomes exacerbated as σ increases. Thus, smaller σ values may help locate the corners more accurately. The corner response image needs to be further processed for the detection of corner locations. Most often a simple thresholding should be sufficient to detect the regions of high response in the corner response image.

Another measure of local differential structures based on the structure tensor **M** has been suggested and used in the literature [5,6]. This is known as the structure coherence measure and is given by

$$C = (\lambda_1 - \lambda_2)^2 \qquad (2.50)$$

where λ_i are the eigenvalues of the structure tensor. C is going to be large at edges where one of the eigenvalues is larger than the other. However, it will be small at corners where both eigenvalues are equally large. Figure 2.35 shows the coherence image of the lumbar disk computed as per Equation (2.50).

The structure tensor **M** in 3-D can be written as

$$\mathbf{M} = \begin{bmatrix} I_x \\ I_y \\ I_z \end{bmatrix} \begin{bmatrix} I_x & I_y & I_z \end{bmatrix} = \begin{pmatrix} I_x^2 & I_x \cdot I_y & I_x \cdot I_z \\ I_y \cdot I_x & I_y^2 & I_y \cdot I_z \\ I_z \cdot I_x & I_z \cdot I_y & I_z^2 \end{pmatrix} \qquad (2.51)$$

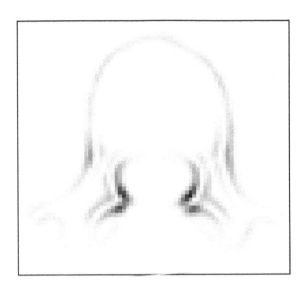

FIGURE 2.35
The coherence image of the vertebra.

This 3-D structure tensor can be used to compute the features in volumetric images.

2.10.8 Other Differential Structure Measures for Multispectral Images

In this section, we will define the image gradient differently, and discuss how this definition can be applied to multispectral images for which the calculation of the gradient is not straightforward. Di Zenzo has proposed measures based on our structure tensor for the purpose of edge detection in multispectral images [7]. Let us denote our structure tensor for a multispectral image by **M** again. We can express the gradient of our multispectral image **I** as

$$\| \nabla I \| = \begin{pmatrix} dx \\ dy \end{pmatrix} \mathbf{M}(dx \quad dy) \tag{2.52}$$

where $\mathbf{M} = \sum_{i=1}^{m} \nabla I_i \nabla I_i^T$. For a 2-D image we can write **M** more explicitly in terms of the gradients in the x and y directions as

$$\mathbf{M} = \begin{pmatrix} m_{11} = \sum_{i=1}^{m} I_{yi}^2 & m_{12} = \sum_{i=1}^{m} I_{xi} \cdot I_{yi} \\ m_{21} = \sum_{i=1}^{m} I_{xi} \cdot I_{yi} & m_{22} = \sum_{i=1}^{m} I_{yi}^2 \end{pmatrix} \tag{2.53}$$

It is straightforward to show that the eigenvalues and eigenvectors of **M** are given by

$$\lambda_{1,2} = \frac{m_{11} + m_{22} \pm \sqrt{\Delta}}{2} \tag{2.54}$$

where $\Delta = (m_{11} - m_{22})^2 + 4m_{12}^2$, and the corresponding eigenvectors are $v_{1,2} = [\cos\theta_{1,2}, \sin\theta_{1,2}]$ [8, 9] where

$$\theta_1 = \frac{1}{2}\arctan\frac{2m_{12}}{m_{11} - m_{12}} \tag{2.55}$$

$$\theta_2 = \theta_1 + \pi/2$$

respectively, where $\Delta = (m_{11} - m_{22})^2 + 4m_{12}^2$.

We will show how norms based on the structure tensor can be used to identify differential structures in a multispectral image. Recall that we discussed one of the norms in the context of corner detection. The application of these norms is not limited to multispectral images; it can also be applied to scalar-valued images. Although they can be applied to scalar-valued images, we will call these norms *vector-gradient norms*.

The first norm is

$$\sqrt{\lambda_1} \tag{2.56}$$

This norm is the largest of the eigenvalues of **M**. We already know it corresponds to the eigenvector pointing in the direction of maximum variation.

The second norm is

$$\sqrt{\lambda_1 + \lambda_2} \tag{2.57}$$

This is the sum of eigenvalues. It will be large at edges and corners. With simple algebra it can be shown that this norm is equal to

$$trace(M)^{1/2} = \sqrt{I_x^2 + I_y^2} \tag{2.58}$$

Thus, it does not require the calculation of eigenvalues.

The third norm can be given by

$$\sqrt{\lambda_1 - \lambda_2} \tag{2.59}$$

This is also called the *coherence measure* and is equal to

$$(\Delta)^{1/4} = \left(\left(I_x^2 + I_y^2\right) + 4I_x I_y\right)^{1/4} \tag{2.60}$$

The gradients given in the above equations are, in fact, computed using approaches discussed earlier. We have already discussed how we can compute the norm of these vector gradients. Remember, we suggested three different vector norms that can be employed to combine the gradients of individual channels.

Let us demonstrate these norms on our color image of islets. We will use the L-inf to calculate the norm of vector gradients. The function `mipstructuretensor` in the Medical Image Processing Toolbox can be used to calculate the structure tensor M. The following script shows how to compute these norms using the structure tensor function given the input image I:

```
M = mipstructuretensor(I,1,0.5,'linf');
[r,c,z]=size(I)
E=zeros(r,c);  I
for i=1:r
   for j=1:c
      E(i,j,1:2) = eig([M(i,j,1) M(i,j,2);M(i,j,2) M(i,j,3)]);
   end
end
MaxE = max(E,[],3);
N = sqrt(M(:,:,1) + M(:,:,3));
N = (M(:,:,1) + M(:,:,3)).^2 +4*M(:,:,2);
```

Figure 2.36 illustrates the vector gradient norms of the islet image. It is difficult to see the differences among these norms as differences appear to be very small for this particular color image. For the application of these

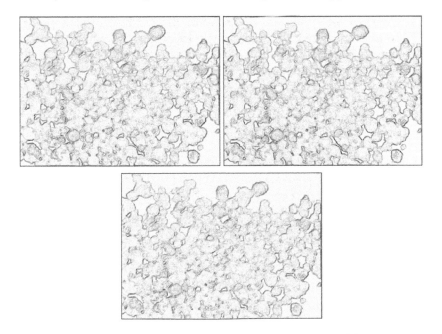

FIGURE 2.36

Vector gradient norms of the islet image. Top left: $\sqrt{\lambda_1}$. Top right: $\sqrt{\lambda_1 + \lambda_2}$. Bottom: $\sqrt{\lambda_1 - \lambda_2}$.

norms in the context of anisotropic diffusion filtering, the reader can refer to Tschumperlé and Deriche [10].

Problems

1. Write a MATLAB function that generates a synthetic image of a Gaussian point source image. The input parameters are pixel size, with possibly different full width at half maximum (FWHM) of the Gaussian in both x and y directions, and image size.

2. Use the function written in problem 1 to create an image with three Gaussian point sources. The locations of the point sources are the center, on the positive x axis 10 cm from the center, and on the positive y axis 10 cm from the center. The off-center point sources will have different FWHM values (e.g., 7 and 10 mm) for the x and y directions, that is, they will have radially elongated shapes. The image should be a 256×256 matrix with a pixel size of 2.24 mm.

3. Use the image generated in problem 2 to create a synthetic image of a cylindrical phantom with three line sources whose cross sections will be the same as the image created in problem 2.

4. Create a 3-D phantom image with three 3-D Gaussian point sources arranged as shown in the following diagram. The volume is 256×256×256 with a pixel size of 2.24 mm. The FWHM of the point sources should be 9 mm.

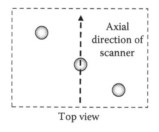

Top view

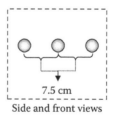

Side and front views

5. Create a sigmoid image and
   a. Compute the partial derivative images I_x, I_{xx}, I_{xy}, and I_{yy}.
   b. Compute the Hessian matrix for each pixel.
   c. Find and mark the maximum, minimum, and saddle points on the image using the criteria discussed in the chapter.

6. Show that the domain of the Gaussian should be at least as large as the range $x \in [\mu - 3\sqrt{2}\sigma, \mu + 3\sqrt{2}\sigma]$.

7. Convolve the vertebra image provided in the image database with a LoG kernel and develop an algorithm to detect the zero crossings in the image.

8. Write a function that will bin n×m pixels of an image, but each resulting binned pixel will be the average of the n×m block. Hint: use blockproc function.

9. Write a function code that implements the Harris corner response function.

10. Find the possible range of values for k in Equation (2.49) assuming that $R \geq 0$ for a corner to exist.

11. Create an image with rectangular regions of different intensity contrasts (e.g., 5, 10, 15, 25, 75, 250). Process the image with the Harris corner response function implemented in problem 9. Observe the impact of the parameter k by changing it within the range found in problem 10.

References

1. R. M. Haralick and L. G. Shapiro, *Computer and Robot Vision (1)*, New York: Addison-Wesley, 1992.
2. A. K. Jain, *Fundamentals of Digital Image Processing*. Englewood Cliffs, NJ: Prentice-Hall, 1989.
3. D. Marr and E. C. Hildreth, Theory of edge detection, presented at Proceedings of the Royal Society, London B, 1980.
4. C. Harris and M. Stephens, A combined corner and edge detector, presented at Proceedings of the 4th Alvey Vision Conference, 1988.
5. D. Tschumperlé and R. Deriche, Diffusion PDE's on vector-valued images. *IEEE Signal Processing Magazine* 19: 16–25, 2002.
6. G. G. Medioni, M.-S. Lee, and C.-K. Tang, *A Computational Framework for Feature Extraction and Segmentation*. Elsevier Science, March 2000.
7. S. D. Zenzo, A note on the gradient of a multi-image. *Computer Vision, Graphics, Image Process* 33: 116–125, 1986.
8. G. Sapiro and D. L. Ringach, "Anisotropic diffusion of multivalued images with application to color filtering," *IEEE Trans. on Image Processing,* 5: 1582–1586, 1996.
9. A. Cumani, "Edge detection in multispectral images," *Computer Vision, Graphics, and Image Processing,* 53: 40–51, 1991.
10. D. Tschumperlé and R. Deriche, "Constrained and Unconstrained PDE's for Vector Image Restoration," in *The Scandinavian Conference of Image Analysis*, Bergen, Norway, 2001, 153–160.

3

Probability Theory for Stochastic Modeling of Images

CONTENTS

3.1 Introduction

The objective of modeling in image analysis and image segmentation is to capture the intrinsic characteristics of images in a few parameters so as to understand the nature of the phenomenon generating the images. Image models are useful in quantitatively specifying natural constraints and general assumptions about the physical world and the imaging process. The introduction of stochastic models in image analysis has led to the development of many practical algorithms that would not have been realized with ad hoc processing. By approaching problems in image analysis from the modeling viewpoint, one focuses on the key issues of model selection, sampling, parameter estimation, and goodness-of-fits.

Formal mathematical image models have long been used in the design of image algorithms for applications such as compression and restoration, and such models have traditionally been low stochastic models of limited complexity. In recent years, however, important theoretical advances and increasingly powerful computers have led to more complex and sophisticated image models. Depending on the applications, researchers have proposed both low-level and high-level models.

High-level models are generally used to describe a more restrictive class of images. These models explicitly describe larger structures in an image, rather than describing individual pixel interactions such as Gibb's random field (GRF) and Markov random field (MRF).

Many well-known image modeling techniques for the analysis and segmentation of images have their roots in probability theory and mathematical statistics. In the following sections, we will describe some important concepts and techniques that will be used in the other chapters of this book. Much of the materials for this chapter was extracted from a forthcoming book by Sahoo [1].

3.2 Probability Measure

A random experiment is an experiment whose outcomes cannot be predicted with certainty. However, in most cases, every possible outcome of a random experiment can be listed. A sample space of a random experiment is the collection of all possible outcomes. Each element of the sample space is called a *sample point*. If the sample space consists of a countable number of sample points, then the sample space is said to be a *countable sample space*. If a sample space contains an uncountable number of sample points, then it is called a *continuous sample space*.

An event A is a subset of the sample space S. It seems obvious that if A and B are events in sample space S, then $A \cup B$, A^c, and $A \cap B$ are also entitled to be events, where A^c represents the complement of the event A. Thus, we precisely define an event as follows:

DEFINITION 3.1
A subset A of the sample space S is said to be an event if it belongs to a collection $\Im$ of subsets of S satisfying the following three rules: (a) $S \in \Im$; (b) if $A \in \Im$, then $A^c \in \Im$; and (c) if $A_j \in \Im$ for $j \geq 1$, then $\bigcup_{j=1}^{\infty} A_j \in \Im$. The collection $\Im$ is called an event space or a σ-field. If A is the outcome of an experiment, then we say that the event A has occurred.

DEFINITION 3.2
Let S be the sample space of a random experiment. A probability measure $P : \Im \to [0, 1]$ is a set function that assigns real numbers to the various events of S satisfying the following:

(P1) $P(A) \geq 0$ for all events $A \in \Im$

(P2) $P(S) = 1$

(P3) $P\left(\bigcup_{k=1}^{\infty} A_k\right) = \sum_{k=1}^{\infty} P(A_k)$ if A_1, A_2,..., A_k,... are mutually disjoint events of S

Any set function with the previously mentioned three properties is a probability measure for S. For a given sample space S, there may be more than one probability measure. The probability of an event A is the value of the probability measure at A, that is, $\text{Prob}(A) = P(A)$.

THEOREM 3.1
If $\varnothing$ is an empty set (that is, an impossible event), then $P(\varnothing) = 0$.
The proof of this theorem follows from (P1) and (P2). This theorem states that the probability of an impossible event is zero. Note that if the probability of an event is zero, that does not mean the event is empty (or impossible). There are random experiments in which there are infinitely many events, each with probability 0. Similarly, if A is an event with probability 1, then it does not mean A is the sample space S. In fact there are random experiments in which one can find infinitely many events each with probability 1.

THEOREM 3.2
Let $\{A_1, A_2,..., A_n\}$ be a finite collection of n events such that $A_i \cap E_j = \varnothing$ for $i \neq j$. Then

$$P\left(\bigcup_{i=1}^{n} A_i\right) = \sum_{i=1}^{n} P(A_i).$$

When $n = 2$, this theorem yields $P(A_1 \cup A_2) = P(A_1) + P(A_2)$, where A_1 and A_2 are disjoint (or mutually exclusive) events.

In the following theorem, we give a method for computing the probability of an event A by knowing the probabilities of the elementary events of the sample space S. The proofs of the following results are elementary and thus they are omitted.

THEOREM 3.3
If A is an event of a discrete sample space S, then the probability of A is equal to the sum of the probabilities of its elementary events.

COROLLARY 3.1
If S is a finite sample space with n sample elements and A is an event in S with m elements, then the probability of A is given by

$$P(A) = \frac{m}{n}$$

Next, we present some theorems that will illustrate the various intuitive properties of a probability measure.

THEOREM 3.4
If A be any event of the sample space S, then $P(A^c) = 1 - P(A)$, where A^c denotes the complement of A with respect to S.

THEOREM 3.5
If $A \subseteq B \subseteq S$, then $P(A) \leq P(B)$.

THEOREM 3.6
If A is any event in S, then $0 \leq P(A) \leq 1$.

THEOREM 3.7
If A and B are any two events, then $P(A \cup B) = P(A) + P(B) - P(A \cap B)$.
   Theorem 3.7 tells us how to calculate the probability that at least one of A and B occurs.

THEOREM 3.8
If A_1 and A_2 are two events such that $A_1 \subseteq A_2$, then

$$P(A_2 \backslash A_1) = P(A_2) - P(A_1)$$

3.3   Conditional Probabilities and Bayes' Theorem

We begin with the definition of a conditional probability of an event.

DEFINITION 3.3
Let S be a sample space associated with a random experiment. The conditional probability of an event A, given that event B has occurred, is defined by

$$P(A/B) = \frac{P(A \cap B)}{P(B)}$$

provided $P(B) > 0$.

This conditional probability measure $P(A/B)$ satisfies all three axioms of a probability measure. That is,

(CP1) $P(A/B) \geq 0$ for all events A

(CP2) $P(B/B) = 1$

(CP3) If A_1, A_2,..., A_k,... are mutually exclusive events, then

$$P\left(\bigcup_{k=1}^{\infty} A_k / B\right) = \sum_{k=1}^{\infty} P(A_k / B).$$

Thus, it is a probability measure with respect to the new sample space B.

DEFINITION 3.4

Two events A, $B \subseteq S$ are said to be independent if and only if

$$P(A \cap B) = P(A)P(B).$$

THEOREM 3.9

Let A, $B \subseteq S$. If A and B are independent events and $P(B) > 0$, then $P(A/B) = P(A)$.

PROOF   The proof follows from the following computation using definitions of conditional probability and the independence of two events:

$$P(A/B) = \frac{P(A \cap B)}{P(B)}$$

$$= \frac{P(A)P(B)}{P(B)}$$

$$= P(A).$$

THEOREM 3.10

If A and B are independent events, then A^c and B are independent. Similarly, A and B^c are independent.

PROOF   We know that A and B are independent, that is, $P(A \cap B) = P(A)P(B)$, and we want to show that A^c and B are independent, that is,

$$P(A^c \cap B) = P(A^c)P(B).$$

Because

$$P(A^c \cap B) = P(A^c/B)P(B)$$

$$= [1 - P(A/B)]P(B)$$

$$= P(B) - P(A/B)P(B)$$

$$= P(B) - P(A \cap B)$$

$$= P(B) - P(A)P(B)$$

$$= P(B)[1 - P(A)]$$

$$= P(B)P(A^c)$$

the events A^c and B are independent. Similarly, it can be shown that A and B^c are independent, and the proof is now complete.

THEOREM 3.11
Two possible mutually exclusive events are always dependent (that is, not independent).

THEOREM 3.12
Two possible independent events are not mutually exclusive.
   If the possible events A and B are exclusive, it implies that A and B are not independent; and if A and B are independent, it implies that A and B are not exclusive.
   There are many situations where the ultimate outcome of an experiment depends on what happens in various intermediate stages. This issue is resolved by the Bayes' theorem.

DEFINITION 3.35
Let S be a set, and let $\{A_i\}_{i=1}^m$ be a collection of subsets of S. The collection $\{A_i\}_{i=1}^m$ is called a partition of S if

(a) $$S = \bigcup_{i=1}^m A_i$$

(b) $A_i \cap A_j = \varnothing$ for $i \neq j$

THEOREM 3.13
If the events $\{B_i\}_{i=1}^m$ constitute a partition of the sample space S, and $P(B_i) \neq 0$ for $i = 1, 2, ..., m$, then for any event A in S

$$P(A) = \sum_{i=1}^{m} P(B_i)P(A/B_i).$$

PROOF Let S be a sample space and A be an event in S. Let $\{B_i\}_{i=1}^{m}$ be any partition of S. Then

$$A = \bigcup_{i=1}^{m}(A \cap B_i).$$

Thus

$$P(A) = \sum_{i=1}^{m} P(A \cap B_i)$$

$$= \sum_{i=1}^{m} P(B_i)P(A/B_i).$$

THEOREM 3.14
If the events $\{B_i\}_{i=1}^{m}$ constitute a partition of the sample space S and $P(B_i) \neq 0$ for $i = 1, 2, ..., m$, then for any event A in S such that $P(A) \neq 0$

$$P(B_k) = \frac{P(B_k)P(A/B_k)}{\sum_{i=1}^{m} P(B_i)P(A/B_i)}, \quad k = 1, 2, ..., m.$$

PROOF Using the definition of conditional probability, we get

$$P(B_k/A) = \frac{P(A \cap B_k)}{P(A)}.$$

Using Theorem 3.13, we get

$$P(B_k/A) = \frac{P(A \cap B_k)}{\sum_{i=1}^{m} P(B_i)P(A/B_i)}.$$

This completes the proof.
  This last theorem is called Bayes' theorem. The probability $P(B_k)$ is called *prior probability*. The probability $P(B_k/A)$ is called the *posterior probability*.

3.4 Random Variable

In many random experiments, the elements of sample space are not necessarily numbers. For example, in a coin-tossing experiment, the sample space consists of

$$S = \{\text{Head, Tail}\}.$$

Statistical methods involve primarily numerical data. Hence, one has to "mathematize" the outcomes of the sample space. This mathematization, or quantification, is achieved through the notion of random variables.

DEFINITION 3.6
Consider a random experiment whose sample space is S. A random variable X is a function from the sample space S into the set of real numbers $\mathbb{R}$ such that for each interval I in $\mathbb{R}$, the set $\{s \in S \mid X(s) \in I\}$ is an event in S.

In a particular experiment a random variable X would be some function that assigns a real number $X(s)$ to each possible outcome s in the sample space. Given a random experiment, there can be many random variables. This is due to the fact that given two (finite) sets A and B, the number of distinct functions one can come up with is $|B|^{|A|}$. Here, $|A|$ means the cardinality of the set A.

A random variable is not a variable. Also, it is not random. Thus, someone named it inappropriately. The following analogy speaks to the role of the random variable. A random variable is like the Holy Roman Empire—it was not holy, it was not Roman, and it was not an empire. A random variable is neither random nor variable; it is simply a function. The values it takes on are both random and variable.

DEFINITION 3.7
The set $\{x \in \mathbb{R} \mid x = X(s),\ s \in S\}$ is called the space of the random variable X.

The space of the random variable X will be denoted by R_X. The space of the random variable X is actually the range of the function $X : S \to \mathbb{R}$. Now, we introduce some notations. By $(X = x)$ we mean the event $\{s \in S \mid X(s) = x\}$. Similarly, $(a < X < b)$ means the event $\{s \in S \mid a < X < b\}$ of the sample space S.

DEFINITION 3.8
If the space of random variable X is countable, then X is called a *discrete random variable*.

DEFINITION 3.9
If the space of random variable X is uncountable, then X is called a *continuous random variable*.

In the case of a continuous random variable, the space is either an interval or a union of intervals. A random variable is characterized through its probability density function. First, we consider the discrete case, and then we examine the continuous case.

3.4.1   Distribution Function of Discrete Random Variables

DEFINITION 3.10
Let R_X be the space of the random variable X. The function $f : R_X \to \mathbb{R}$ defined by

$$f(x) = P(X = x)$$

is called the *probability density function* (pdf) of X.
    The probability density function $f(x)$ of a random variable X completely characterizes it. Some basic properties of a discrete probability density function are now summarized.

THEOREM 3.15
If X is a discrete random variable with space R_X and probability density function $f(x)$, then

(a) $f(x) \geq 0$ for all x in R_X, and

(b) $\sum_{x \in R_X} f(x) = 1$.

DEFINITION 3.11
The cumulative distribution function $F(x)$ of a random variable X is defined as

$$F(x) = P(X \leq x)$$

for all real numbers x

THEOREM 3.16
If X is a random variable with the space R_X, then

$$F(x) = \sum_{t \leq x} f(t)$$

for $x \in R_X$.
    The cumulative distribution function $F(x)$ represents the accumulation of $f(t)$ up to $t \leq x$.

THEOREM 3.17
Let X be a random variable with cumulative distribution function $F(x)$. Then the cumulative distribution function satisfies the following:

(a) $F(-\infty) = 0$,

(b) $F(\infty) = 1$, and

(c) $F(x)$ is an increasing function; that is, if $x < y$, then $F(x) \le F(y)$ for all reals x, y.

The proof of this theorem is trivial, and we leave it to the reader.

THEOREM 3.18
If the space R_X of X is given by $R_X = \{x_1 < x_2 < \cdots < x_n\}$, then

$$f(x_1) = F(x_1)$$
$$f(x_2) = F(x_2) - F(x_1)$$
$$f(x_3) = F(x_3) - F(x_2)$$
$$\cdots \quad = \quad \cdots \quad \cdots$$
$$f(x_n) = F(x_n) - F(x_{n-1})$$

Theorem 3.16 tells us how to find the cumulative distribution function from the probability density function, whereas Theorem 3.18 tells us how to find the probability density function given the cumulative distribution function.

We close this subsection with an example showing that there is no one-to-one correspondence between a random variable and its distribution function. Consider a coin-tossing experiment with the sample space consisting of a head and a tail; that is, $S = \{$ head, tail $\}$. Define two random variables X_1 and X_2 from S as follows:

$$X_1(\text{head}) = 0 \quad \text{and} \quad X_1(\text{tail}) = 1$$

and

$$X_2(\text{head}) = 1 \quad \text{and} \quad X_2(\text{tail}) = 0.$$

It is easy to see that both these random variables have the same distribution function, namely,

$$F_{X_i}(x) = \begin{cases} 0 & \text{if } x < 0 \\ \dfrac{1}{2} & \text{if } 0 \le x < 1 \\ 1 & \text{if } 1 \le x \end{cases}$$

for $i = 1, 2$. Hence, there is no one-to-one correspondence between a random variable and its distribution function.

3.4.2 Distribution Functions of Continuous Random Variables

Recall that a random variable X is said to be continuous if its space is either an interval or a union of intervals.

DEFINITION 3.12
Let X be a continuous random variable whose space is the set of real numbers $\mathbb{R}$. A nonnegative real-valued function $f : \mathbb{R} \to \mathbb{R}$ is said to be the probability density function for the continuous random variable X if it satisfies the following:

(a) $\int_{-\infty}^{\infty} f(x)dx = 1$, and
(b) if A is an event, then $P(A) = \int_A f(x)dx$.

DEFINITION 3.13
Let $f(x)$ be the probability density function of a continuous random variable X. The cumulative distribution function $F(x)$ of X is defined as

$$F(x) = P(X \leq x) = \int_{-\infty}^{x} f(t)dt.$$

The cumulative distribution function $F(x)$ represents the area under the probability density function $f(x)$ on the interval $(-\infty, x)$.

As in the discrete case, the cdf is an increasing function of x, and it takes value 0 at negative infinity and 1 at positive infinity.

THEOREM 3.19
If $F(x)$ is the cumulative distribution function of a continuous random variable X, the probability density function $f(x)$ of X is the derivative of $F(x)$; that is,

$$\frac{d}{dx}F(x) = f(x).$$

PROOF By the fundamental theorem of calculus, we get

$$\frac{d}{dx}F(x) = \frac{d}{dx}\left(\int_{-\infty}^{x} f(t)dt \right)$$

$$= f(x)\frac{dx}{dx}$$

$$= f(x).$$

This theorem tells us that if the random variable is continuous, then we can find the pdf given cdf by taking the derivative of the cdf. Recall that for a discrete random variable, the pdf at a point in space of the random variable can be obtained from the cdf by taking the difference between the cdf at the point and the cdf immediately below the point.

Next, we briefly discuss the problem of finding probability when the cdf is given. We summarize our results in the following theorem.

THEOREM 3.20
Let X be a continuous random variable whose cdf is $F(x)$. Then, the following are true:

(a) $P(X < x) = F(x)$,

(b) $P(X > x) = 1 - F(x)$,

(c) $P(X = x) = 0$, and

(d) $P(a < X < b) = F(b) - F(a)$.

3.5 Moments of Random Variables

In this section, we introduce the concepts of various moments of a random variable. Further, we examine the expected value and the variance of random variables in detail.

DEFINITION 3.14
The nth moment about the origin of a random variable X, as denoted by $E(X^n)$, is defined to be

$$E(X^n) = \begin{cases} \displaystyle\sum_{x \in R_X} x^n f(x) & \text{if } X \text{ is discrete} \\[2em] \displaystyle\int_{-\infty}^{\infty} x^n f(x)dx & \text{if } X \text{ is continuous} \end{cases}$$

for $n = 0, 1, 2, \ldots$ provided the right side converges absolutely.

If $n = 1$, then $E(X)$ is called the *first moment* about the origin. If $n = 2$, then $E(X^2)$ is called the *second moment* of X about the origin. In general, these moments may or may not exist for a given random variable. If, for a random variable, a particular moment does not exist, then we say that the random variable does not have that moment. For these moments to exist, absolute convergence of the sum or the integral is required. Next, we shall define two important characteristics of a random variable, namely, the expected value and variance. Occasionally, $E(X^n)$ will be written as $E[X^n]$.

3.5.1 Expected Value of Random Variables

A random variable X is characterized by its probability density function, which defines the relative likelihood of assuming one value over the others. In Section 3.4, we saw that given a probability density function f of a random variable X, one can construct its distribution function F through summation or integration. Conversely, the density function $f(x)$ can be obtained as the marginal value or derivative of $F(x)$. The density function can be used to infer a number of characteristics of the underlying random variable. The two most important attributes are measures of location and dispersion. In this, we treat the measure of location and treat the other measure in the next subsection.

DEFINITION 3.15
Let X be a random variable with space R_X and probability density function $f(x)$. The mean μ_X of the random variable X is defined as

$$\mu_X = \begin{cases} \displaystyle\sum_{x \subset R_X} x\,f(x) & \text{if } X \text{ is discrete} \\[2em] \displaystyle\int_{-\infty}^{\infty} x\,f(x)dx & \text{if } X \text{ is continuous} \end{cases}$$

if the right-hand side exists.

The mean of a random variable is a composite of its values weighted by the corresponding probabilities. The mean is a measure of central tendency: the value that the random variable takes "on average." The mean is also called the expected value of the random variable X and is denoted by $E(X)$. The symbol E is called the expectation operator. The expected value of a random variable may or may not exist.

3.5.2 Variance of Random Variables

The spread of the distribution of a random variable X is its variance.

DEFINITION 3.16
Let X be a random variable with mean μ_X. The variance of X, denoted by $Var(X)$, is defined as

$$Var(X) = E([X - \mu_X])$$

It is also denoted by σ_X^2. The positive square root of the variance is called the *standard deviation* of the random variable X. Similar to variance, the standard deviation also measures the spread. The following theorem tells us how to compute the variance in an alternative way.

THEOREM 3.21

If X is a random variable with mean μ_X and variance σ_X^2, then

$$\sigma_X^2 = E(X^2) - (\mu_X)^2.$$

PROOF

$$\sigma_X^2 = E([X - \mu_X]^2)$$
$$= E(X^2 - 2\mu_X X + \mu_X^2)$$
$$= E(X^2) - 2\mu_X E(X) + (\mu_X)^2$$
$$= E(X^2) - 2\mu_X \mu_X + (\mu_X)^2$$
$$= E(X^2) - (\mu_X)^2$$

THEOREM 3.22

If X is a random variable with mean μ_X and variance σ_X^2, then

$$Var(aX + b) = a^2 Var(X),$$

where a and b are arbitrary real constants.

PROOF

$$Var(aX + b) = E([(aX + b) - \mu_{aX+b}]^2)$$
$$= E([aX + b - E(aX + b)]^2)$$
$$= E([aX + b - a\mu_X - b]^2)$$
$$= E(a^2[X - \mu_X]^2)$$
$$= a^2 E([X - \mu_X]^2)$$
$$= a^2 Var(X).$$

The following MATLAB script finds the mean and variance of the image in Figure 3.1:

```
% Image_stat.m
% This script computes the mean and variance of an image.
%
clear all
close all
clc
```

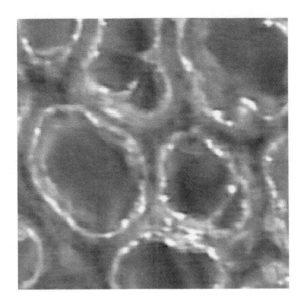

FIGURE 3.1
The mean and variance of the cell image are 75.15 and 1786.34, respectively.

```
%
A = imread('cell.jpg');
A = A(:,:,1);
I = double(A);
I_mean = mean(I(:));
I_var = var(I(:));
%
fprintf('Mean of the Image = %3.8f \n\n',I_mean)
fprintf('Variance of the Image = %3.8f \n\n',I_var)
%
figure
subplot(1,1,1)
imshow(A);
title(sprintf('Cell image with mean %5.2f and variance...
  %5.2f \n', I_mean, I_var))
%
% To print the figure uncomment the command "print my_
% figure.ps"
% The figure will be saved in postscript format in a file
% called "my_figure.ps"
%
print my_figure.ps
%
% End of the script
```

3.6 Some Common Probability Distributions

In this section, we explore some frequently encountered discrete and continuous probability distributions in imaging sciences and study their important characteristics.

3.6.1 Discrete Distributions

First, we consider the commonly used discrete distributions such as the Bernoulli distribution, the binomial distribution, the geometric distribution, and the Poisson distribution.

3.6.1.1 Bernoulli Distribution

A Bernoulli trial is a random experiment in which there are precisely two possible outcomes, which we conveniently call "failure" (F) and "success" (S). We can define a random variable from the sample space $\{S, F\}$ into the set of real numbers as follows:

$$X(F) = 0 \quad \text{and} \quad X(S) = 1.$$

The probability density function of this random variable is

$$f(0) = P(X = 0) = 1 - p$$

$$f(1) = P(X = 1) = p,$$

where p is the probability of success. Hence

$$f(x) = p^x(1-p)^{1-x}, \quad x = 0, 1.$$

DEFINITION 3.17
The random variable X is called the Bernoulli random variable if its probability density function is of the form

$$f(x) = p^x(1-p)^{1-x}, \quad x = 0, 1$$

where p is the probability of success.

We denote the Bernoulli random variable by writing $X \sim BER(p)$. If X is a Bernoulli random variable with parameter p, then the mean and variance are respectively given by

$$\mu_X = p$$

$$\sigma_X^2 = p(1-p).$$

In MATLAB, the Bernoulli pdf for $x = 10$ and $p = 0.8$ can be computed using the command `binopdf(10,1,0.8)`.

3.6.1.2 Binomial Distribution

Consider a fixed number n of mutually independent Bernoulli trails. Suppose these trials have the same probability of success, say p. A random variable X is called a binomial random variable if it represents the total number of successes in n independent Bernoulli trials.

Now, we determine the probability density function of a binomial random variable. Recall that the probability density function of X is defined as

$$f(x) = P(X = x).$$

Thus, to find the probability density function of X, we have to find the probability of x successes in n independent trials.

If we have x successes in n trials, then the probability of each n-tuple with x successes and $n - x$ failures is

$$p^x (1-p)^{n-x}.$$

However, there are $\binom{n}{x}$ tuples with x successes and $n - x$ failures in n trials. Hence,

$$P(X = x) = \binom{n}{x} p^x (1-p)^{n-x}.$$

Therefore, the probability density function of X is

$$f(x) = \binom{n}{x} p^x (1-p)^{n-x}, \quad x = 0, 1, 2, ..., n.$$

DEFINITION 3.18
The random variable X is called the binomial random variable with parameters p and n if its probability density function is of the form

$$f(x) = \binom{n}{x} p^x (1-p)^{n-x}, \quad x = 0, 1, 2, ..., n$$

where $0 < p < 1$ is the probability of success.

In MATLAB, the binomial pdf for $x = 10$, $n = 15$, and $p = 0.8$ can be computed using the command `binopdf(10,15,0.8)`.

We will denote a binomial random variable with parameters p and n as $X \sim BIN(n, p)$. If X is a binomial random variable with parameters p and n, then the mean and variance are respectively given by

$$\mu_X = np$$

$$\sigma_X^2 = np\,(1-p).$$

The binomial distribution can arise whenever we select a random sample of n units with replacement. Each unit in the population is classified into one of two categories according to whether it does or does not possess a certain property. For example, the unit may be a person, and the property may be whether he intends to vote "yes." If the unit is a machine part, the property may be whether the part is defective, and so on. If the proportion of units in the population possessing the property of interest is p, and if Z denotes the number of units in the sample of size n that possess the given property, then

$$Z \sim BIN(n, p).$$

3.6.1.3 Geometric Distribution

Let X denote the trial number on which the first success occurs. Hence, the probability that the first success occurs on xth trial is given by

$$f(x) = P(X = x) = (1-p)^{x-1}p.$$

Hence, the probability density function of X is

$$f(x) = (1-p)^{x-1}p \quad x = 1, 2, 3, \ldots, \infty,$$

where p denotes the probability of success in a single Bernoulli trial.

DEFINITION 3.19
A random variable X has a geometric distribution if its probability density function is given by

$$f(x) = (1-p)^{x-1}p \quad x = 1, 2, 3, \ldots, \infty,$$

where p denotes the probability of success in a single Bernoulli trial.

In MATLAB, the geometric pdf for $x = 10$ and $p = 0.8$ can be computed using the command geopdf(10,0.8).

If X has a geometric distribution, we denote it as $X \sim GEO(p)$. If X is a geometric random variable with parameter p, then the mean and variance are, respectively, given by

$$\mu_X = \frac{1}{p}$$

$$\sigma_X^2 = \frac{1-p}{p^2}.$$

The difference between the binomial and the geometric distributions is the following. In the binomial distribution, the number of trials was predetermined, whereas in the geometric distribution it is the random variable.

3.6.1.4 Poisson Distribution

In this section, we define an important discrete distribution that is widely used for modeling many real-life situations.

DEFINITION 3.20
A random variable X is said to have a Poisson distribution if its probability density function is given by

$$f(x) = \frac{e^{-\lambda}\lambda^x}{x!}, \qquad x = 0, 1, 2, ..., \infty,$$

where $0 < \lambda < \infty$ is a parameter.

In MATLAB, the Poisson pdf for $x = 10$ and $\lambda = 5$ can be computed using the command `poisspdf(10,5)`.

We denote such a random variable by $X \sim POI(\lambda)$. If $X \sim POI(\lambda)$, then

$$E(X) = \lambda$$

$$Var(X) = \lambda.$$

3.6.2 Some Continuous Distributions

Now we present some well-known continuous probability density functions that arise in many applications in imaging sciences. We begin with the simplest probability density function.

3.6.2.1 Uniform Distribution

Let the random variable X denote the outcome when a point is selected at random from an interval $[a, b]$. We want to find the probability of the event $X \leq x$; that is, we would like to determine the probability that the point selected from $[a, b]$ would be less than or equal to x. To compute this probability, we need a probability measure μ that satisfies the three axioms of Kolmogorov (namely, nonnegativity, normalization, and countable additivity). For continuous variables, the events are the interval or union of intervals. The length of the interval when normalized satisfies all the three axioms and, thus, it can be used as a probability measure for one-dimensional random variables. Hence

$$P(X \leq x) = \frac{\text{length of } [a, x]}{\text{length of } [a, b]}.$$

Thus, the cumulative distribution function F is

$$F(x) = P(X \leq x) = \frac{x - a}{b - a}, \qquad a \leq x \leq b,$$

where a and b are any two real constants with $a < b$. To determine the probability density function from the cumulative density function, we calculate the derivative of $F(x)$. Hence

$$f(x) = \frac{d}{dx} F(x) = \frac{1}{b - a}, \qquad a \leq x \leq b.$$

DEFINITION 3.21
A random variable X is said to be uniform on the interval $[a, b]$ if its probability density function is of the form

$$f(x) = \frac{1}{b - a}, \qquad a \leq x \leq b.$$

where a and b are constants.

In MATLAB, the uniform pdf for $x = 10$, $a = 5$, and $b = 15$ can be computed using the command unifpdf(10,5,15).

We denote a random variable X with the uniform distribution on the interval $[a, b]$ as $X \sim UNIF(a, b)$. If X is uniform on the interval $[a, b]$, then the mean and variance of X are given by

$$E(X) = \frac{b + a}{2}$$

$$Var(X) = \frac{(b - a)^2}{12}.$$

The uniform distribution provides a probability model for selecting points at random from an interval $[a, b]$. An important application of uniform distribution lies in random number generation.

THEOREM 3.23
If X is a continuous random variable with a strictly increasing cumulative distribution function $F(x)$, then the random variable Y, defined by $Y = F(X)$, has the uniform distribution on the interval $[0, 1]$.

PROOF Because F is strictly increasing, the inverse $F^{-1}(x)$ of $F(x)$ exists. We want to show that the probability density function $g(y)$ of Y is $g(y) = 1$. First, we find the cumulative distribution $G(y)$ function of Y. The cdf of Y is

$$G(y) = P(Y \le y)$$
$$= P(F(X) \le y)$$
$$= P(X \le F^{-1}(y))$$
$$= F(F^{-1}(y))$$
$$= y.$$

Hence, the probability density function of Y is given by

$$g(y) = \frac{d}{dy} G(y) = \frac{d}{dy} y = 1.$$

3.6.2.2 *Gamma Distribution*

The gamma distribution involves the notion of the gamma function. First, we develop the notion of the gamma function and study some of its well-known properties. The gamma function, $\Gamma(z)$, is a generalization of the notion of factorial. The gamma function is defined as

$$\Gamma(z) = \int_0^\infty x^{z-1} e^{-x} dx,$$

where z is a positive real number (that is, $z > 0$). The condition $z > 0$ is assumed for the convergence of the integral. Although the integral does not converge for $z < 0$, it can be shown by using an alternative definition of the gamma function that it is defined for all $z \in \mathbb{R} \setminus \{0, -1, -2, -3, \cdots\}$.

The integral on the right side of the preceding expression is called Euler's second integral, after the Swiss mathematician Leonhard Euler (1707–1783).

The gamma function has the following properties: (a) $\Gamma(1) = 1$, (b) the gamma function $\Gamma(z)$ satisfies the equation $\Gamma(z) = (z-1)\Gamma(z-1)$ for all real numbers $z > 1$, (c) $\Gamma(1/2) = \sqrt{\pi}$, and (d) $\Gamma(-1/2) = -2\sqrt{\pi}$.

DEFINITION 3.22

A continuous random variable X is said to have a gamma distribution if its probability density function is given by

$$f(x) = \begin{cases} \dfrac{1}{\Gamma(\alpha)\,\theta^\alpha} x^{\alpha-1} e^{-\frac{x}{\theta}} & \text{if } 0 < x < \infty \\ 0 & \text{otherwise,} \end{cases}$$

where $\alpha > 0$ and $\theta > 0$.

In MATLAB, the gamma pdf for $x = 10$, $\alpha = 5$, and $\beta = 7$ can be computed using the command gampdf(10,5,7).

We denote a random variable with gamma distribution as $X \sim GAM(\theta, \alpha)$. If $X \sim GAM(\theta, \alpha)$, then

$$E(X) = \theta\,\alpha$$

$$Var(X) = \theta^2\,\alpha.$$

DEFINITION 3.23

A continuous random variable is said to be an exponential random variable with parameter θ if its probability density function is of the form

$$f(x) = \begin{cases} \dfrac{1}{\theta} e^{-\frac{x}{\theta}} & \text{if } x > 0 \\ 0 & \text{otherwise,} \end{cases}$$

where $\theta > 0$. If a random variable X has an exponential density function with parameter θ, then we denote it by writing $X \sim EXP(\theta)$.

An exponential distribution is a special case of the gamma distribution. If the parameter $\alpha = 1$, then the gamma distribution reduces to the exponential distribution. Hence, most of the information about an exponential distribution can be obtained from the gamma distribution.

DEFINITION 3.24
A continuous random variable X is said to have a chi-square distribution
with r degrees of freedom if its probability density function is of the form

$$f(x) = \begin{cases} \dfrac{1}{\Gamma\left(\dfrac{r}{2}\right) 2^{\frac{r}{2}}} x^{\frac{r}{2}-1} e^{-\frac{x}{2}} & \text{if } 0 < x < \infty \\ 0 & \text{otherwise,} \end{cases}$$

where $r > 0$. If X has a chi-square distribution, then we denote it by writing $X \sim \chi^2(r)$.
The gamma distribution reduces to the chi-square distribution if $\alpha = 1/2$
and $\theta = 2$. Thus, the chi-square distribution is a special case of the gamma
distribution. Further, if $r \to \infty$, then the chi-square distribution tends to
the normal distribution.
The chi-square distribution originated in the works of British statisti-
cian Karl Pearson (1857–1936), but this distribution was originally discovered by German physicist F. R. Helmert (1843–1917).

DEFINITION 3.25
A continuous random variable X is said to have n-Erlang distribution if its
probability density function is of the form

$$f(x) = \begin{cases} \lambda\, e^{-\lambda x} \dfrac{(\lambda x)^{n-1}}{(n-1)!} & \text{if } 0 < x < \infty \\ 0 & \text{otherwise,} \end{cases}$$

where $\lambda > 0$ is a parameter.
The gamma distribution reduces to n-Erlang distribution if $\alpha = n$, where
n is a positive integer and $\theta = 1/\lambda$. The gamma distribution can be generalized to include the Weibull distribution. We call this generalized distribution the unified distribution. The form of this distribution is the following:

$$f(x) = \begin{cases} \dfrac{\alpha}{\theta^{\alpha\psi} \Gamma(\alpha\psi + 1)} x^{\alpha-1} e^{-\frac{x^{-(\alpha\psi - \alpha - 1)}}{\theta}} & \text{if } 0 < x < \infty \\ 0 & \text{otherwise,} \end{cases}$$

where $\theta > 0$, $\alpha > 0$, and $\psi \in \{0, 1\}$ are parameters.

If $\psi = 0$, the unified distribution reduces to

$$f(x) = \begin{cases} \dfrac{\alpha}{\theta} x^{\alpha-1} e^{-\frac{x^\alpha}{\theta}} & \text{if } 0 < x < \infty \\ 0 & \text{otherwise,} \end{cases}$$

which is known as the Weibull distribution. For $\alpha = 1$, the Weibull distribution becomes an exponential distribution. The Weibull distribution provides probabilistic models for life-length data of components or systems. The mean and variance of the Weibull distribution are given by

$$E(X) = \theta^{\frac{1}{\alpha}} \, \Gamma\left(1 + \frac{1}{\alpha}\right)$$

$$Var(X) = \theta^{\frac{2}{\alpha}} \left\{ \Gamma\left(1 + \frac{2}{\alpha}\right) - \left[1 + \frac{1}{\alpha}\right]^2 \right\}.$$

From this Weibull distribution, one can get the Rayleigh distribution by taking $\theta = 2\sigma^2$ and $\alpha = 2$. The Rayleigh distribution is given by

$$f(x) = \begin{cases} \dfrac{x}{\sigma^2} e^{-\frac{x^2}{2\sigma^2}} & \text{if } 0 < x < \infty \\ 0 & \text{otherwise.} \end{cases}$$

If $\psi = 1$, the unified distribution reduces to the gamma distribution.

3.6.2.3 Beta Distribution

The beta distribution is one of the basic distributions in statistics. It has many applications in classical as well as Bayesian statistics. It is a versatile distribution and, as such, it is used in modeling the behavior of random variables that are positive but bounded in possible values proportions and percentages fall in this category.

The beta distribution involves the notion of beta function. First, we explain the notion of the beta integral and present some of its simple properties. Let α and β be any two positive real numbers. The beta function $B(\alpha, \beta)$ is defined as

$$B(\alpha, \beta) = \int_0^1 x^{\alpha-1} (1-x)^{\beta-1} dx.$$

For any two positive numbers, α and β, the beta function can be written as

$$B(\alpha, \beta) = \frac{\Gamma(\alpha)\Gamma(\beta)}{\Gamma(\alpha + \beta)},$$

where $\Gamma(z)$ denotes the gamma function.

DEFINITION 3.26
A random variable X is said to have the beta density function if its probability density function is of the form

$$f(x) = \begin{cases} \dfrac{1}{B(\alpha, \beta)} x^{\alpha-1}(1-x)^{\beta-1} & \text{if } 0 < x < 1 \\ 0 & \text{otherwise} \end{cases}$$

for every positive α and β.

The graph of the beta distributions (pdf and cdf) for $\alpha = 7$ and $\beta = 17$ is shown in figure 3.2.

Figure 3.2 was generated using the following MATLAB script:

```
% MATLAB Script: beta_distribution.m
% This script generates plots of beta pdf and cdf
clear all
close all
clc
%
alpha = input('Please enter a positive value for the...
   parameter alpha: ');
beta = input('Please enter a positive value for the...
   parameter beta: ');
```

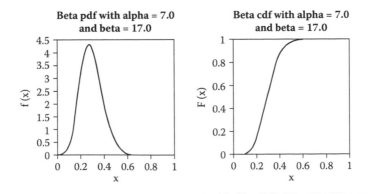

FIGURE 3.2
The pdf and cdf of the beta distribution with $\alpha = 7$ and $\beta = 17$.

```
%
x = [0:0.01:1];
f = betapdf(x, alpha, beta);
F = betacdf(x, alpha, beta);
%
figure
subplot(1,2,1)
plot(x,f)
axis('square')
xlabel('x')
ylabel('f(x)')
title(sprintf('Beta pdf with alpha = %2.1f and beta =...
  %2.1f \n', alpha, beta))
subplot(1,2,2)
plot(x,F)
axis('square')
xlabel('x')
ylabel('F(x)')
title(sprintf('Beta cdf with alpha = %2.1f and beta =...
  %2.1f \n', alpha, beta))
%
% The figure will be saved in a postscript file called
% "beta_figure.ps"
%
print beta_figure.ps
%
% End of the script
```

The beta distribution reduces to the uniform distribution over (0, 1) if $\alpha = 1 = \beta$. If X has a beta distribution, then we symbolically denote this by writing $X \sim BETA(\alpha, \beta)$. If $X \sim BETA(\alpha, \beta)$,

$$E(X) = \frac{\alpha}{\alpha + \beta}$$

$$Var(X) = \frac{\alpha\beta}{(\alpha + \beta)^2(\alpha + \beta + 1)}.$$

The beta distribution can be generalized to any bounded interval $[a, b]$. This generalized distribution is called the generalized beta distribution. If a random variable X has this generalized beta distribution, we denote it by writing $X \sim GBETA(\alpha, \beta, a, b)$. The probability density of the generalized beta distribution is given by

$$f(x) = \begin{cases} \dfrac{1}{B(\alpha, \beta)} \dfrac{(x-a)^{\alpha-1}(b-x)^{\beta-1}}{(b-a)^{\alpha+\beta-1}} & \text{if } a < x < b \\ 0 & \text{otherwise} \end{cases}$$

where α, β, $a > 0$. If $X \sim GBETA(\alpha, \beta, a, b)$, then

$$E(X) = (b - a)\frac{\alpha}{\alpha + \beta} + a$$

$$Var(X) = (b - a)^2 \frac{\alpha\beta}{(\alpha + \beta)^2(\alpha + \beta + 1)}.$$

3.6.2.4 Normal Distribution

Among continuous probability distributions, the normal distribution is very well known because it arises in many applications. The normal distribution was discovered by a French mathematician, Abraham DeMoivre (1667–1754). DeMoivre wrote two important books. *Annuities upon Lives*, the first book on actuarial sciences and the second book, *Doctrine of Chances*, is one of the early books on probability theory. Pierre Simon Laplace (1749–1827) applied the normal distribution to astronomy. Carl Friedrich Gauss (1777–1855) used the normal distribution in his studies of problems in physics and astronomy. Adolphe Quetelet (1796–1874) demonstrated that man's physical traits (such as height, chest expansion, weight etc.) as well as social traits follow the normal distribution. The main importance of the normal distribution is due to the central limit theorem, which states that the standardized sample mean has a standard normal distribution if the sample size is large.

DEFINITION 3.27
A random variable X is said to have a normal distribution if its probability density function is given by

$$f(x) = \frac{1}{\sqrt{2\pi\sigma^2}} e^{-\frac{1}{2}\left(\frac{x-\mu}{\sigma}\right)^2} \qquad -\infty < x < \infty,$$

where $-\infty < \mu < \infty$ and $0 < \sigma^2 < \infty$ are arbitrary parameters.

If X has a normal distribution with parameters μ and σ^2, then we write $X \sim N(\mu, \sigma^2)$. If $X \sim N(\mu, \sigma^2)$, then

$$E(X) = \mu$$

$$Var(X) = \sigma^2.$$

DEFINITION 3.28
A normal random variable is said to be standard normal if its mean is zero and its variance is one. We denote a standard normal random variable X by $X \sim N(0, 1)$.

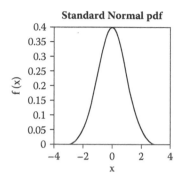
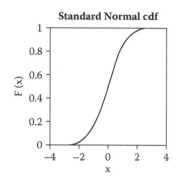

FIGURE 3.3
The pdf and cdf of the standard normal distribution. This figure was generated using a script similar to the script used for generating Figure 3.2 (beta_distribution.m).

The probability density function of standard normal distribution is the following:

$$f(x) = \frac{1}{\sqrt{2\pi}} e^{-\frac{1}{2}x^2} \qquad -\infty < x < \infty.$$

Figure 3.3 illustrates the pdf and cdf of a standard normal distribution. The following theorem is very important and allows us to find probabilities by using the standard normal table.

THEOREM 3.24
If $X \sim N(\mu, \sigma^2)$, then the random variable $Z = \frac{X-\mu}{\sigma} \sim N(0, 1)$.

PROOF We will show that Z is standard normal by finding the probability density function of Z. We compute the probability density of Z by the cumulative distribution function method:

$$F(z) = P(Z \le z)$$

$$= P\left(\frac{X-\mu}{\sigma} \le z\right)$$

$$= P(X \le \sigma z + \mu)$$

$$= \int_{-\infty}^{\sigma z+\mu} \frac{1}{\sqrt{2\pi\sigma^2}} e^{-\frac{1}{2}\left(\frac{x-\mu}{\sigma}\right)^2} dx$$

$$= \int_{-\infty}^{z} \frac{1}{\sqrt{2\pi\sigma^2}} \sigma\, e^{-\frac{1}{2}w^2} dw \qquad \text{where } w = \frac{x-\mu}{\sigma}.$$

Hence

$$f(z) = \frac{d}{dz} F(z) = \frac{1}{\sqrt{2\pi}} e^{-\frac{1}{2}z^2}.$$

The following theorem can be proved in a similar manner as the previous theorem.

THEOREM 3.25
If $X \sim N(\mu, \sigma^2)$, then the random variable $\left(\frac{X-\mu}{\sigma}\right)^2 \sim \chi^2(1)$.
A generalization of the normal distribution is the following:

$$g(x) = \frac{\nu \, \phi(\nu)}{2\sigma \, \Gamma(1/\nu)} \, e^{-\left(\frac{\phi(\nu)}{\sigma}|x-\mu|\right)^{\nu}}$$

where

$$\phi(\nu) = \sqrt{\frac{\Gamma(3/\nu)}{\Gamma(1/\nu)}}$$

and ν and σ are real positive constants and $-\infty < \mu < \infty$ is a real constant. The constant μ represents the mean, and the constant σ represents the standard deviation of the generalized normal distribution. If $\nu = 2$, the generalized normal distribution reduces to the normal distribution. If $\nu = 1$, the generalized normal distribution reduces to the Laplace distribution, whose density function is given by

$$f(x) = \frac{1}{2\theta} e^{-\frac{|x-\mu|}{\theta}}$$

where $\theta = \sigma/\sqrt{2}$. The generalized normal distribution is very useful in signal processing and, in particular, modeling of the discrete cosine transform (DCT) coefficients of a digital image.

3.6.2.5 Lognormal Distribution

The study of the lognormal distribution was initiated by Galton [2] and McAlister [3] in 1879. They came across this distribution while studying the use of the geometric mean as an estimate of location. Later, Kapteyn [4] discussed the genesis of this distribution. This distribution can be defined as the distribution of a random variable whose logarithm is normally distributed. Often, the size distribution of organisms, the distribution of species, the distribution of the number of persons in a census occupation class, the distribution of stars in the universe, and the distribution of the size of incomes are modeled by lognormal distributions. The lognormal distribution is used in biology, astronomy, economics, pharmacology, and engineering. This distribution is sometimes known as the Galton–McAlister distribution. In economics, the lognormal distribution is called the Cobb–Douglas distribution.

DEFINITION 3.29

A random variable X is said to have a lognormal distribution if its probability density function is given by

$$f(x) = \begin{cases} \dfrac{1}{x\sigma\sqrt{2\pi}} e^{-\frac{1}{2}\left(\frac{\ln x - \mu}{\sigma}\right)^2} & \text{if } 0 < x < \infty \\ 0 & \text{otherwise,} \end{cases}$$

where $-\infty < \mu < \infty$ and $0 < \sigma^2 < \infty$ are arbitrary parameters.

If X has a lognormal distribution with parameters μ and σ^2, then we write $X \sim \Lambda(\mu, \sigma^2)$. If $X \sim \Lambda(\mu, \sigma^2)$, then

$$E(X) = e^{\mu + \frac{1}{2}\sigma^2}$$

$$Var(X) = \left[e^{\sigma^2} - 1\right] e^{2\mu + \sigma^2}.$$

3.6.2.6 *Inverse Gaussian Distribution*

If a sufficiently small macroscopic particle is suspended in a fluid that is in thermal equilibrium, the particle will move about erratically in response to natural collisional bombardments by the individual molecules of the fluid. This erratic motion is called Brownian motion after the botanist Robert Brown (1773–1858), who first observed this erratic motion in 1828. Independently, Einstein [5] and Smoluchowski [6] gave the mathematical description of Brownian motion. The distribution of the first passage time in Brownian motion is the inverse Gaussian distribution. This distribution was systematically studied by Tweedie [7] in 1945. The interpurchase times of toothpaste of a family, the duration of labor strikes in a geographical region, word frequency in a language, conversion time for convertible bonds, length of employee service, and crop field size follow inverse Gaussian distribution. An inverse Gaussian distribution is very useful for analysis of certain skewed data.

DEFINITION 3.30
A random variable X is said to have an inverse Gaussian distribution if its probability density function is given by

$$f(x) = \begin{cases} \sqrt{\dfrac{\lambda}{2\pi}}\, x^{-\frac{3}{2}}\, e^{-\frac{\lambda(x-\mu)^2}{2\mu^2 x}} & \text{if } 0 < x < \infty \\[2mm] 0 & \text{otherwise,} \end{cases}$$

where $0 < \mu < \infty$ and $0 < \lambda < \infty$ are arbitrary parameters.

If X has an inverse Gaussian distribution with parameters μ and λ, then we write $X \sim IG(\mu, \lambda)$. If $X \sim IG(\mu, \lambda)$, then

$$E(X) = \mu$$

$$Var(X) = \frac{\mu^3}{\lambda}.$$

The distribution function $F(x)$ of the inverse Gaussian random variable X with parameters μ and λ was computed by Shuster (1968) as

$$F(x) = \Phi\left(\sqrt{\frac{\lambda}{\mu}}\left[\frac{x}{\mu} - 1 \right] \right) + e^{\frac{2\lambda}{\mu}}\,\Phi\left(-\sqrt{\frac{\lambda}{\mu}}\left[\frac{x}{\mu} + 1 \right] \right),$$

where Φ is the distribution function of the standard normal random function.

3.7 Bivariate Distributions

There are many random experiments that involve more than one random variable. For example, an educator may study the joint behavior of grades and time devoted to study; a physician may study the joint behavior of blood pressure and weight. Similarly, an economist may study the joint behavior of business volume and profit. In fact, most real problems we come across will have more than one underlying random variable of interest.

3.7.1 Bivariate Discrete Random Variables

In this section, we develop all the necessary terminologies for studying bivariate discrete random variables.

DEFINITION 3.31
A discrete *bivariate random variable* (X, Y) is an ordered pair of discrete random variables.

DEFINITION 3.32
Let (X, Y) be a bivariate random variable, and let R_X and R_Y be the range spaces of X and Y, respectively. A real-valued function $f : R_X \times R_Y \to \mathbb{R}$ is called a *joint probability density function* for X and Y if and only if

$$f(x,y) = P(X = x, \ Y = y)$$

for all $(x,y) \in R_X \times R_Y$. Here, the event $(X = x, \ Y = y)$ means the intersection of the events $(X = x)$ and $(Y = y)$.

DEFINITION 3.33
Let (X, Y) be a discrete bivariate random variable. Let R_X and R_Y be the range spaces of X and Y, respectively. Let $f(x, y)$ be the joint probability density function of X and Y. The function

$$f_1(x) = \sum_{y \in R_Y} f(x,y)$$

is called the *marginal probability density function* of X. Similarly, the function

$$f_2(x) = \sum_{x \in R_X} f(x,y)$$

is called the *marginal probability density function* of Y.
    The following theorem follows from the definition of the joint probability density function.

THEOREM 3.26
A real-valued function f of two variables is a joint probability density function of a pair of discrete random variables X and Y (with range spaces R_X and R_Y, respectively) if and only if

(a) $f(x,y) \geq 0$ for all $(x,y) \in R_X \times R_Y$;

(b) $\sum_{x \in R_X} \sum_{y \in R_Y} f(x,y) = 1$.

3.7.2 Bivariate Continuous Random Variables

In this subsection, we shall extend the idea of probability density functions of one random variable to that of two continuous random variables.

DEFINITION 3.34
The *joint probability density function* of the random variables X and Y is an integrable function $f(x, y)$ satisfying

(a) $f(x,y) \geq 0$ for all $(x,y) \in \mathbb{R}^2$; and

(b) $\int_{-\infty}^{\infty} \int_{-\infty}^{\infty} f(x,y) dx dy = 1.$

If we know the joint probability density function f of the random variables X and Y, then we can compute the probability of the event A from

$$P(A) = \iint_A f(x,y)\, dx\, dy.$$

3.7.3 Conditional Distributions

The conditional probability density function of two random variables X and Y is defined as follows.

DEFINITION 3.35
Let X and Y be any two random variables with joint density $f(x, y)$ and marginals $f_1(x)$ and $f_2(y)$. The *conditional probability density function g of X*, given (the event) $Y = y$, is defined as

$$g(x/y) = \frac{f(x,y)}{f_2(y)} \qquad f_2(y) > 0.$$

Similarly, the *conditional probability density function h of Y*, given (the event) $X = x$, is defined as

$$h(y/x) = \frac{f(x,y)}{f_1(x)} \qquad f_1(x) > 0.$$

In the next two subsections, we define various product moments of a bivariate random variable. The main concept we introduce is the notion of covariance between two random variables. Using this notion, we study the statistical dependence of two random variables.

3.7.4 Covariance of Bivariate Random Variables

First, we define the notion of product moment of two random variables and then, using this product moment, we give the definition of covariance between two random variables.

DEFINITION 3.36

Let X and Y be any two random variables with joint density function $f(x,y)$. The product moment of X and Y, denoted by $E(XY)$, is defined as

$$E(XY) = \begin{cases} \displaystyle\sum_{x \in R_X} \sum_{y \in R_Y} xy\, f(x,y) & \text{if } X \text{ and } Y \text{ are discrete} \\[2em] \displaystyle\int_{-\infty}^{\infty}\int_{-\infty}^{\infty} xy\, f(x,y)\, dxdy & \text{if } X \text{ and } Y \text{ are continuous.} \end{cases}$$

Here, R_X and R_Y represent the range spaces of X and Y, respectively.

DEFINITION 3.37

Let X and Y be any two random variables with joint density function $f(x,y)$. The covariance between X and Y, denoted by $Cov(X,Y)$ (or σ_{XY}), is defined as

$$Cov(X,Y) = E([X - \mu_X][Y - \mu_Y]),$$

where μ_X and μ_Y are the means of X and Y, respectively.

Note that the covariance of X and Y is really the product moment of $X - \mu_X$ and $Y - \mu_Y$. Further, the mean of μ_X is given by

$$\mu_X = E(X) = \int_{-\infty}^{\infty} x f_1(x)\, dx = \int_{-\infty}^{\infty}\int_{-\infty}^{\infty} x f(x,y)\, dxdy,$$

and, similarly, the mean of Y is given by

$$\mu_Y = E(Y) = \int_{-\infty}^{\infty} y f_2(y)\, dy = \int_{-\infty}^{\infty}\int_{-\infty}^{\infty} y f(x,y)\, dydx.$$

THEOREM 3.27

Let X and Y be any two random variables. Then

$$Cov(X,Y) = E(XY) - E(X)E(Y).$$

PROOF

$$C(X,Y) = E([X - \mu_X][Y - \mu_Y])$$

$$= E(XY - \mu_X Y - \mu_Y X + \mu_X \mu_Y)$$

$$= E(XY) - \mu_X E(Y) - \mu_Y E(X) + \mu_X \mu_Y$$

$$= E(XY) - \mu_X \mu_Y - \mu_X \mu_Y + \mu_X \mu_Y$$

$$= E(XY) - \mu_X \mu_Y$$

$$= E(XY) - E(X)E(Y).$$

For an arbitrary random variable, the product moment and covariance may or may not exist. Further, note that unlike variance, the covariance between two random variables may be negative.

THEOREM 3.28
If X and X are any two random variables and a, b, c, and d are real constants, then

$$Cov(aX + b, \ cY + d) = ac \ Cov(X,Y).$$

PROOF

$$Cov(aX + b, \ cY + d) = E((aX + b)(cY + d)) - E(aX + b)E(cY + d)$$

$$= E(acXY + adX + bcY + bd) - (aE(X) + b)(cE(Y) + d)$$

$$= acE(XY) + adE(X) + bcE(Y) + bd$$

$$- \left[acE(X)E(Y) + adE(X) + bcE(Y) + bd] \right]$$

$$= ac\left[E(XY) - E(X)E(Y) \right]$$

$$= acCov(X,Y).$$

THEOREM 3.29
If X and Y are independent random variables, then

$$E(XY) = E(X) \ E(Y).$$

PROOF   Recall that X and Y are independent if and only if

$$f(x,y) = f_1(x)f_2(y).$$

Let us assume that X and Y are continuous. Therefore

$$E(XY) = \int_{-\infty}^{\infty}\int_{-\infty}^{\infty} xy\, f(x,y)\, dxdy$$

$$= \int_{-\infty}^{\infty}\int_{-\infty}^{\infty} xy\, f_1(x)f_2(y)\, dxdy$$

$$= \left(\int_{-\infty}^{\infty} x f_1(x)\, dx\right)\left(\int_{-\infty}^{\infty} y f_2(y)\, dy\right)$$

$$= E(X)\, E(Y).$$

If X and Y are discrete, then replace the integrals by appropriate sums to prove the same result. The following theorem follows easily from the previous theorem.

THEOREM 3.30
If X and Y are independent random variables, then the covariance between X and Y is always zero, that is

$$Cov(X,Y) = 0.$$

THEOREM 3.31
$Cov(X,X) = \sigma_X^2$

PROOF
$$Cov(X,X) = E(XX) - E(X)E(X)$$
$$= E(X^2) - \mu_X^2$$
$$= Var(X)$$
$$= \sigma_X^2.$$

Given two random variables, X and Y, we determine the variance of their linear combination, that is, $aX + bY$.

THEOREM 3.32
Let X and Y be any two random variables, and let a and b be any two real numbers. Then

$$Var(aX + bY) = a^2 \ Var(X) + b^2 \ Var(Y) + 2ab \ Cov(X,Y).$$

PROOF $\quad Var(aX + bY)$

$$= E\left(\left[aX + bY - E(aX + by)\right]^2\right)$$

$$= E\left(\left[aX + bY - aE(X) - bE(Y)\right]^2\right)$$

$$= E\left(\left[a(X - \mu_X) + b(Y - \mu_Y)\right]^2\right)$$

$$= E\left(a^2(X - \mu_X)^2 + b^2(Y - \mu_Y)^2 + 2ab(X - \mu_X)(Y - \mu_Y)\right)$$

$$= a^2 E((X - \mu_X)^2) + b^2 E((Y - \mu_Y)^2) + 2ab E((X - \mu_X)(Y - \mu_Y))$$

$$= a^2 Var(X) + b^2 Var(Y) + 2abCov(X,Y).$$

THEOREM 3.33
If X and Y are independent random variables with $E(X) = 0 = E(Y)$, then

$$Var(XY) = Var(X) \ Var(Y).$$

PROOF $\quad\quad Var(XY) = E([XY]^2) - \left[E(X)E(Y)\right]^2$

$$= E\left(X^2 Y^2\right)$$

$$= E\left(X^2\right) E\left(Y^2\right)$$

$$= Var(X) \ Var(Y).$$

3.7.5 Correlation

The dependency of the random variable Y on the random variable X can be obtained by examining the correlation coefficient. The definition of the correlation coefficient ρ between X and Y is as follows.

DEFINITION 3.38
Let X and Y be two random variables with variances σ_X^2 and σ_Y^2, respectively. Let the covariance of X and Y be $Cov(X,Y)$. Then, the correlation coefficient P between X and Y is given by

$$\rho = \frac{Cov(X,Y)}{\sigma_X \sigma_Y}.$$

The proof of the following theorem is straightforward.

THEOREM 3.34
If X and Y are independent, the correlation coefficient between X and Y is zero.

THEOREM 3.35
If X^* and Y^* are the standardizations of the random variables X and Y, respectively, the correlation coefficient between X^* and Y^* is equal to the correlation coefficient between X and Y.

PROOF   Let ρ^* be the correlation coefficient between X^* and Y^*. Further, let ρ denote the correlation coefficient between X and Y. We will show that $\rho^* = \rho$. This follows from

$$\rho^* = \frac{Cov(X^*, Y^*)}{\sigma_{X^*} \, \sigma_{Y^*}}$$

$$= Cov(X^*, Y^*)$$

$$= Cov\left(\frac{X - \mu_X}{\sigma_X}, \frac{Y - \mu_Y}{\sigma_Y} \right)$$

$$= \frac{Cov(X - \mu_X, Y - \mu_Y)}{\sigma_X \, \sigma} = \frac{Cov(X,Y)}{\sigma_X \, \sigma_Y} = \rho.$$

This lemma states that the value of the correlation coefficient between two random variables does not change as a result of their standardization.

THEOREM 3.36
For any random variables X and Y, the correlation coefficient ρ satisfies

$$-1 \le \rho \le 1,$$

and $\rho = 1$ or $\rho = -1$ implies that the random variable $Y = aX + b$, where a and b are arbitrary real constants with $a \ne 0$.

PROOF Let μ_X be the mean of X and μ_Y be the mean of Y, and σ_X^2 and σ_Y^2 be the variances of X and Y, respectively. Further, let

$$X^* = \frac{X - \mu_X}{\sigma_X} \quad \text{and} \quad Y^* = \frac{Y - \mu_Y}{\sigma_Y}$$

be the standardization of X and Y, respectively. Then

$$\mu_{X^*} = 0 \quad \text{and} \quad \sigma_{X^*}^2 = 1,$$

and

$$\mu_{Y^*} = 0 \quad \text{and} \quad \sigma_{Y^*}^2 = 1.$$

Thus

$$Var(X^* - Y^*) = Var(X^*) + Var(Y^*) - 2Cov(X^*, Y^*)$$
$$= \sigma_{X^*}^2 + \sigma_{Y^*}^2 - 2\rho^* \sigma_{X^*} \cdot \sigma_{Y^*}$$
$$= 1 + 1 - 2\rho^*$$
$$= 1 + 1 - 2\rho$$
$$= 2(1 - \rho).$$

Because the variance of a random variable is always positive, we get

$$2(1 - \rho) \geq 0,$$

which is $\rho \leq 1$. By a similar argument, using $Var(X^* + Y^*)$, one can show that $-1 \leq \rho$. Hence, we have $-1 \leq \rho \leq 1$. Now, we show that if $\rho = 1$ or $\rho = -1$, Y and X are related through an affine transformation. Consider the case $\rho = 1$; then

$$Var(X^* - Y^*) = 0.$$

However, if the variance of a random variable is 0, then all the probability mass is concentrated at a point (that is, the distribution of the corresponding random variable is degenerate). Thus, $Var(X^* - Y^*) = 0$ implies $X^* - Y^*$ takes only one value. However, $E(X^* - Y^*) = 0$. Thus, we get

$$X^* - Y^* \equiv 0$$

or

$$X^* \equiv Y^*.$$

Hence

$$\frac{X - \mu_X}{\sigma_X} = \frac{Y - \mu_Y}{\sigma_Y}.$$

Solving this for Y in terms of X, we get

$$Y = aX + b$$

where

$$a = \frac{\sigma_Y}{\sigma_X} \qquad \text{and} \qquad b = \mu_Y - a\mu_X.$$

Thus, if $\rho = 1$, then Y is a linear in X. Similarly, we can show for the case $\rho = -1$, the random variables X and Y are linearly related. This completes the proof of the theorem.

3.8 Finite Mixture Probability Densities

A finite mixture probability distribution is a compounding of a finite number of statistical distributions that arise by sampling from inhomogeneous populations with different probability density functions in each component. If X is a random variable that takes values in a sample space Ω and its distribution can be represented by a probability density function of the form

$$f(x) = \pi_1 f_1(x) + \pi_2 f_2(x) + \cdots + \pi_c f_c(x)$$

where

$$0 \leq \pi_i \leq 1, \qquad i = 1, 2, \ldots, c, \qquad \pi_1 + \pi_2 + \cdots + \pi_c$$

then the random variable X is said to have a finite mixture distribution. The probability density function $f(x)$ is said to be a finite mixture density function. The parameters $\pi_1, \pi_2, \ldots, \pi_c$ are called the mixing weights, or mixing proportions, and $f_1(x), f_2(x), \ldots, f_c(x)$ are called the component densities of the mixture. In many science and engineering applications, one is given a random variable X with the mixture distribution $f(x)$, and the goal is to find the component distributions $f_i(x)$ and the mixing proportions π_i. This is the finite mixture model. Hence, for a random variable X, a finite mixture model decomposes a probability density function $f(x)$ into the sum of c class probability density functions. The finite mixture model with c components expands as

$$f(x) = \sum_{i=1}^{c} \pi_i f_i(x).$$

The mixing proportion π_i may be interpreted as the prior probability of observing a sample from class i, that is, $\pi_i = P(\{x_i\}/\text{class } i)$.

The following MATLAB script generates the plots used in Figures 3.4 and 3.5 for $f(x)$ with $c = 3$, $f_1(x) = \Phi(x, -4, 0.5)$, $f_2(x) = \Phi(x, 0, 1)$, $f_3(x) = \Phi(x, 3, 0.7)$, $\pi_1 = 0.3$, $\pi_2 = 0.3$, and $\pi_3 = 0.4$. Here Φ is the pdf of the standard normal random variable.

```
% MATLAB Script: mixture_plot.m
% This script plot mixture of normal distributions
clear all
close all
clc
%
```

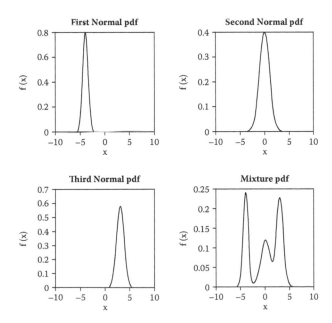

FIGURE 3.4
Plot of the three normal densities and their mixture density. The plot was generated using the MATLAB script mixture _ plot.m.

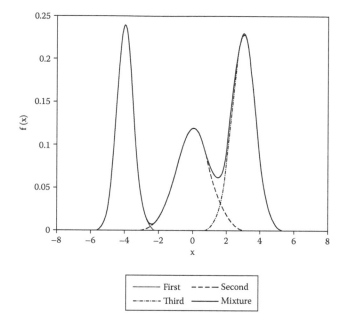

FIGURE 3.5

Plot of the three terms in the mixture density and the mixture density. The plot was generated using the MATLAB script `mixture _ plot.m`.

```
x = [-7:0.01:7];
pi1 = 0.3;
pi2 = 0.3;
pi3 = 0.4;
mu1 = -4; mu2 = 0; mu3 = 3;
sig1 = 0.5; sig2 = 1.0; sig3 = 0.7;
y1 = normpdf(x,mu1,sig1);
y2 = normpdf(x,mu2,sig2);
y3 = normpdf(x,mu3,sig3);
y = pi1*y1+pi2*y2+pi3*y3;
% plot each component distribution and also the mixture
figure
subplot(2,2,1)
plot(x,y1)
axis('square')
xlabel('x')
ylabel('f(x)')
title('first normal pdf')
subplot(2,2,2)
plot(x,y2)
axis('square')
xlabel('x')
ylabel('f(x)')
```

```
title('second normal pdf')
subplot(2,2,3)
plot(x,y3)
axis('square')
xlabel('x')
ylabel('f(x)')
title('third normal pdf')
subplot(2,2,4)
plot(x,y)
axis('square')
xlabel('x')
ylabel('f(x)')
title('mixture pdf')
%
print -depsc mixture_figure1 % for color figure
%
% plot mixture distribution along with each of its term.
%
figure
name = {'First','Second','Third', 'Mixture'};
plot(x,pi1*y1,'r', x,pi2*y2,'m', x,pi3*y3,'b', x, y, 'g')
xlabel('x')
ylabel('f(x)')
legend(name(:))
%
%
print -depsc mixture_figure2 % for color figure
% print mixture_figure2.ps % for black and white figure
%
% End of the script
```

There is no requirement that the component densities should all belong to the same parametric family, but in this section we will restrict our attention to the simplest case, where $f_1(x), f_2(x), ..., f_c(x)$ have a common functional form but different parameters. We will denote $f_i(x) = f(x / \theta_i)$, where θ_i denotes the parameters occurring in $f_i(x)$. Then, the finite mixture density function can be written as

$$f(x / \Psi) = \sum_{i=1}^{c} \pi_i f(x / \theta_i),$$

where $\Psi = (\pi_1, \pi_2, ..., \pi_c, \theta_1, \theta_2, ..., \theta_c)$ is the complete collection of all distinct parameters occurring in the mixture model. To fit finite mixture distributions, one needs to estimate all the parameters in the mixture models. There are several estimation methods such as the moment method, maximum likelihood method, minimum chi-square method, and least squares method. In this section, we focus only on the maximum likelihood method.

Let $x_1, x_2, ..., x_n$ be a random sample of size n from a mixed population X. Then, a complete data is defined as

$$\{y_j \mid j = 1, 2, ..., n\} = \{(x_j, z_j) \mid j = 1, 2, ..., n\}$$

where each $z_j = (z_{1j}, z_{2j}, ..., z_{cj})$ is an indicator vector of length c with 1 in the position corresponding to the appropriate category and 0s elsewhere. For a complete data set $(y_1, y_2, ..., y_n)$, the log likelihood function can be written as

$$\ln L(\Psi) = \sum_{j=1}^{n} \sum_{i=1}^{c} z_{ij} \ln \pi_i + \sum_{j=1}^{n} \sum_{i=1}^{c} z_{ij} \ln f(x_j / \theta).$$

For a complete data set, the likelihood estimation is straightforward if there are no constraints on the parameters. However, for incomplete data, the log likelihood function is given as

$$\ln L(\Psi) = \sum_{j=1}^{n} \ln \left(\sum_{i=1}^{c} \pi_i f(x_j / \theta_i) \right).$$

From the preceding formula, one can see that incomplete data result in a complicated log likelihood function, and it is difficult to obtain the maximum likelihood estimates. In many practical applications, such as image segmentation, the data sets are not complete, and the maximum likelihood estimates are obtained by an iterative process known as expectation maximization (EM) algorithm due to Dempster, Laird, and Rubin [8].

3.8.1 EM Algorithm

For an incomplete data set, the maximization of $\ln L(\Psi)$ can be achieved by the Gauss–Newton method. However, it requires heavy preliminary analytical work to obtain the required derivatives (gradient or Hessian). The EM algorithm, on the other hand, can often be reduced to a very simple reestimation procedure without much analytical work. Before we describe the EM algorithm, we first explain what the incomplete data problem is.

Let Ω_X and Ω_Y be two sample spaces, and let $H : \Omega_X \rightarrow \Omega_Y$ be a many-to-one transformation. Suppose the observed random variable y in Ω_Y is related to an unobserved random variable x by $y = H(x)$. That is, there is some complete data x that is only partially observed in the form of the incomplete data y. Let $p(x/\theta)$ be the parametric distribution of x, where θ is a vector of parameters taking its values in the parameter space Θ. The distribution of y, denoted by $q(y/\theta)$, is also parametrized by θ because

$$q(y/\theta) = \int_{H(x)=y} q(x/\theta)\, dx.$$

Estimation of θ from y is an incomplete data problem.

The maximum likelihood estimator $\hat{\theta}$ of θ is obtained from

$$\hat{\theta} = \arg\max_{\theta \in \Theta} L(\theta),$$

where

$$L(\theta) = \ln q(y/\theta).$$

Because only the incomplete data y are available, it is not possible to perform directly the optimization of the complete data likelihood $\ln p(x/\theta)$. Instead, it seems intuitively reasonable to estimate $\ln p(x/\theta)$ from y and use this estimated likelihood function to obtain the maximizer of $\hat{\theta}$. Because estimating the complete data likelihood $\ln p(x/\theta)$ requires θ, it is necessary to use an iterative approach: first, estimate the complete data likelihood given the current value of θ; then maximize this likelihood function over θ; and iterate, hoping for convergence. The best estimate of $\ln p(x/\theta)$ given a current value θ' of the parameters and y is the conditional expectation

$$Q(\theta, \theta') = E(\ln p(x/\theta)/y, \theta').$$

The EM algorithm is then given by
E-step: compute

$$Q(\theta, \theta^{(p)}) = E\left(\ln p(x/\theta)/y, \theta^{(p)}\right),$$

M-step: choose

$$\theta^{(p+1)} \in \arg\max_{\theta \in \Theta} Q\left(\theta, \theta^{(p)}\right)$$

where $\theta^{(p)}$ denotes the value of the parameter obtained at the pth iteration.

Now we illustrate how the EM algorithm can be used for estimating of parameters in the mixture model. Let $y = (y_1, y_2, ..., y_n)$ be a sequence of independent and identically distributed (i.i.d) random variables, observations drawn from a mixture of two univariate Gaussians with means μ_1

and μ_2, variances σ_1^2 and σ_2^2, and mixing proportions π_1 and π_2. That is, $y_k \sim q(y)$, where

$$q(y) = \pi_1\, q_1(y) + \pi_2\, q_2(y), \qquad y \in \mathbb{R}$$

with $\pi_1 + \pi_2 = 1$ and

$$q_j(y) = \frac{1}{\sqrt{2\pi\sigma_j^2}}\, \exp\left(-\frac{1}{2}\left(\frac{y - \mu_j}{\sigma_j}\right)^2\right), \qquad j = 1, 2.$$

For simplicity, assume that the variances and mixing proportions are known. The unknown parameters that have to be estimated from y are the means, that is, $\theta = \{\mu_1, \mu_2\}$. The log-likelihood of θ is given by

$$\ln p(y / \theta) = \sum_{k=1}^{n} \ln q(y_k / \theta).$$

The maximization of the preceding can be easily performed by casting the mixture problem as an incomplete data problem and by using the EM algorithm. Drawing a sample y of a random variable with mixture pdf $q(y)$ can be interpreted as a two-step process. First, a Bernoulli random variable i taking value 1 with probability π_1 or value 2 with probability $\pi_2 = 1 - \pi_1$ is drawn. According to the value of i, y is then drawn from one of the two populations with pdf $q_1(y)$ and $q_2(y)$. Of course, the selector variable i is not directly observed. The complete data are thus $x = (x_1, x_2, ..., x_n)$ with $x_k = (y_k, i_k)$, and the associated complete data log-likelihood is

$$\ln p(x / \theta) = \sum_{k=1}^{n} \ln p((y_k, i_k) / \theta).$$

with

$$p(x_k / \theta) = \pi_{i_k} q_{i_k}(y_k)$$

$$= \pi_1\, q_1(y_k)\, 1_{i_k=1} + \pi_2\, q_2(y_k)\, 1_{i_k=2}$$

where 1_A is the indicator function for the event A. Then

$$Q(\theta, \theta') = E\left(\ln p(x / \theta) / y, \theta' \right)$$

$$= \sum_{k=1}^{n} \sum_{j=1}^{2} \left[\ln \pi_j + \ln q_j(y_k) \right] P(i_k = j / y, \theta').$$

From the last expression, it is straightforward to show that the EM algorithm reduces to a pair of iterative formulas for the means of the mixture of two Gaussians:

$$\mu_1^{(p+1)} = \frac{1}{n} \sum_{k=1}^{n} y_k \, P\left(i_k = 1/y_k, \theta^{(p)} \right)$$

$$\mu_2^{(p+1)} = \frac{1}{n} \sum_{k=1}^{n} y_k \, P\left(i_k = 2/y_k, \theta^{(p)} \right),$$

where the a posteriori probabilities $P(i_k = j / y_k, \theta^{(p)})$ can be obtained using Bayes' rule:

$$P(i_k = j/y_k, \theta^{(p)}) = \frac{\pi_j \, q_j(y_k/\theta^{(p)})}{\pi_1 \, q_1(y_k/\theta^{(p)}) + \pi_2 \, q_2(y_k/\theta^{(p)})}, \quad j = 1, 2.$$

3.8.2 Estimation of Parameters for the Mixture Model

In this subsection, we explain how EM can be used to find the maximum likelihood estimates of the parameters Ψ in the mixture model

$$q(y/\theta) = \sum_{j=1}^{c} \pi_j \, q_j(y/\theta_j), \quad y \in \mathbb{R}^d$$

where $0 \le \pi_j \le 1$, $\pi_1 + \pi_2 + \cdots + \pi_c = 1$, $q_j(y/\theta_j)$ is itself a density parametrized by θ_j, and $\Psi = (\pi_1, \pi_2, ..., \pi_c, \theta_1, \theta_2, ..., \theta_c)$. The complete data are formulated as the combination of observations y, with multinomial random variables i acting as selectors for the component densities $q_j(y/\theta_i)$. Let $y = (y_1, y_2, ..., y_n)$ be a sample of i.i.d. observations, $y_k \sim q(y/\theta)$. It can be shown that the EM algorithm for the maximum likelihood estimation of θ reduces to the set of iterative formulas

$$\pi_j^{(p+1)} = \frac{1}{n} \sum_{k=1}^{n} \frac{\pi_j^{(p)} q_j(y_k/\theta_j^{(p)})}{q(y_k/\theta^{(p)})},$$

$$\theta_j^{(p+1)} \in \arg\max_{\theta_j} \sum_{k=1}^{n} \left[\ln q_j(y_k/\theta_j) \, \frac{\pi_j^{(p+1)} q_j(y_k/\theta_j^{(p)})}{q(y_k/\theta^{(p)})} \right],$$

for $j = 1, 2, ..., c$.

Suppose each $q_j(y/\theta_j)$ is multivariate normal, that is

$$q_j(y/\theta_j) = \frac{1}{(2\pi)^{d/2}\,|\Sigma_j|^{1/2}} \exp\left\{-\frac{1}{2}(y-\mu_j)^T\,\Sigma^{-1}(y-\mu_j)\right\}$$

$$=: \phi(y;\mu_j,\Sigma_j),$$

where y is a d-component column vector, μ_j is the $d \times 1$ column vector of means, and Σ_j is the $d \times d$ covariance matrix. The superscript T represents the transpose on an array, and the notation $|\Sigma_j|$ denotes the determinant of the covariance matrix Σ_j. Here $\theta_j = (\mu_j, \Sigma_j)$. Then the posterior probabilities are given by

$$\tau_{kj}^{(p+1)} = \frac{\pi_j^{(p)}\phi\left(y_k;\mu_j^{(p)};\Sigma_j^{(p)}\right)}{\displaystyle\sum_{j=1}^{c}\pi_j^{(p)}\phi\left(y_k;\mu_j^{(p)};\Sigma_j^{(p)}\right)}, \qquad j=1,2,...,c,\ k=1,2,...,n.$$

From the last equation, we can compute the iterative EM update equations for the mixing coefficients, the means, and the covariance matrices. These are

$$\pi_k^{(p+1)} = \frac{1}{n}\sum_{j=1}^{n}\tau_{kj}^{(p+1)}$$

$$\mu_k^{(p+1)} = \frac{1}{n}\sum_{j=1}^{n}\frac{\tau_{kj}^{(p+1)}y_j}{\pi_k^{(p)}}$$

$$\Sigma_k^{(p+1)} = \frac{1}{n}\sum_{j=1}^{n}\frac{\tau_{kj}^{(p+1)}\left(y_j-\mu_k^{(p+1)}\right)\left(y_j-\mu_k^{(p+1)}\right)^T}{\pi_k^{(p)}}.$$

Note that if $d=1$, then the update equation of variance is

$$\sigma_k^{2(p+1)} = \frac{1}{n}\sum_{j=1}^{n}\frac{\tau_{kj}^{(p+1)}\left(y_j-\mu_k^{(p+1)}\right)^2}{\pi_k^{(p)}}.$$

The steps of the EM algorithm to estimate the parameters for a finite mixture with multivariate normal components are the following:

1. Determine the number of terms or component densities c in the mixture.

2. Determine an initial guess at the component parameters. These are the mixing coefficients, means, and covariance matrices for each normal density.

3. For each point y_j, calculate the posterior probability using the preceding formula.

4. Update the mixing coefficients, the means, and the covariance matrices for the individual components using the last three equations.

5. Repeat step 3 through step 4 until the estimates converge.

Typically, step 5 is implemented by continuing the iteration until the changes in the estimates at each iteration are less than some preset tolerance.

We close this section with the following remarks. First, EM iteration can be shown to increase the likelihood of the observed data given the model parameters. Second, EM converges to local maxima (not necessarily global maxima). For more on mixture model and expectation-maximization algorithms, readers are encourage to see Couvreur [9], Dellaert [10], Martinez and Martinez [11], Martinez and Martinez [12], and Moon [13].

Problems

1. A die is loaded in such a way that the probability of the face with j dots turning up is proportional to j for j=1, 2, ..., 6. What is the probability, in one roll of the die, that an odd number of dots will turn up?

2. If $P(A)=0.25$ and $P(B) = 0.8$, then show that $0.05 \leq P(A \cap B) \leq 0.25$.

3. Mr. Flowers plants 10 rose bushes in a row. Eight of the bushes are white and two are red, and he plants them in random order. What is the probability that he will consecutively plant seven or more white bushes?

4. Sixty percent of new drivers have had driver education. During their first year, new drivers without driver education have probability 0.08 of having an accident, but new drivers with driver education have only a 0.05 probability of an accident. What is the probability a new driver has had driver education, given that the driver has had no accident the first year?

5. An urn contains 10 balls numbered 1 through 10. Five balls are drawn at random without replacement. Let A be the event that "exactly two odd-numbered balls are drawn and they occur on odd-numbered draws from the urn." What is the probability of event A?

6. A box contains five colored balls, two black, and three white. Balls are drawn successively without replacement. If the random variable X is the number of draws until the last black ball is obtained, find the probability density function for the random variable X.

7. An urn contains five balls numbered 1 through 5. Two balls are selected at random without replacement from the urn. If the random variable X denotes the sum of the numbers on the two balls, then what are the space and the probability density function of X?

8. If $X \sim BIN(n, p)$, then prove that $E(X) = np$ and $Var(X) = np(1 - p)$.

9. If X is a geometric random variable with parameter p, then prove that $E(X) = \frac{1}{p}$ and $Var(X) = \frac{1-p}{p^2}$.

10. If $X \sim POI(\lambda)$, then prove that $E(X) = \lambda$ and $Var(X) = \lambda$.

11. If $X \sim GAM(\theta, \alpha)$, then prove that $E(X) = \theta\alpha$ and $Var(X) = \theta^2\alpha$.

12. If $X \sim BETA(\alpha, \beta)$, then prove that $E(X) = \frac{\alpha}{\alpha+\beta}$ and
$$Var(X) = \frac{\alpha\beta}{(\alpha+\beta)^2(\alpha+\beta+1)}.$$

13. If $X \sim N(\mu, \sigma^2)$, then prove that $E(X) = \mu$ and $Var(X) = \sigma^2$.

14. If $X \sim \Lambda(\mu, \sigma^2)$, then prove that $E(X) = e^{\mu+\frac{1}{2}\sigma^2}$ and $Var(X) = \left[e^{\sigma^2} - 1\right]e^{2\mu+\sigma^2}$.

15. Ron and Glenna agree to meet between 5 p.m. and 6 p.m. Suppose that each of them arrives at a time distributed uniformly at random in this time interval, independent of the other. Each will wait for the other at most 10 minutes (and if other does not show up they will leave). What is the probability that they actually go out?

16. A bus and a passenger arrive at a bus stop at a uniformly distributed time over the interval 0 to 1 hour. Assume that the arrival times of the bus and passenger are independent of one another and that the passenger will wait up to 15 minutes for the bus to arrive. What is the probability that the passenger will catch the bus?

17. Suppose the random variables X and Y are independent and identically distributed. Let $Z = aX + Y$. If the correlation coefficient between X and Z is $\frac{1}{3}$, then what is the value of the constant a?

18. Let X and Y be two random variables. Suppose $E(X) = 1$, $E(Y) = 2$, Var (X) = 1, Var (Y) = 2, and Cov (X, Y) = 0.5. For what values of the constants a and b, does the random variable $aX + bY$, whose expected value is 3, have minimum variance?

19. Let the joint density function of X and Y be

$$
f(x,y) = \begin{cases} \dfrac{1}{36} & \text{if } 1 \le x = y \le 6 \\[2mm] \dfrac{2}{36} & \text{if } 1 \le x < y \le 6. \end{cases}
$$

What is the correlation coefficient of X and Y?

20. Write a MATLAB function to compute the parameters of a univariate Gaussian mixture model for a given c.

References

1. Sahoo, P. K., *Probability and Mathematical Statistics*. Lecture Notes, Department of Mathematics, University of Louisville, 2008.
2. Galton, F., The geometric mean in vital and social statistics. *Proc. Roy. Soc* 29: 365–367, 1879.
3. McAlister, D., The law of the geometric mean. *Proc. Roy. Soc* 29: 367–375, 1879.
4. Kapteyn, J. C., Skew frequency curves in biology and statistics. Astronomical Laboratory, Noordhoff, Groningen 1903.
5. Einstein, A., Uber die von der molekularkinetischen theorie der Warme geforderte bewegung von in ruhenden flussigkeiten suspendierten teilchen. *Annalen der Physik* 17: 549–560, 1905.
6. Smoluchowski, M., Zur kinetischen theorie der Brownschen molekularbewegung und der suspensionen. *Ann. Phys.* 1906 21: 756–780, 1906.
7. Tweedie, M. C. K., Inverse statistical variates. *Nature* 155–453, 1945.
8. Dempster, A. P., N. M. Laird and D. B. Rubin, Maximum likelihood from incomplete data via the EM algorithm. *J. Roy. Stat. Soc* B 39: 1–38, 1977.
9. Couvreur, C., The EM algorithm: A guided tour. In *Proc. 2nd IEEE European Workshop on Computationaly Intensive Methods in Control and Signal Processing (CMP'96)* 115–120, Prague, Czech Republic, August, 1996.
10. Dellaert, D., The Expectation Maximization Algorithm. College of Computing, Georgia Institute of Technology, Technical Report No GIT-GVU-02-20, February 2002.
11. Martinez, W. L. and A. R. Martinez, *Computational Statistics Handbook with MATLAB*. Boca Raton, FL: Chapman and Hall/CRC, 2002.
12. Martinez, W. L. and A. R. Martinez, *Exploratory Data Analysis with MATLAB*. Boca Raton, FL: Chapman and Hall/CRC, 2005.
13. Moon, T. K., The Expectation-Maximization Algorithm. *IEEE Signal Processing Magazine*, 1996, November, 47–60.

4

Two-Dimensional Fourier Transform

CONTENTS

4.1   Introduction

We include a short discussion of this relatively classical subject of image processing for the sake of completeness. Because there is already a wealth of literature on the topic, our coverage will be somewhat limited. Here, we will assume that the reader is already familiar with the topic of sinusoidal signals and the one-dimensional (1-D) Fourier transform (FT). For a good refresher on this topic, we recommend the famous *Signals and Systems* book by Oppenheim, Willsky, and Nawab [1]. The idea behind the FT is to represent the temporal (time) or spatial (space) variations in signals in terms of some sinusoidal basis functions (i.e., sinusoidal signals of different frequencies). This way, the information contained in the signal (in the original domain) could be exactly transformed into spectral information in the frequency domain. Going back and forth between these two domains is possible with the forward and inverse FTs, which we will discuss shortly.

What could be the benefit of looking at the signal or image at the frequency domain rather than the spatial domain? Some image processing systems may pass or process certain frequencies, whereas block or limit others. This is a well-known topic in linear system theory, that is, the frequency-selective nature of the systems. Generally speaking, too much variation cannot be handled by most natural systems. For instance, in the case of our eyes, we cannot differentiate more than 20 frames per second, which is simply the idea behind motion pictures. Similarly, optical systems allow only a range of frequencies to pass through. We call this range the *bandwidth* of the system. Therefore, if we know the behavior of the system at different frequencies in advance, we can always have a good idea about how the system will respond to a certain input by performing a Fourier analysis of the signal to see its spectral components. This will enable us to directly understand what the system will do to that kind of input.

Inversely, to carry out some frequency-selective image processing operations, we can switch to the frequency domain via the FT and select (suppress or emphasize) the frequency components that we want, and go back to the spatial or image domain by the inverse FT. This type of direct processing, or filtering in the frequency domain, is more intuitive or instructional. However, for image processing tasks that demand more speed, the extra cost of FT and inverse FT operations should also be kept in perspective.

4.2   Two-Dimensional Discrete Fourier Transform

In what follows, we will give the definition of FT and discuss how it is obtained in discrete space. We will then directly go into the study of its applications in image processing. For a more detailed discussion of this powerful tool of signal and system analysis, we refer the reader to the excellent textbooks in the literature [1,2].

Given an $M{\times}N$ image $I[m,n]$ of two discrete spatial variables m (row direction or axis) and n (column direction), its two-dimensional (2-D) discrete Fourier transform (DFT) $X[k,l]$ is given by

$$X[k,l] = \sum_{m=1}^{M} \sum_{n=1}^{N} I[m,n]e^{-j2\pi[(k-1)(m-1)/M+(l-1)(n-1)/N]} \tag{4.1}$$

where $k = 1,2,...,M$ and $l = 1,2,...,N$ are spatial frequency variables, in units of "per sample," and $j = \sqrt{-1}$ is the unit imaginary number. We note here that, in the preceding 2-D DFT formula, we have adopted MATLAB's convention of indexing vectors or matrices by starting from 1, rather than 0. In many other textbooks, because there is not a concern of a particular computational platform, indexing starts from 0; for example, the whole image is scanned by letting m and n vary from 0 to $M-1$ and $N-1$, respectively.

We note that the 2-D DFT is separable in row and column directions. We can easily see this by rewriting the double sum in Equation (4.1) as

$$X[k,l] = \sum_{m=1}^{M} e^{-j2\pi(k-1)(m-1)/M} \sum_{n=1}^{N} I[m,n]e^{-j2\pi(l-1)(n-1)/N}$$

or

$$X[k,l] = \sum_{n=1}^{N} e^{-j2\pi(l-1)(n-1)/N} \sum_{m=1}^{M} I[m,n]e^{-j2\pi(k-1)(m-1)/M}$$

which simply tells us that, to obtain the 2-D DFT, we can take the 1-D FFT of the image matrix in the horizontal (column, n) direction first and take another 1-D DFT along the vertical (row, m) direction or vice versa.

The inverse 2-D DFT, which lets us recover the image from its transform, is given by

$$I[m,n] = \frac{1}{MN} \sum_{k=1}^{M} \sum_{l=1}^{N} X[k,l] e^{j2\pi[(k-1)(m-1)/M+(l-1)(n-1)/N]} \qquad (4.2)$$

Here, we observe that through Equation (4.2), our image is simply expressed as a weighted sum of some 2-D complex exponential basis functions of the following form:

$$B_{k,l}[m,n] = e^{j2\pi(k-1)(m-1)/M} e^{j2\pi(l-1)(n-1)/N} \qquad (4.3)$$

For each different (k, l) combination, we have a new basis function and the corresponding weights are the 2-D DFT values or coefficients, that is, $X[k, l]$. The basis function corresponding to $k = l = 1$ has a flat value of 1. Figure 4.1 gives a plot of the real and imaginary parts of the basis functions for several (k, l) pairs. The MATLAB script that we have used to generate this figure is as follows:

```
M = 20; N = 10;
[nspace,mspace] = meshgrid(1:N,1:M);
% meshgrid(x,y) operates in the regular cartesian space
% where x is the column and y is the row index in the
% image space
for k = 1:2
    for l = 1:2
        B = exp(j*2*pi*(k-1)*(mspace-1)/M).* ...
            exp(j*2*pi*(l-1)*(nspace-1)/N);
        figure, colormap(gray)
        subplot(121), imagesc(real(B)), axis image
        set(gca,'fontsize',12)
        xlabel('n'), ylabel('m') % n (col) is the x...
          direction
        title(sprintf('Real part of B(m,n) (k=%d,...
          l=%d)',k,l))
        subplot(122), imagesc(imag(B)), axis image
        set(gca,'fontsize',12)
        xlabel('n'), ylabel('m') % m (row) is the y...
          direction
        title(sprintf('Imaginary part of B(m,n) (k=%d,...
          l=%d)',k,l))
    end
end
```

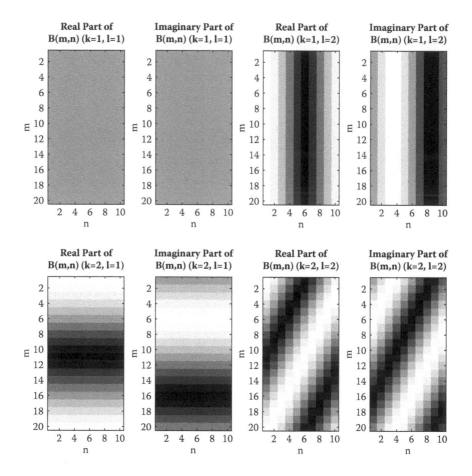

FIGURE 4.1

First four basis functions of the 2-D DFT (given by Equation [4.3]) for $M = 20$. and $N = 10$. Upper left: $k = l = 1$. Upper right: $k = 1$, $l = 2$. Lower left: $k = 2$, $l = 1$. Lower right: $k = l = 2$. The left and right panels, respectively, display real and imaginary parts of the spatial basis functions.

We observe that when $k = 1$, $l = 2$, there is a spatial variation in the column direction. Similarly, when $k = 2$, $l = 1$, there is a spatial variation in the row direction. When $k = l = 2$, there is a variation in both directions. Thus, if we construct a linear combination of these 2-D complex spatial basis functions or undulations, where the weights $X[k, l]$ are the 2-D DFT coefficients for an image, we will obtain or recover the image.

We can verify that the $B_{k,l}[m,n]$ are indeed basis functions in the image domain, where $m = 1, 2, ..., M$ and $n = 1, 2, ..., N$, by observing that the orthogonality condition is satisfied. That is,

$$\sum_{m=1}^{M} \sum_{n=1}^{N} B_{k,l}[m, n] B_{u,v}[m, n] = MN\delta[k - u, l - v],$$

where $\delta[k - u, l - v]$ is the Kronecker-Delta function (in 2-D discrete space), which is 0 everywhere except at the origin, that is, $[k - u, l - v] = [0, 0]$, when $k = u$ and $l = v$.

At the first glance, we may think that as k or l increases, the frequency of spatial variation in the basis functions $B_{k,l}[m, n]$ will increase. This is indeed a tricky point that needs some attention. Let us first discuss the equivalent case in 1-D for ease of understanding. The corresponding basis functions in 1-D are given as

$$\Phi_k[m] = e^{j2\pi(k-1)(m-1)/M}; \quad k = 1, 2, ..., M \tag{4.4}$$

These basis functions are also known as the *discrete space harmonically related complex exponentials*. We will observe that as k increases, the spatial frequency increases up to a certain point, then it starts decreasing. Before we verify this property, let us first note that $\Phi_k[m]$s are all periodic or cyclic with period M, because

$$\Phi_k[m + M] = e^{j2\pi(k-1)(m+M-1)/M} = \underbrace{e^{j2\pi(k-1)M/M}}_{1} e^{j2\pi(k-1)(m-1)/M}$$

$$= e^{j2\pi(k-1)(m-1)/M} = \Phi_k[m]$$

Here, we have used the fact that $e^{j2\pi(k-1)} = \cos(2\pi(k-1)) + j\sin(2\pi(k-1)) = 1$, because $k - 1$ is an integer. Therefore, the index m runs from 0 to $M - 1$, or from 1 to M in MATLAB.

We can also show that $\Phi_k[m] = \Phi_{k+M}[m]$ by following a similar treatment. This implies that we can have only M distinct basis functions of period or length M. Therefore, we can use any set of indices $k = u + 1, ..., u + M$, where u is an integer, that scan M consecutive values of k to express the same set of M basis functions of length M.

In Equation (4.4), for ease of indexing, we assumed that $u = 0$, and consequently, k was $1, 2, ..., M$. This same result can also be stated as

$$\Phi_k[m] = \Phi_{k\pm vM}[m] \tag{4.5}$$

where v is an integer. Therefore, if the index k is scanning the values $1, 2, ..., M$, until it hits the midrange, the frequency of the basis functions $\Phi_k[m]$s will keep on increasing, after which it will start decreasing. Indeed, from Equation (4.5) we obtain

$$\Phi_{M-k}[m] = \Phi_{M-k-M}[m] = \Phi_{-k}[m],$$

which means that when k hits $M - k$, we get the same frequency as at k, because $\Phi_k[m]$ and $\Phi_{-k}[m]$ are conjugate symmetric, that is, $\Phi_k[m] = \Phi^*_{-k}[m]$ or $\text{Re}\{\Phi_k[m]\} = \text{Re}\{\Phi_{-k}[m]\}$; $\text{Im}\{\Phi_k[m]\} = -\text{Im}\{\Phi_{-k}[m]\}$. Essentially, $\Phi_k[m]$ and $\Phi_{-k}[m]$ consist of cosine and sine functions of the same frequency; therefore, they represent the same frequency. However, for ease of reference or for mathematical convenience, the basis functions $\Phi_{-k}[m]$s corresponding to negative k values are typically specified as having a negative frequency.

The peak frequency for $\Phi_k[m]$s will occur at either $k-1 = M/2$ or $k-1 = (M-1)/2$, depending on whether M is even or odd, respectively. At this peak frequency, the basis function $\Phi_k[m]$ will become either

$$\Phi_k[m] = e^{j2\pi(k-1)(m-1)/M} = e^{j2\pi(M/2)(m-1)/M} = e^{j\pi(m-1)} \text{ for } k-1 = M/2, M \text{ is even,}$$

or

$$\Phi_k[m] = e^{j2\pi(k-1)(m-1)/M} = e^{j2\pi((M-1)/2)(m-1)/M} = e^{j\pi(M-1)(m-1)/M} \text{ for}$$
$$k-1 = (M-1)/2, M \text{ is odd.}$$

We note that the peak angular frequency is exactly π for M even, or $\pi(M-1)/M$ (which is very close to π when M is large) for M odd. These points can easily be demonstrated by the following piece of MATLAB code, where $M = 4$ so that the peak frequency is obtained at $k-1 = M/2 = 2$ or $k = 3$. The corresponding result is given in Figure 4.2.

```
M = 4; % Period of harmonically related exponentials
m = 1:M; % Spatial index
w0 = 2*pi/M;
for k = 1:M % k is the frequency index
    figure(k)
    Phi_km = exp(j*w0*(k-1)*(m-1));
    subplot(2,1,1), stem(m,real(Phi_km))
    set(gca,'xtick',m,'fontsize',12), xlabel('m')
    axis([.5 M+.5 -1.1 1.1]),title(sprintf ...
        ('Real part of \\Phi_%d(m)',k))
    subplot(2,1,2), stem(m,imag(Phi_km))
    set(gca,'xtick',m,'fontsize',12), xlabel('m')
    axis([.5 M+.5 -1.1 1.1]),title(sprintf ...
        ('Imaginary part of \\Phi_%d(m)',k))
end
```

We observe that $\Phi_1[m]$ corresponds to DC (0 frequency), $\Phi_2[m]$ and $\Phi_4[m]$ are conjugate symmetric, and $\Phi_3[m]$ has the highest frequency. This discussion shows that the angular frequency of $\Phi_k[m]$ increases in the first half of the frequency index k; it then decreases toward zero in the second half of the index. Because of this cyclic nature of the basis functions, sometimes the first and second halves of the DFT coefficients are swapped before they are plotted. This way, the plot will extend from the negative peak frequency to the positive peak frequency, and the zero-frequency component (i.e., $k = 1$) will be right in the middle of the range. The fft-shift function does this swapping of DFT coefficients. We can easily check these new or shifted ranges for the case of even and odd M values by the following lines of code:

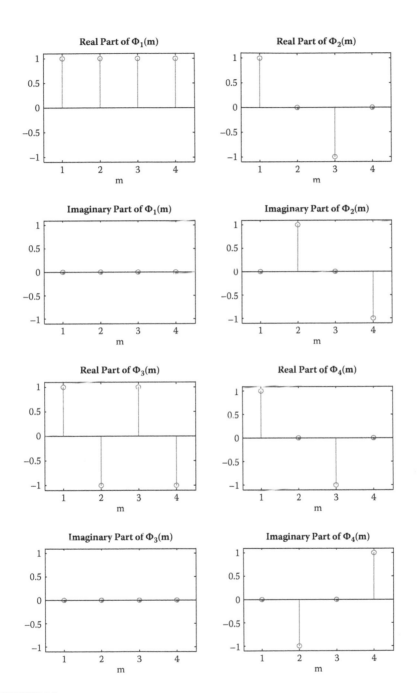

FIGURE 4.2

Demonstration of cyclic nature of harmonically related discrete space complex exponentials $\Phi_k[m] = e^{j2\pi(k-1)(m-1)/4}$; $k = 1, 2, 3, 4$ over $m = 1, 2, 3, 4$. Upper left panel: $\Phi_1[m]$. Upper right panel: $\Phi_2[m]$. Lower left panel: $\Phi_3[m]$. Lower right panel: $\Phi_4[m]$. Upper and lower plots in each panel respectively show real and imaginary parts.

```
M = 4; % example for M even
k = 1:M % regular range
shifted_k = fftshift(k)
% k = 1, 2, 3, 4
% shifted_k = 3, 4, 1, 2
% Peak frequency occurs at k = 3
% which is at the left-most position of the shifted
% spectrum

M = 5; % example for M odd
k = 1:M % regular range
shifted_k = fftshift(k)
% k = 1, 2, 3, 4, 5
% shifted_k = 4, 5, 1, 2, 3
% Peak frequency occurs at k = 3 or k = 4
% which are at the left- and right-most positions of the
% shifted spectrum
```

We can extend this discussion into 2-D as well. From the defining equation of 2-D DFT Equation (4.1), we observe that $X[k, l]$ is periodic in both row and column directions with periods M and N, respectively. Therefore, by using the fftshift function again, we can have the zero-frequency component moved into the center of the transform matrix, instead of having it at the (1, 1) position. Figure 4.3 nicely explains what is achieved by the fftshift operation in 2-D. The inverse operation of the fftshift is done through the ifftshift function.

Without further delay, let us compute our first 2-D DFT for the following test image, which consists of a simple square:

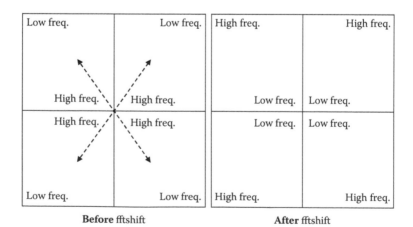

Before fftshift   **After** fftshift

FIGURE 4.3
Moving of low-frequency content in the 2-D DFT into the center- and high-frequency content on the outsides of the transform matrix by the fftshift operation.

```
I = zeros(51);
I(22:31,22:31) = 1;
X = fft2(I);
```

The name of the MATLAB function that does the 2-D DFT is `fft2`; fft stands for fast Fourier transform, which is just the name of a fast (optimized) algorithm that exploits the inherent symmetries in the basis functions. With the FFT method, the DFT is computed in an efficient (less demanding) manner, in terms of storage requirements (memory) and number of computations [2,3].

The entry of the X matrix at $k = l = 1$ is the strength or weight of the DC frequency (i.e., zero spatial frequency in both directions) component, which corresponds to the sum of all image pixel values. We can easily see this by putting $k = l = 1$ in Equation (4.1),

$$X[1,1] = \sum_{m=1}^{M} \sum_{n=1}^{N} I[m,n] \cdot$$

We can have MATLAB verify this for us by simply issuing the following command:

```
>> [X(1,1) sum(I(:))]
ans =
   100 100
```

The DC value is typically the largest value in X (the 2-D DFT of I), magnitude-wise. Therefore, while viewing the 2-D DFT of an image, suppressing this relatively unimportant value (i.e., pulling it down to 0) is usually a good idea to improve the visibility of other more interesting coefficients. Images that we deal with are typically obtained to convey to us the information visually in the best possible way. However, the 2-D DFT coefficients of an image are not generated for our viewing pleasure; they have a totally different function or meaning. First and foremost, they are complex numbers corresponding to the weights of complex 2-D spatial exponential basis functions. Nevertheless, considering or viewing them as an image, because they are already in matrix format, is still very practical. Another technique to improve the visibility of these coefficients is to take the log transform that compresses their dynamic range.

We will now `fftshift` the X matrix and view its magnitude and phase separately along with the original image. The result is shown in Figure 4.4.

```
X = fftshift(X); % Place the zero frequency in the
% center through fftshift
Mag = abs(X);    % Magnitude of 2D DFT
Pha = angle(X);  % Phase of 2D DFT
```

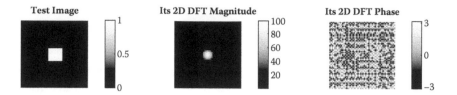

FIGURE 4.4

A test image consisting of a square box (left) and its 2-D DFT (middle magnitude, right phase in radians). Before viewing the DFT matrix, we have used the fftshift command to shift the zero frequency into the middle of the plot.

```
subplot(131), imshow(I,[]), title('Test image'), colorbar
subplot(132), imshow(Mag,[]), title('Its 2D DFT Magnitude')
  colorbar
subplot(133), imshow(Pha,[]),...
  title('Its 2D DFT Phase'),colorbar
colormap(gray)
```

We observe that the 2-D DFT angle or phase image (in radians) has only three distinct values, which are 0, $-\pi$, and π. This indicates that the 2-D DFT of our box image is real-valued. This is because the box image is symmetrical, about the center of the image space. (For a complete list/ discussion of symmetry properties of the 2-D DFT, we refer the reader to [1].) Instead of magnitude and phase, viewing real and imaginary parts of the transform matrix reveals this point readily (see Figure 4.5).

```
subplot(131), imshow(I,[]), title('Test image'), colorbar
subplot(132), imshow(real(X),[])
title('Its 2-D DFT (Real part)'), colorbar
subplot(133), imshow(imag(X),[])
title('Its 2-D DFT (Imaginary part)'), colorbar,...
  colormap(gray)
```

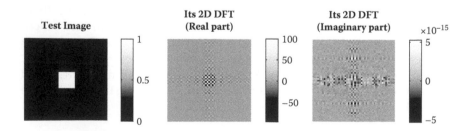

FIGURE 4.5

The test image (left panel) and its 2-D DFT (middle panel: real part; right panel: imaginary part).

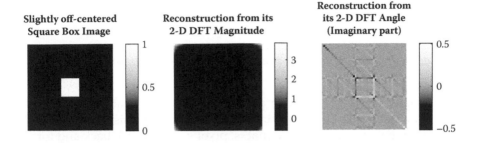

FIGURE 4.6
Left: Slightly off-centered square box image. Middle: Image reconstructed from its 2-D DFT magnitude, assuming that the phase is 0 everywhere. Right: Imaginary part of the image reconstructed from its 2-D DFT phase, assuming that the magnitude is 1 everywhere.

We note that, within MATLAB's numerical tolerances, the imaginary part of the 2-D DFT is 0 everywhere. However, in the more general case, 2-D DFT coefficients are complex numbers; their phase as well as magnitude do carry some important information about the corresponding image. It may be easier to appreciate the meaning of 2-D DFT magnitude, as it represents the strength of the 2-D sinusoidal basis functions. The phase, on the other hand, carries information about the delays or phases, as the name implies, of the 2-D sinusoidal basis functions or undulations.

In order to recognize the importance of the information in the phase, let us first create another image with some proper phase information, take its 2-D DFT. (Recall that our current image, which is a symmetrical square box, has practically zero phase.) We will then do an inverse transform using the magnitude of the 2-D DFT only, assuming that the phase is 0 everywhere. The resultant image will be real-valued and even symmetrical around the center of the image, owing to the even symmetry of the 2-D FFT magnitude. We can also carry out an inverse transform on the phase of the 2-D DFT only, assuming that the magnitude is constant (e.g., 1) everywhere. In contrast to the previous case, the resultant image will be purely imaginary in this case. Therefore, we will view its imaginary part only. The following lines of code implement these ideas. The result is presented in Figure 4.6. We note that the edges of the box in the original image are clearly visible in the imaginary part of the image reconstructed from the phase (the right panel in Figure 4.5), which proves that the phase information also has a crucial role.

```
I = zeros(51); I(21:31,21:31) = 1; X = fft2(I);
Ir_mag = ifft2(abs(X)); % Reconstruction using 2D DFT ...
% Magnitude only
Ir_ang = ifft2(angle(X)); % Reconstruction using 2D DFT ...
% Angle only
subplot(131), imshow(I,[]), colorbar
```

```
title('Slightly off-centered square box image')
subplot(132), imshow(Ir_mag,[]), colorbar
title('Reconstruction from its 2D DFT Magnitude')
subplot(133), imshow(imag(Ir_ang),[]), colorbar
title('Reconstruction from its 2D DFT Angle (Imaginary part)'),...
   colormap(gray)
```

Let us now create images with patterns of different spatial frequencies and view their 2-D DFTs. We start with an image consisting of vertical stripes of maximum frequency, that is, pixel values switch back and forth between two values (1 and –1 in this case) as we move from one pixel to the next in the horizontal direction. Note how we generate this pattern using the cosine function. We first generate an index idx vector that runs from 0 to 50, and then compute cos(pi*idx), which is a cosine with the maximum frequency (i.e., π) in the discrete space. We then repeat this row 51 times to complete the image. The next few lines take the 2-D DFT of this image and prepare or process the transform matrix for better viewing.

```
L = 51; % Size of the square image
idx = 0:L-1; % Row index
one_row = cos(pi*idx); % Cosine with the max frequency,...
   i.e. pi
I = repmat(one_row,L,1); % Repeat the row L many times
X = fft2(I); % 2D DFT
X = fftshift(X); % Place the zero frequency in the center
% View the original image
subplot(121), imshow(I,[]), title('Original Image'),...
   colorbar
% View the magnitude of transform image
subplot(122), imshow(abs(X),[]), title('Its 2D DFT...
   Magnitude')
colorbar, colormap(cool)
```

The resultant image is shown in Figure 4.7. We observe that there is only one significant component in the image's spectrum, that is, in its 2-D FFT plot, and this component is at the maximum available horizontal spatial frequency, and all other frequency components have 0 magnitude.

If we make the stripes two pixels wide and in the horizontal direction instead of vertical, the peaks in the spectrum will appear at around half of the maximum available spatial frequency in the vertical direction. This is demonstrated in Figure 4.8 with the following lines of code. Compared to the previous case, where the stripes were one pixel wide, the spectral peaks are spread out this time. This is because our new pattern, consisting of two-pixel–wide bars, is not purely sinusoidal; it is similar to a square pulse, which has a rich spectral content.

```
I = zeros(50); % Fill image with zeros
I(1:4:end,:) = 1; % Make rows 1,5, 9,..,49 ones
```

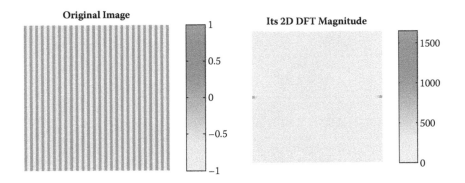

FIGURE 4.7
A test image consisting of a maximum sinusoidal variation in the horizontal direction (left)
and its 2-D DFT magnitude (right).

```
I(2:4:end,:) = 1; % Make rows 2,6,10,..,50 ones
X = fft2(I); % 2D DFT
X(1,1) = 0; % Suppress the DC component
X = fftshift(X); % Place the zero frequency in the center
subplot(121), imshow(I,[]), title('Original Image'), colorbar
subplot(122), imshow(abs(X),[]), title('Its 2D DFT Magnitude')
colorbar, colormap(cool)
```

We assume that the following block of code will be self-explanatory. The
resultant images are given in Figure 4.9. Here, we demonstrate the linear
nature of the 2-D DFT. Note that the images I1 through I5 in the following
are even-symmetric about their centers. Therefore, their corresponding

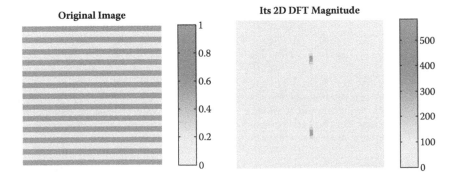

FIGURE 4.8
A test image with 2 pixel-wide square-wave type of variation in the vertical direction (left)
and its 2-D DFT magnitude (right).

Image	Its 2D DFT Magnitude

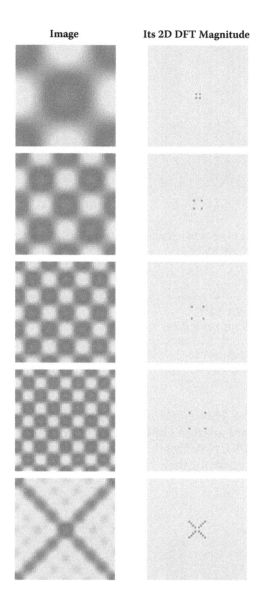

FIGURE 4.9

Top four rows: Left columns show symmetrical images of increasing spatial variation in both directions. Right columns show their 2-D DFT magnitudes. The last row: Sum of the images in the first four rows and corresponding 2-D DFT magnitude. We observe that the 2-D DFT of the sum image is similar to the sum of 2-D DFT images.

2-D DFT matrices are purely real. This is why we have displayed only the 2-D DFT magnitudes in the figure.

```
L = 51; % Size of the square image
idx = 0:L-1; % Index
```

```
one_row = cos(2*pi*idx/L)'; %Cosine with lowest spatial...
% freq.(1/L)
I1 = one_row*one_row'; % Outer multiplication to obtain...
% a matrix

one_row = cos(4*pi*idx/L)'; % Cosine with higher...
% frequency (2/L)
I2 = one_row*one_row'; % Outer multiplication to obtain...
% a matrix

one_row = cos(6*pi*idx/L)'; % Cosine with higher...
% frequency (3/L)
I3 = one_row*one_row'; % Outer multiplication to obtain...
% a matrix

one_row = cos(8*pi*idx/L)'; % Cosine with higher...
% frequency (4/L)
I4 = one_row*one_row'; % Outer multiplication to obtain...
% a matrix

I5 = I1+I2+I3+I4; % Sum of images I1... I4

for i = 1:5
    eval(['I = I' num2str(i) ';'])
    X = fft2(I); X(1,1) = 0; X = fftshift(abs(X));
    figure(i)
    subplot(121), imshow(I,[]), title('Image')
    subplot(122), imshow(X,[]), title('Its 2D DFT Magnitude')
    colormap(cool)
end
```

4.3   Applications of 2-D DFT to Image Processing

In this section, we will briefly mention some applications of the FT in the field of image processing. A typical application is low-pass or high-pass filtering of images in the frequency domain either to remove the noise or to enhance the small structures or edges. The other area in which FT has been used and still used today is tomographic image reconstruction.

Tomographic image reconstruction methods can be grouped under two main categories: filtered backprojection (FBP) and iterative reconstruction methods. It is not our intention to discuss these two types of methods in detail here. Nonetheless, we would like to describe how FT is employed within the FBP reconstruction method. Today, the FBP method is still the choice of image reconstruction in modalities such as MR and CT. Iterative reconstruction methods are gaining ground in SPECT and PET, owing to their superior performance in the case of noisy or fewer number of projections, and their ability to incorporate imaging system models to improve the contrast and resolution.

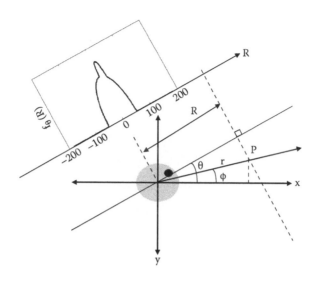

FIGURE 4.10
Projection of the image in the center consisting of two circles. The projection $f_\theta(R)$ was computed at $\theta = 60$.

If we regard simple backprojection as a process or a system, its effect on the output image is known as $1/r$ blurring. It can be shown that after simple backprojection, the resultant image function $f_b(x, y)$ is the convolution of the original image function $f(x, y)$ with $(x^2 + y^2)^{-1/2}$ 2-D blur function [4]. That is,

$$f_b(x, y) = f(x, y) \oplus \oplus (x^2 + y^2)^{-1/2} \tag{4.6}$$

where the $\oplus\oplus$ sign denotes a 2-D convolution operation. In polar coordinates, this can be written as

$$f_b(r, \phi) = f(r, \phi) \oplus \oplus \frac{1}{r} \xrightarrow{\text{2D Fourier Transform}} F_b(\rho, \theta) = \frac{F(\rho, \theta)}{\rho} \tag{4.7}$$

where $r = (x^2 + y^2)^{1/2}$ and (ρ, θ) denote the frequency domain corresponding to the polar coordinates. (It can be shown that the FT of $1/r$ is equal to $1/\rho$.) This means that each point in the image is blurred radially by the point spread function (PSF) of the simple backprojection operation. However, correcting for this blurring effect requires 2-D FT.

Figure 4.10 shows the projection $f_\theta(R)$ of the 2-D function (image) consisting of two circles that was computed at $\theta = 60$. The image and the projection can be computed using the following script:

```
% Define the circles
E = [0.3 0.4 0.4 0 0 0;0.5 0.08 0.08 0.2 0.2 0];
% Create the phantom image
```

```
Img = phantom (E,256);
% Display the image
figure;imagesc(Img);
% Compute the projection for theta = 120
% 60 degree in figure 4.10 corresponds to 120 in MATLAB's radon
[ftheta,R] = radon(Img,120);
% Plot the profile
figure;plot(R,ftheta)
```

It can also be shown that the backprojection process weighs the FT of each 1-D projection $f_\theta(R)$ signal $F_\theta(\rho,\theta)$, with $1/\rho$ along the radial line defined by θ in the (ρ, θ) domain [4,5]. Here, R denotes the distance from the image center along the direction perpendicular to the projection direction. Due to this property of the backprojection, the radial blurring effect can be corrected by taking the FT of the 1-D projection $f_\theta(R)$, and multiplying it by $|\rho|$ before the backprojection. This reconstruction method is known as *filtered backprojection*. Figure 4.11 shows the flow diagram of the FBP operation.

The 1-D filter function, used to correct for the blurring and known as the ramp function due to its shape, is defined in the frequency domain as

$$H(f) = |f|. \tag{4.8}$$

Here we use f instead of ρ because the former is used more widely to denote frequency. Unfortunately, the ramp filter has the undesired trade-off between the deblurring and boosting high-frequency noise. In order to alleviate this problem, the ramp filter is multiplied by a window function, which is in essence a low-pass filter. These window functions are also known as *apodizing windows*. Table 4.1 includes some of these functions utilized in FBP. We know that the convolution operation in the spatial domain corresponds to simple multiplication in the frequency domain.

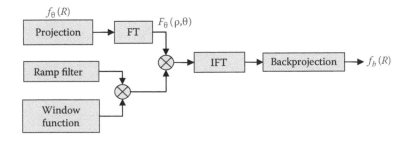

FIGURE 4.11
Flow diagram of the filtered backprojection process. FT and IFT refer to the Fourier and inverse Fourier transforms, respectively. The symbol ⊗ denotes multiplication performed in the frequency domain.

TABLE 4.1

Window functions and low-pass filters used in FBP

Shepp–Logan	$H(f) = \dfrac{2f_c}{\pi}\sin\dfrac{\lvert f\pi\rvert}{2f_c}$
Hamming	$H(f) = 0.54 + 0.46\cos\dfrac{\lvert f\rvert\,\pi}{f_c}$
Hann	$H(f) = 0.5\,\lvert f\rvert\left[1 + \cos\dfrac{\lvert f\rvert\,\pi}{f_c}\right]$
Butterworth	$H(f) = \left[1 + \left(\dfrac{\lvert f\rvert}{f_c}\right)^{2p}\right]^{-\frac{1}{2}}$

Note: The f_c refers to the cut-off frequency. The p is the order that determines the shape of the Butterworth filter.

The deblurred projection is transformed using the inverse FT back to image space before the backprojection process.

The following script, some of which is modified from `iradon` function of MATLAB, creates the ramp and the windowing functions in the frequency domain rather than the spatial domain, and plots them together. Their graphs for a cut-off frequency of $f_c = 0.5$ and for a projection signal length of $L \le 128$ are given in Figure 4.12. Note that the window functions are multiplied with the ramp function. These plots clearly demonstrate how the different windowing functions suppress the high frequency

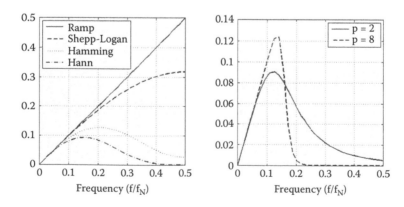

FIGURE 4.12

Left: Graphs of the ramp and the window functions for a cut-off frequency of $f_c = 0.5$. Right: Butterworth filter with orders of $p = 2$ for $f_c = 0.5$.

signals. The right graph illustrates the plot of the Butterworth filter, again multiplied with the ramp, for two different orders. The order p is a shape factor that determines the steepness of the filter's roll-off; the higher the order, steeper the roll-off.

```
% projection length L and cut-off frequency fc
L = 128; fc = 0.5;
figure;hold on;

% Ramp function
ramp = 2*(0:(L/2))./L;
w = 2*pi*(0:size(ramp,2)-1)/L;
% below cut-off frequency
INDX = (w <= pi*fc);
ramp = ramp(INDX);
w = w(INDX);
plot (w/pi,ramp);

% Shepp-Logan window
shepplog = zeros(1,length(ramp));
shepplog(2:end) = ramp(2:end).* sin(w(2:end)/(2*fc))./...
  (w(2:end)/(2*fc)));
plot (w/pi,shepplog)

% Hamming window
hamm = zeros(1,length(ramp));
hamm(2:end) = ramp(2:end).* (.54 + .46 * cos(w(2:end)/fc));
plot (w/pi,hamm)

% Hamming window
hann = zeros(1,length(ramp));
hann(2:end) = ramp(2:end) .*(1+cos(w(2:end)./fc)) / 2;
plot (w/pi,hann);axis square
legend ('Ramp','Shepp-Logan','Hamming','Hann','Fontsize',14);

% Butterworth filter
figure; hold on;
fc = 0.5; p = 2;
bworth = ramp.*(1./(1 + (w/fc).^(2*p)));
plot(w/pi,bworth);
p = 8;
bworth = ramp.*(1./(1 + (w/fc).^(2*p)));
plot (w/pi,bworth);
legend ('p = 2 ','p = 8','Fontsize',14);
set (gca,'Fontsize',14);
xlabel ('frequency (f/f_N)');
grid on; box on; axis square
```

Figure 4.13 shows the images of an anthropomorphic phantom that includes the lung; the heart inserts were scanned using a SPECT/CT

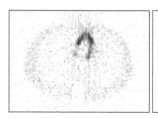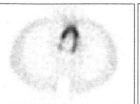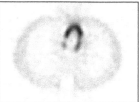

FIGURE 4.13

Image of the anthropomorphic phantom acquired using a dual-head SPECT/CT system. The images were reconstructed using the Ramp (left), Shepp–Logan (middle) and Butterworth (right) filters. The cut-off frequency and the order of the Butterworth filter were 0.5 and 8, respectively.

system. The images show the impact of the filter or the window function used within the FBP.

In our image library we have included a sinogram from this data set, so the reader can try out different parameters and filters to observe their influence on the reconstructed image. The tomographic image from the provided sinogram can be reconstructed by issuing the following commands:

```
simg = imread('anthropomorphic_proj.tif');
theta = 0:3:359;
I = iradon(double(simg), theta, 'Shepp-logan', 0.5);
```

The first line reads the sinogram data saved in the file anthropomorphic_proj.tif in TIF format. Then the image is reconstructed using the `iradon` function. The theta specifies the angles at which the projections were taken.

Problems

1. Take the 2-D DFT of the following test image I that we have used previously in the text and call it X, that is,

   ```
   I = zeros(51); I(22:31,22:31) = 1; X = fft2(I);
   ```

   Then, take the 2-D DFT of the X matrix this time and call it I2. Compare I and I2. Do they look similar? (I2 may have an ignorable/small imaginary part; therefore, you may want to take its real part before comparison.) What do you observe? This property is called *the duality of the Fourier transform*. That is, except for some scaling factors, the spectrum (2-D DFT) of an image's spectrum restores the original image back. What is the scaling factor in this case?

2. Consider the following lines of code that we have introduced before to generate Figure 4.7.

```
L = 51; % size of the square image
idx = 0:L-1; % Row index
one_row = cos(pi*idx); % Cosine with the max
% frequency, i.e. pi
I = repmat(one_row,L,1); % Repeat the row L many times
X = fft2(I); % 2D DFT
X = fftshift(x); % Place the zero frequency in the center
subplot(121), imshow(I,[]), title('Original Image'),...
   colorbar
subplot(122), imshow(abs(x), []),...
   title('Its 2D DFT Magnitude')
```

Now change the size of the square image to 50 (i.e., make L = 50) and rerun the code. Observe the resultant 2-D DFT image, why do we have only one peak at $-\pi$? What happened to the symmetric frequency component that needs to appear at π? (Hint: Remember that 2-D DFT is periodic.)

3. Develop a MATLAB script/code that demonstrates convolution in the image domain corresponds to multiplication in the Fourier domain, and vice versa.

4. Develop a MATLAB script/code that demonstrates the 2-D DFT of a shifted image is same as that of the original image, except for a linearly varying phase factor.

5. Develop a MATLAB script/code that demonstrates the *scaling property* of the 2-D DFT; that is, a contraction in the image domain produces a proportional expansion in the Fourier domain, or vice versa.

6. Develop a MATLAB script/code that demonstrates the *rotation property* of the 2-D DFT; that is, if an image is rotated, then its Fourier transform rotates an equal amount.

7. Develop a MATLAB script/code which demonstrates that the 2-D DFT of an $M \times M$ image $I[m, n]$ with a 2-D Gaussian intensity variation, for example,

$$I[m,n] = e^{-\frac{[(m-M/2)^2+(n-M/2)^2]}{2\sigma^2}},$$

is an another 2-D Gaussian in the Fourier domain. (Let $\sigma = M / 4$.)

8. Prove the *projection slice theorem*, which states that the 1-D Fourier transform of the projection of a 2-D object/image is the central slice of the 2-D Fourier transform of that image.

9. Study the effect of different filters on the reconstructed image using our sinogram data provided in our image database. See Section 4.3 about reading sinogram data.

References

1. A. V. Oppenheim, A. S. Willsky, and S. H. Nawab, *Signals and Systems*, 2nd ed. Englewood Clifts, NJ: Prentice Hall, 1996.
2. A. V. Oppenheim, R. W. Schafer, and J. R. Buck, *Discrete-Time Signal Processing*, 2nd ed. Englewood Cliffs, NJ: Prentice Hall, 1999.
3. R. C. Gonzalez and R. E. Woods, *Digital Image Processing*, Addison-Wesley, Reading, MA, 1992.
4. A. Macovski, *Medical Imaging Systems*. Englewood Cliffs, NJ: Prentice Hall, 1983.
5. A. K. Jain, *Fundamentals of Digital Image Processing*. Englewood Cliffs, NJ: Prentice Hall, 1989.

5

Nonlinear Diffusion Filtering

CONTENTS

5.1   Introduction

Linear filtering techniques (e.g., Gaussian filtering) are perhaps the most frequently used filtering techniques in image processing, but they suffer from two major drawbacks. First, they smooth image features such as edges and unwanted noise indiscriminately. Second, they dislocate image features (such as edges). To tackle the latter problem, the notion of scale-space was introduced by Witkin [1] and Koenderick [2] (see also Chapter 9). Scale-space representation consists of a set of images filtered with a Gaussian kernel with varying σ to change the resolution from coarse to fine. In scale-space analysis, to find the correct location of a feature, one tracks the feature in the scale-space from the coarse level back to the fine level. To alleviate the previously mentioned disadvantages of linear filtering, nonlinear diffusion filtering methods have been proposed. The lead work in this area is the seminal work of Perona and Malik [3], in which they proposed a nonlinear diffusion filtering method for scale-space representation, enhancement, and segmentation (edge detection) of images. The filters in this category address the two important disadvantages of linear filtering. This particular class of filters has found widespread application in medical image processing [4–17] owing to their superb performance in removing noise while preserving edge sharpness. Noise is a major problem in almost all medical imaging modalities, and these filters have provided a solution to the problem of resolution loss when removing noise with linear filtering methods. In this chapter we will discuss some of these nonlinear diffusion filtering techniques that have been applied in medical and biological image processing and analysis.

5.2 Diffusion as a Physical Phenomenon

In the context of particle movement, diffusion is the movement of particles from a place of higher to lower concentration. It is the rate of change (the concentration gradient) across the medium that causes the diffusion of particles. Thus, the flux density j is proportional to the concentration gradient

$$j = -D\nabla u \tag{5.1}$$

where the constant D is the diffusion coefficient, and ∇u denotes the gradient of the concentration u.

This equation is known as Fick's first law of diffusion, which states that the change in concentration is the driving force for the movement (flux) of particles. The continuity equation,

$$\partial_t u = -div\, j \tag{5.2}$$

where t is the time and *div* denotes the divergence operator, is a consequence of the fact that the number of particles remains constant or is conserved.

We know from basic calculus that the divergence of a function $f(x, y, z)$ is equal to the dot product of the divergence operator ∇ and the function f:

$$div\, f = \nabla \cdot f = \frac{\partial f}{\partial x} + \frac{\partial f}{\partial y} + \frac{\partial f}{\partial z} \tag{5.3}$$

In other words, the continuity equation states that the number of particles entering a region is equal to the number of particles that leave the surrounding regions.

If we substitute Fick's first law into the continuity equation, we obtain Fick's second law of diffusion:

$$\partial_t u = -div\ (D\nabla u) \tag{5.4}$$

$$\partial_t u = D\left(\frac{\partial^2 u}{\partial x^2} + \frac{\partial^2 u}{\partial y^2} + \frac{\partial^2 u}{\partial z^2}\right) \tag{5.5}$$

The second law states that the change in the flux with position determines how the concentration changes with time. This is the general diffusion equation for many physical transport processes such as heat transfer or the transfer of charged particles. In the context of heat transfer, this is known as the heat equation. In Equation (5.5), the term in parenthesis on the right hand side is called the Laplacian of u and is often abbreviated as $\nabla^2 u$ (see Chapter 2):

$$\partial_t u = -D\nabla^2 u \tag{5.6}$$

The heat equation has been much studied, and it can be shown by substitution that the Gaussian function is a solution of the heat equation (see Problem 1). The `pdedemo5` program in the MATLAB PDE Toolbox solves the heat equation. Although it is not necessary for understanding of the remainder of this chapter, we ask the reader to design and solve a heat transfer (diffusion) problem using `pdetool` in MATLAB (see Problem 3). Seeing the heat transfer or diffusion process in action will help you understand some of the notions discussed here, which may otherwise be difficult.

5.3 Application of the Concept of Diffusion to Image Filtering

If we regard image intensities as particles in two- or higher-dimensional image space, then the diffusion of particles is equivalent to filtering. Because the Gaussian function is a solution of the heat equation, linear filtering of images with a Gaussian kernel is equivalent to solving the heat equation over an image space or domain. If the diffusion coefficient D is a constant, then we are talking about a linear diffusion, and if D is a function of differential characteristics (e.g., edge gradient) of images, then the diffusion is said to be nonlinear, but still isotropic. That is,

$$D = \begin{cases} \text{Constant} & \text{linear} \\ g(|\nabla u|) & \text{nonlinear} \end{cases} \tag{5.7}$$

If D is a tensor-valued function, the diffusion is said to be an anisotropic nonlinear diffusion. Here, the term anisotropic refers to the direction-dependent characteristic of the diffusion process.

5.4 Perona–Malik Diffusion

Anisotropic diffusion filtering (ADF) was first proposed by Perona and Malik [3] for multiscale description, enhancement, and segmentation of images. Let a gray-scale and 2-D (scalar-valued) image u be represented by a real-valued mapping $u : \mathbb{R}^2 \to \mathbb{R}$. In Perona–Malik (PM) diffusion, the initial image u_0 is modified through the anisotropic diffusion equation:

$$\partial u_t = div(g(\|\nabla u\|)\nabla u)$$
$$u(0) = u_0$$
(5.8)

where div denotes the divergence operator, u is the smoothed image at time step t, $\|\nabla u\|$ is the gradient magnitude of u, and $g(\|\nabla u\|)$ is the diffusivity function. $g(x)$ should be a nonnegative, monotonically decreasing function approaching zero at infinity so that the diffusion process will take place only in the interior of regions and will not affect edges, where the gradient magnitude is sufficiently large. In this chapter, only scalar-valued diffusivities will be discussed.

The behaviors of the various anisotropic filtering techniques have been extensively studied [4]. PM diffusion has been shown to be ill-posed in the sense that images close to one another (e.g., repeated images of the same object) may diverge as the diffusion process evolves [4]. This stability issue was addressed by biasing the algorithm toward the original image with an additional bias term [5] given by

$$\partial u_t = div(g(\|\nabla u\|)\nabla u) + \beta(u - u_0) \quad u(0) = u_0.$$
(5.9)

PM diffusion may also produce false step edges. More importantly, PM diffusion cannot distinguish high-gradient oscillations of the noise from real edges causing high-gradient spurious edges to be preserved in the final diffused image.

5.5 Edge Enhancement

Nonlinear diffusion techniques not only preserve the edge sharpness, they may also enhance it. Let us assume that our steplike edge is parallel to the y-axis and the intensity profile along the x axis is represented by $I(x)$.

Let us define the flux function $\Phi(x) = g(x) \cdot x$, where $g(x)$ is the diffusivity function. Instead of the diffusivity, the flux function is often used for ease of understanding.

To study edge enhancement, we need to understand how and under which condition the slope of the edge evolves with time t. In other words, we need to find the function of $\partial(I_x)/\partial t$. Here, the time refers to the iteration step.

In the case of a 1-D signal, the diffusion equation can be rewritten in terms of the flux as

$$\partial I_t = \Phi'(I_x) I_{xx} \tag{5.10}$$

Let us expand the right-hand side of Equation (5.8) as

$$div(g(x,t)I_x) = \frac{\partial}{\partial x}(g(x,t)I_x) = \frac{\partial g(I_x)}{\partial x}I_x + g(I_x)I_{xx} \tag{5.11}$$

The derivative of the edge gradient or the slope with respect to t is given by

$$\frac{d}{dt}(I_x) = \frac{d}{dt}(\Phi'(I_x) \cdot I_{xx}) \tag{5.12}$$

If the edge function is sufficiently smooth, the order of differentiation can be changed as

$$\frac{d}{dx}(I_t) = \frac{d}{dt}(I_x) = \frac{d}{dx}(\Phi'(I_x) \cdot I_{xx}) \tag{5.13}$$

Then the rate of change of the slope can be expressed as

$$\frac{dI_x}{dt} = \Phi''(I_x) \cdot I_{xx}^2 + \Phi'(I_x) \cdot I_{xxx} \tag{5.14}$$

If the edge is positioned along the x direction as shown in Figure 5.1 (top left), then around the inflection point the second derivative $I_{xx} = 0$ and $I_{xxx} \ll 0$ (bottom-left). So the sign of $\Phi'(I_x)$ determines the behavior of the edge around the inflection point. If $\Phi'(I_x) > 0$, the slope of the edge decreases, and if $\Phi'(I_x) < 0$, the slope increases with time.

One of the two diffusivity functions proposed by Perona and Malik in their seminal paper has the following form:

$$g(x) = 1/(1+(x/\delta)^2) \tag{5.15}$$

where δ is the noise threshold or contrast parameter; the derivative of the flux function is negative when $\Phi'(I_x) < \delta$ and positive when $\Phi'(I_x) > \delta$. Figure 5.2 shows the plots of the flux and its derivative for $\delta = 10$. As seen in the figure, the derivative of the flux for the values less than the threshold is positive and it is negative when it is larger than the threshold.

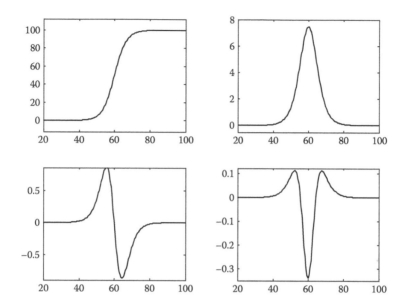

FIGURE 5.1

The edge function and its first, second, and third derivatives, in the top left, top right, bottom left, and bottom right, respectively.

Let us demonstrate how the edge gradient or slope behaves around the inflection point with time or (i.e., as we iterate the diffusion equation) using the Symbolic Math Toolbox.

Let us first define our symbolic variables for the space variable x, the diffusivity function $g(x)$, the flux function $\Phi(x)$, the noise threshold k, and edge profile $I(x)$, respectively, as:

```
% Define symbolic variables
syms x g phi k I
```

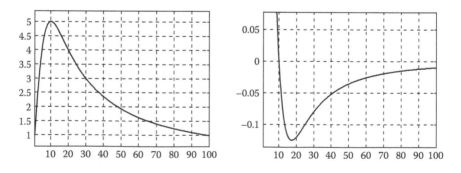

FIGURE 5.2

The flux function (left) and its derivative (right).

The following script creates and plots the expressions for the edge function that represents an edge profile in an image and its first, second, and third derivatives.

```
% Define edge function
I = 100./(1+exp(-0.3*(x-60)));
% First derivative of the edge
Ix = diff(I);
% Second derivative of the edge
Ixx = diff(Ix);
% Third derivative of the edge
Ixxx = diff(Ixx);
% ----------------------------- ---------
% Plot the 1st and 2nd and 3rd derivatives
% for the range [20,100]
figure;
subplot(221);ezplot(I,[20 100]);
subplot(222);ezplot(Ix,[20 100]);
subplot(223);ezplot(Ixx,[20 100]);
subplot(224);ezplot(Ixxx,[20 100]);
```

Their graphs are given in Figure 5.1. Next, we can create the expressions for the diffusivity and flux functions for a threshold of 10 using the following script:

```
% Let us define the diffusivity
g    = 1/(1+(x/k)^2);
% Differentiate g with respect to x
gx   = diff(g);
% Compute 2nd derivative of g
gxx = diff(gx);
% Obtain phi (flux) by multiplying g by x
phi = g*x;
k    = 10;
% Substitute k noise threshold in phi
phi = subs(phi);
```

The graph of the diffusivity is presented later in this chapter. We compute the first and second derivatives of the flux and plot (see Figure 5.2) them using in the following script:

```
% Compute the 1st and 2nd derivative of phi
phix  = diff(phi);
phixx = diff(phix);
% Plot phi and phix
figure; ezplot(phi,[1 100]); set(gca,'Xtick',[0:10:100])
% Plot the 1st derivative of phi
figure; ezplot(phix,[1 100]); set(gca,'Xtick',[0:10:100])
```

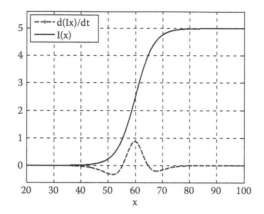

FIGURE 5.3
An edge function and the rate of change of the edge gradient or the slope with time.

As we see from the expression of the edge function, it is a 1-D sigmoid function centered at position 60. Now, we can create the expression given in Equation (5.14) and plot it together with the edge function using the following script. Note that we scale both the $\partial(I_x)/\partial t$ function and the edge function to be able to display them on the same figure:

```
% Compute derivative of the edge slope Ix with respect to
% time (i.e., iteration step), that is, d(Ix)/dt
dIxdt = phixx*Ixx^2 + phix*Ixxx;
% Plot the edge I and d(Ix)/dt
% Note that both signals are scaled for
% better visualization only
figure;
ezplot(100*dIxdt,[20 100]);
hold on; grid on;
ezplot(I/20,[20 100]);
```

Figure 5.3 shows the plots of the edge profile and the change of its slope with time as a function of position. On the $\partial(Ix)/\partial t$ curve, denoted by the dashed line, the positive center lobe denotes that the slope of the edge is increasing at and around the inflection point of the edge as the diffusion process continues, whereas negative lobes signify a decrease in slope.

5.6 Linear versus Nonlinear Diffusion

If we use a constant diffusivity function (i.e., $g(x) = 1$), then the diffusion will be linear, and the diffusion equation will be of the following form:

$$\partial u_t = \nabla^2 u \tag{5.16}$$

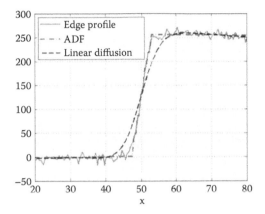

FIGURE 5.4
Plots of the 1-D sigmoid function (solid) and its filtered versions. Anisotropic diffusion filtering (ADF) (dot-dash) and linear diffusion filtering (dashed).

The right-hand side of this equation is simply the Laplacian of u.

Here, we would like to show the difference between the linear and anisotropic diffusion filtering methods and their impact on edge sharpness. The following script creates an edge profile using the sigmoid function and adds a normally distributed noise to it. The functions `mipadfoned` and `miplinoned` perform 1-D anisotropic diffusion and linear filtering, respectively. The former function performs an anisotropic diffusion, whereas the latter function implements the linear diffusion given by Equation (5.16).

```
[S,sx]  = mipsigmoidoned(256,0.8,100);
Sn      = S + 7*randn(1,length(S));
adf     = mipadfoned(Sn, 5000, 10, 0.05);
lindif  = miplinoned(Sn, 1000, 0.05);
plot(sx,Sn,sx,adf,sx,lindif);
```

The function `mipadfoned` discretizes Equation (5.8) as suggested in Perona and Malik [3], except that it is a 1-D version. We will discuss the discretization of partial differential equations (PDEs) in detail later in this chapter.

Figure 5.4 shows the plots of the noisy 1-D sigmoid function and its filtered versions. As seen in the figure, the linear filtering blurs the edge, whereas the ADF preserves edge sharpness.

5.7 Diffusivity Functions

The edge-enhancing ability of the ADF depends on the diffusivity function and the noise threshold, which is also known as the contrast threshold. The following code implements the diffusivity function given by

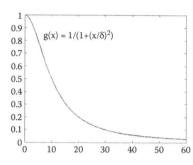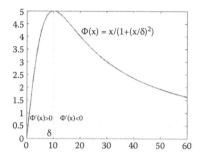

FIGURE 5.5
The diffusivity and flux functions.

Equation (5.15) and its flux for $\delta = 10$:

```
x = 0:0.5:60;
k = 10;
t = x/k;
g = 1./(1 + t.*t);
flux = x.*g;
```

Figure 5.5 shows that this diffusivity function is positive, monotonically decreasing. It approaches 0 as x approaches ∞, and its flux function reaches its maximum at the noise threshold. Recall that $\Phi'(x) > 0$ when $\Phi(x) < \delta$ and $\Phi'(x) < 0$ when $\Phi(x) > \delta$. Therefore, the diffusion is a forward diffusion for $\Phi(x) < \delta$, and it is a backward diffusion for $\Phi(x) > \delta$.

Diffusivity functions play a critical role in the performance of anisotropic diffusion filtering, so different diffusivity functions have been proposed. The decay (fall) time, in particular, of a diffusivity function impacts its ability to enhance edges. The most commonly used diffusivity functions are listed in Table 5.1. The MATLAB codes for other frequently used diffusivities are also provided in the function library, The Medical Image Processing Toolbox. The function $g_3(x)$ given in Table 5.1 can be generalized [6] as

$$g(x) = \begin{cases} 1 - \exp[-C_m/(x/\delta)^m] & x > 0 \\ 1 & x \le 0 \end{cases} \tag{5.17}$$

The constant C_m, which depends on the value of m, can be determined such that the flux reaches its maximum at the noise threshold δ (see the related problem). The exponent m affects the rise and fall times of the flux function in the neighborhood of the noise threshold (see Problems). This function code implements $g_3(x)$:

```
function g = diffusivityWeickert(k,Img)
g        = ones(size(Img));
indx     = (Img > 0);
Imgindx  = Img(indx);
g(indx)  = 1-exp(-3.15./((Imgindx/k).^4));
```

TABLE 5.1

Some diffusivity functions suggested in the literature

Function	Reference
$g_1(x) = 1 / (1 + x^2 / \delta^2)$	[3]
$g_2(x) = \exp(-x^2 / \delta^2)$	[3]
$g_3(x) = \begin{cases} 1 - \exp[-3.15/(x/\delta)^4], & x > 0 \\ 1 & x \leq 0 \end{cases}$	[6]
$g_4(x) = 0.5 \cdot ((\tan h(0.2 \cdot (\delta - x))) + 1)$	[7]
$g_5(x) = \begin{cases} \dfrac{1}{2}[1 - (x/\delta)^2]^2, & \lvert x \rvert > \delta \\ 0 & \text{otherwise} \end{cases}$	[8]
$g_6(x) = \begin{cases} \dfrac{p(T + \varepsilon)^{p-1}}{T}, & x < T \\ \dfrac{p(x + \varepsilon)^{p-1}}{x}, & x \geq T \end{cases}$	[4]
$g_7(x) = \begin{cases} \dfrac{p(T + \varepsilon)^{p-1}}{T} + \dfrac{1}{T}, & x < T \\ \dfrac{p(x + \varepsilon)^{p-1}}{x} + \dfrac{1}{x}, & x \geq T \end{cases}$	[4]

Note: δ is known as the noise threshold or the contrast parameter. T and P are parameters used to meet the requirements of the well-posedness.

5.8 Numerical Implementation

Nonlinear diffusion equations of the form given in Equation (5.8) do not have an analytical or open-form solution. These equations have to be solved using numerical methods. A finite-difference–based approach is the most common approach used to solve these PDEs. Readers can refer to the References [6,9–11] for further discussion of the descritization of the PDEs.

We will demonstrate this for a 1-D case first and then generalize it for 2-D and 3-D images. Let us choose equally spaced points in the x-axis (see Figure 5.6), and in time t and denote them by

$$x_i = i\Delta x, \quad i = 1, \dots N$$
$$t_k = k\Delta t, \quad k = 1, \dots n$$

Let us approximate the smooth signal $u(x_i, t_k)$ at time t_k by I_i^k. Then, the left-hand side of Equation (5.8) can be approximated using the first-order difference in time:

$$\frac{I_i^{k+1} - I_i^k}{\Delta t} \tag{5.18}$$

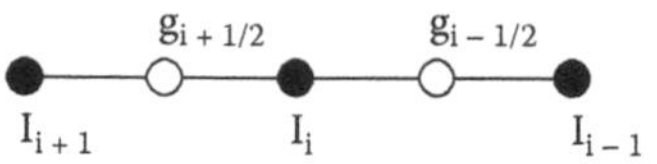

FIGURE 5.6
Neighborhood system in 1-D. Dark circles denote the pixel centers, and the empty ones denote the halfway point between the centers.

This is known as the forward Euler differencing (see Chapter 2). This scheme is first-order accurate in time t.

Let us now rewrite the right-hand side as

$$\frac{\partial}{\partial x}[g\Delta I] = (g\Delta I)_{i+1/2} - (g\Delta I)_{i-1/2} \tag{5.19}$$

Using again the same finite differencing scheme, the right-hand side can be discretized as

$$= (g_{i+1/2})\frac{\left(I_{i+1}^k - I_i^k\right)}{\Delta x} - (g_{i-1/2})\frac{\left(I_i^k - I_{i-1}^k\right)}{\Delta x} \tag{5.20}$$

Then our discrete equation becomes

$$\frac{I_i^{k+1} - I_i^k}{\Delta t} = \frac{g_{j+1/2}\left(I_{i+1}^k - I_i^k\right) - g_{j-1/2}\left(I_i^k - I_{i-1}^k\right)}{\Delta x} \tag{5.21}$$

The diffusivities in the center of the nodes can be calculated by averaging the diffusivities at the adjoining nodes [9]:

$$g(x_{i+1/2}) = \frac{1}{2}\left[\left(g\left(\nabla I_{i+1}^k\right) + g\left(\nabla I_i^k\right)\right)\right]$$
$$g(x_{i-1/2}) = \frac{1}{2}\left[\left(g\left(\nabla I_i^k\right) + g\left(\nabla I_{i-1}^k\right)\right)\right] \tag{5.22}$$

The spatial derivatives or the gradients in the aforementioned equations used to calculate diffusivities are approximated using central differencing (see Chapter 2 for more detail):

$$g_i^k\left(\nabla I_i^k\right) = g\left(\frac{I_{i+1}^k - I_{i-1}^k}{2\Delta x}\right) \tag{5.23}$$

This method is known as the explicit scheme. In other words, each smooth signal is computed directly from the smooth signals computed at previous time steps. There are also implicit methods that are more complicated and require the solution of the systems of equations at each step and are thus computationally expensive. Here, we will only discuss the explicit methods. The implicit schemes are unconditionally stable, whereas the

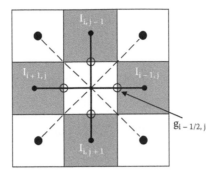

FIGURE 5.7
Pixel neighborhood in 2-D. Dark circles denote the pixel centers, and empty circles denote the halfway point between the centers of the center pixel and its neighbors.

explicit schemes limit the time step size Δt [12]. We will be discussing the stability conditions later in this chapter. Wieckert [12] suggests an efficient implicit discretization scheme with absolute stability based on the additive operator splitting.

5.8.1 Discretization in Multidimensions

Now let us now consider the 2-D case (see Figure 5.7), where sampling intervals are given by

$$
\begin{aligned}
x_i &= ih_1, & i &= 1,\dots N \\
y_j &= jh_2, & j &= 1,\dots M \\
t_k &= k\Delta t, & k &= 1,\dots n
\end{aligned}
\tag{5.24}
$$

The h_1 and h_2 denote the pixel spacing in the x and y directions, respectively. Pixels may be assumed to be isotropic with unit length (i.e., $h_1 = h_2 = 1$).

However, bear in mind that medical images, especially volume images, may have anisotropic pixel or voxel sizes. Let us approximate the smooth image $u(x_i, y_i, t_k)$ at time t_k by $I_{i,j}^k$. Then the left-hand side of Equation (5.8) can be written as

$$
\frac{\partial u}{\partial t} = \frac{I_{i,j}^{k+1} - I_{i,j}^k}{\Delta t}
\tag{5.25}
$$

and the right-hand side becomes

$$
\frac{\partial}{\partial x}[gI_{x,y}] + \frac{\partial}{\partial y}[gI_{x,y}] = [gI_{x,y}]_{i+1/2,j} -
$$
$$
[gI_x]_{i-1/2,j} + [gI_y]_{i,j+1/2} - [gI_y]_{i,j-1/2}
\tag{5.26}
$$

$$\frac{I_{i,j}^{k+1} - I_{i,j}^{k}}{\Delta t} = \frac{g_{i+1/2,j}\left[I_{i+1,j}^{k} - I_{i,j}^{k}\right] - g_{i-1/2,j}\left[I_{i,j}^{k} - I_{i-1,j}^{k}\right]}{h_1^2}$$

$$+ \frac{g_{i,j+1/2}\left[I_{i,j+1}^{k} - I_{i,j}^{k}\right] - g_{i,j-1/2}\left[I_{i,j}^{k} - I_{i,j-1}^{k}\right]}{h_2^2} \tag{5.27}$$

If we substitute g's given in Equation (5.23), then our final equation becomes

$$\frac{I_{i,j}^{k+1} - I_{i,j}^{k}}{\Delta t} = \frac{(g_{i+1,j} + g_{i,j})\left[I_{i+1,j}^{k} - I_{i,j}^{k}\right] - (g_{i,j} + g_{i-1,j})\left[I_{i,j}^{k} - I_{i-1,j}^{k}\right]}{2h_1^2}$$

$$+ \frac{(g_{i,j+1} + g_{i,j})\left[I_{i,j+1}^{k} - I_{i,j}^{k}\right] - (g_{i,j} + g_{i,j-1})\left[I_{i,j}^{k} - I_{i,j-1}^{k}\right]}{2h_2^2} \tag{5.28}$$

The diffusivities are computed as $g_{i,j} = g(\| \nabla u \|_{i,j})$, and the image gradients can be computed using the central differencing scheme given by

$$\| \nabla u \|_{i,j} = \frac{1}{2h}\sqrt{\left|I_{i+1,j}^{k} - I_{i-1,j}^{k}\right|^2 + \left|I_{i,j+1}^{k} - I_{i,j-1}^{k}\right|^2} \tag{5.29}$$

Starting with the initial noisy image $I_{i,j}$, we can compute the smooth image $I_{i,j}^{k+1}$ at a discrete time $t_{k+1} = (k+1) \cdot \Delta t$.

Implementing this finite differencing scheme on a 3-D mesh for volumetric images is fairly straightforward; therefore, we will leave it to the reader to derive the difference equations for 3-D. Our library function `mipisodiffusion3d` implements the 3-D version of the diffusion algorithm.

5.9   Numerical Stability

Numerical stability, in general, refers to the characteristic of the discretization method that it:

- Does not create spurious features and oscillations
- Does not amplify any errors or noise in the image

Let us consider the 1-D diffusion equation where D is a constant:

$$\frac{\partial u}{\partial t} = D\left(\frac{\partial^2 u}{\partial x^2}\right) \tag{5.30}$$

If we discretize it using the explicit scheme

$$u_i^{(k+1)} = u_i^{(k)} + D\frac{\Delta t}{(\Delta x)^2}\left(u_{i+1}^{(k)} - 2u_i^{(k)} + u_{i-1}^{(k)}\right) \tag{5.31}$$

then we can rewrite it in the matrix form as

$$u^{(k+1)} = M * u^{(k)} \tag{5.32}$$

where $M = [D\,\Delta t/h^2 \quad 1 - D2\Delta t/h^2 \quad D\Delta t/h^2]$.

The values of the smooth signal at level $k+1$ can be calculated as a weighted mean of the values of the signal at level k. The averaging mask in this case is given by

$$M = [\varphi \quad 1 - 2\varphi \quad \varphi] \tag{5.33}$$

where $\varphi = D\dfrac{\Delta t}{(\Delta x)^2}$.

Therefore, the filtering can be performed by convolving the signal with the mask M.

Stability can be guaranteed if the individual elements of the averaging mask are larger than or equal to zero. We need to be concerned with only the central element because we know φ is always bigger than zero. So, for a unit spacing, stability requires that $1 - 2\varphi \geq 0$. Finally, for $D = 1$, the inequality becomes

$$1 - \frac{2\Delta t}{(\Delta x)^2} \geq 0 \tag{5.34}$$

and $\Delta t \leq 1/2$ ensures stability for 1-D linear diffusion. It can be shown that the time step size stability limit in 2-D for a unit spacing assuming isotropy is limited by ¼. By isotropy we mean equal spacing in x and y dimensions. We leave the derivation of the time step for stability in 2-D and 3-D to the reader (see Problems).

For an extensive discussion of the stability of nonlinear diffusion, see [9].

5.10 Noise Threshold

The noise threshold, also known as the contrast parameter δ, can be computed for the entire image using the noise estimator described by Canny [13] and used by Perona and Malik [3]. It computes the histogram of the absolute value of the gradient for the entire image and then sets δ equal to the Kth quantile of the cumulative distribution. The smaller the quantile, the slower the diffusion. In medical applications, the quantile is generally adjusted to the problem at hand. Although a global quantile value often works well, K can also be estimated locally if the magnitude of the noise varies with position over the image space. In certain imaging modalities, noise may not be stationary within the image. In this case, estimating K locally may provide better performance. This can be true for PET images. Consider, for instance, the emission image of a cylinder positioned axially in the center of the scanner, and filled with positron-emitting radioisotopes. The magnitude of the noise within the cylinder will decrease radially with increasing radius owing to reduced photon absorption [14]. In this case, applying a different K value to each radial region may be a more effective strategy to reduce the spatially varying noise. The noise contrast δ could also be manually obtained from a uniform region within the image. For most practical applications or imaging modalities, the quantile-based method is in general very effective. It only takes a few trials to obtain a generally applicable value.

Black et al. [8] have introduced the robust estimator median absolute deviation (MAD) into anisotropic diffusion filtering. It was later used by Yu and Acton [15] in their speckle-reducing anisotropic diffusion. The MAD can be written as

$$MAD = 1.4826 \cdot median(abs(\|\nabla I\| - median(\|\nabla I\|))) \qquad (5.35)$$

The constant comes from the fact that the MAD of a normal distribution (with unit variance) is $1/1.4826$. The MAD is a more robust estimator because the intensities that are too large have less influence on the threshold. This estimator may be a good choice if the noise (intensity) distribution is more pulsatile or long-tailed.

The absolute average deviation (AAD) can also be used to calculate the noise threshold. The AAD can be written as

$$AAD = mean(abs(\|\nabla I\| - mean(\|\nabla I\|))) \qquad (5.36)$$

It is straightforward to implement these estimators in MATLAB. The interested reader can implement and investigate their performance on images corrupted by different types of noise distributions.

5.11 Regularization of Perona–Malik Scheme

5.11.1 Gaussian Regularization

To stabilize Perona–Malik diffusion, a Gaussian regularization method has been proposed [16]. In this formulation, the smooth image is the solution of the same diffusion equation, $\partial I = div(g(\|\nabla I_\sigma\|)\nabla I)$, except for the ∇I_σ term. This term denotes the gradient of the smoothed version of the image I and is obtained by convolving the image I with a Gaussian of standard deviation σ:

$$\nabla I_\sigma = \nabla(G_\sigma * I) \qquad (5.37)$$

where $G_\sigma = \dfrac{1}{(2\pi\sigma^2)^{1/2}} \exp\left(-\dfrac{x^2}{2\sigma^2}\right)$.

This method is expected to maintain stability during the iteration process because it obtains its edge estimate from the smoothed image. The existence and uniqueness of the solution have been discussed in detail in [16]. The major drawback of linear filtering before edge estimation is the dislocation of the edge and preservation of the noise in and around the edge. This effect may be more significant for large values of σ. In the next section we will discuss a different regularization method that alleviates the problems of linear filtering and improves edge estimation.

5.11.2 Median Regularization

Instead of Gaussian filtering, we suggest [17] using median filtering to obtain better edge estimation. In this case, the diffusivity function is replaced by $g(|\nabla I_M|)$, where $|\nabla I_M|$ denotes the gradient of the median filtered version of the image I. The median filter neighborhood W is commonly defined as an $N \times N$ (where N is odd) square window chosen around the center pixel (i, j). If $\{x_m\}$ is the sequence representing the ordered pixels of the neighborhood W around pixel (i, j) such that $x_{(1)} \leq x_{(2)} \dots \leq x_{(M)}$, then the mean intensity of the window $I_{i,j} = x_{(M+1)/2}$.

As the window size increases, the level of smoothing also increases. Median filtering eliminates objects smaller than $M/2$ [18], so it is essential to find a window size that is a good compromise between noise suppression and the smallest object to be preserved.

5.11.3 Comparison of the Gaussian and Median Regularization

Let us demonstrate the performance of both regularizations on synthetic images of a hexagon with ideal step edges corrupted by additive Gaussian and salt-and-pepper noise. The noisy image I_n can be expressed as

$$I_n = I_o + \eta \qquad (5.38)$$

where I_o and η are the original (noiseless) image and the additive noise, respectively. We can also show their noise reduction ability on images corrupted by the Weibull noise, whose density function is defined as [19]

$$f(x, a, b) = abx^{b-1} \exp(-ax^b) \quad 0 \leq x \leq \infty \qquad (5.39)$$

where a is the scale and b is the shape parameter.

The expected value of a random variable that has a Weibull distribution is $a^{-1/b}\Gamma(b^{-1}+1)$, where $\Gamma(s) = (s-1)!$ is the gamma function. The median of the distribution is $[a^{-1}\log(2)]^{1/b}$. The right-hand tail of the distribution is heavier than the left-hand one; therefore, this distribution is positively skewed. One can adjust the amount of skewness by changing the shape parameter. As b gets smaller, the tail of the distribution gets heavier and, therefore, the distribution exhibits impulsive behavior. For $b = 1$, the Weibull distribution becomes an exponential distribution.

To draw random samples from the Weibull distribution, the `weibrnd` function of MATLAB may be used.

For quantitative comparison, let us employ the normalized mean square error (NMSE), which is given by

$$NMSE = \sum_{i,j}(I_f(i,j) - I_o(i,j))^2 \bigg/ \sum_{i,j}(I_n(i,j) - I_o(i,j))^2 \qquad (5.40)$$

where I_f is the filtered image. The following MATLAB code computes the NMSE:

```
error1 = If-Io; % filtered - original w/o noise
error2 = In-Io; % original w/ noise - original w/o noise
nmse = sum(sum(error1.^2))/sum(sum(error2.^2));
```

Figure 5.8 shows the performances of both regularization techniques on a hexagon image corrupted by noise. As seen in the graph of NMSE, median regularization removes the noise faster, i.e., in a fewer number of iterations with smaller NMSE.

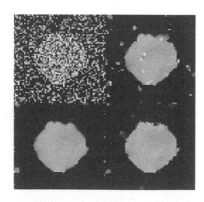
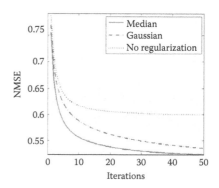

FIGURE 5.8
Original image corrupted by Weibull noise (a = 2, b = 1.9) and filtered images of a hexagon. The parameters of the filters were $\tau = 0.1$, K = 0.7, k = 50, N = 5, and $\sigma = 0.9$. Original (top left). Perona–Malik (top right). Gaussian regularization (bottom left). Median regularization (bottom right). The graph on the right shows NMSEs as a function of number of iterations.

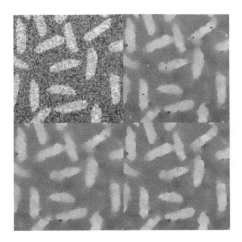

FIGURE 5.9
A subregion from the rice image from the MATLAB image database is used to demonstrate the effect of different regularization schemes. From top left to bottom left, clockwise: original with Gaussian and salt-and-pepper noise added, no regularization, median, and Gaussian regularization, respectively.

As seen again in images in Figure 5.8, median regularization performs better in preserving the edges.

Figure 5.9 shows the images, comparing the application of the two techniques to the rice image available in the MATLAB image database. The edge definition is better preserved with the median regularization. Finally, the images in Figure 5.10 confirm that the ability of the median regularization to preserve edges is greater than that of Gaussian regularization.

The following code can be used to test and demonstrate the differences between the two regularization techniques. If the code is executed with the publish button of MATLAB, then the images can be saved into an html or Word document.

```
% Read and display the rice image
I =imread('rice.png');
imagesc(I);axis off; colormap gray
rect = [21.8333 57.0146 95.0643 93.5673];
% Add Gaussian noise
noisyI1 = imnoise(I,'Gaussian',0,0.02);
imagesc(noisyI1);axis off; colormap gray
% Add salt & pepper noise
noisyI2 = imnoise(noisyI1,'salt & pepper', 0.08);
imagesc(noisyI2);axis off; colormap gray;
drawrect(rect,'r');
% Regularization Methods
% No regularization
dimgPM = mipisodiffusion2d(single(noisyI2),...
```

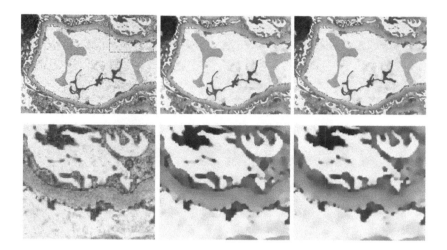

FIGURE 5.10

Images of a glomerulus membrane captured by electron microscopy. Top row shows the original, median, and Gaussian regularized images from left to right. Bottom row shows the images of the inlet denoted by the dashed rectangle on the original image.

```
      'wregion',50,0.1,0.5,3,'n',0.7);
imagesc(dimgPM);axis off; colormap gray
% Median Regularization
dimgM = mipisodiffusion2d(single(noisyI2),...
      'wregion',50,0.1,0.5,3,'m',0.7);
imagesc(dimgM);axis off; colormap gray
% Gaussian Regularization
dimgG = mipisodiffusion2d(single(noisyI2),...
      'wregion',50,0.1,0.5,3,'g',0.7);
imagesc(dimgG);axis off; colormap gray
% Display subregion defined by rect
figure;
subplot(221);
imagesc(imcrop(noisyI1,rect));axis image;axis ...
  off;colormap(gray)
title('Noisy original');
subplot(222);
imagesc(imcrop(dimgPM,rect));axis image;axis ...
  off;colormap(gray)
title('No regularization');
subplot(223);
imagesc(imcrop(dimgG,rect));axis image;axis ...
  off;colormap(gray)
title('Gaussian regularization');
subplot(224);
imagesc(imcrop(dimgM,rect));axis image;axis ...
  off;colormap(gray)
title('Median regularization');
```

5.12 Energy Functional Approach to Diffusion Filtering

In this section, we will discuss the nonlinear diffusion filtering from the energy functional perspective because it helps to better understand its behavior. We will follow the treatment of You et al. [4].

Let us define an energy functional on the space of smooth or piecewise smooth images u as

$$E(u) = \int_\Omega f(|\nabla u|)d\Omega \tag{5.41}$$

where Ω denotes the image domain and $f(|\nabla u|)$ is an increasing function of $|\nabla u|$; that is, $f'(|\nabla u|) > 0$. $f(x)$ is known as the potential function. This energy functional is bounded below, i.e., $E(u) > 0$ and is a measure of image smoothness, so minimization of this energy functional results in smoother images.

The derivative of $E(u)$ can be calculated as [4]

$$\nabla E(u) = -div\left[\frac{f'(|\nabla u|)}{|\nabla u|}\nabla u\right] \tag{5.42}$$

Note that this is the same as PM diffusion. We know that the flux $\phi(x)$ is equal to $g(x)x$. In Equation (5.42), $f'(x)$ is equal to the flux function, so the ratio is the diffusion coefficient, that is,

$$g(|\nabla u|) = \frac{f'(|\nabla u|)}{|\nabla u|} \tag{5.43}$$

The minimization of our energy functional via gradient descent (i.e., moving in the negative direction of $\nabla E(u)$) results in

$$\frac{\partial u}{\partial t} = -\nabla E(u) = div\left[\frac{f'(|\nabla u|)}{|\nabla u|}\nabla u\right] \tag{5.44}$$

Another nonlinear functional of the form [20]

$$\int_\Omega f(\|\nabla u\|)d\Omega \tag{5.45}$$

where $\|\nabla u\|$ is the magnitude of the gradient, with some constraints was proposed for the restoration of images. Their optimization was based on the simulated annealing approach to find the global minimum.

Here, the anisotropic diffusion problem is posed as a cost-functional minimization problem. Therefore, if we know the shape of the surface defined by the energy functional, we can understand the behavior of the diffusion; whether the diffusion process is well-posed or ill-posed.

The boundary, or initial value, problem, defined by our diffusion equation, is said to be well posed if

- There exists a solution.
- The solution is unique and stable.

If the problem is not well-posed, it is said to be ill-posed. We would like to know under what conditions our energy functional minimization is well posed or ill posed. First, it is intuitive that the condition $f'(0) = 0$ has to be met [4]. In other words, the flux $f'(x)$ should be zero when the gradient is zero. Second, to have a unique solution (well-posedness), $E(u)$ has to be convex. This strictly depends on the shape of our potential function $f(x)$; if $f(x)$ is convex, then $E(u)$ will be convex. It can be shown [4] that the energy functional does not have a unique solution if $f'(\infty) = 0$, so the anisotropic diffusion will be ill-posed. The last requirement [4] for a well-posed minimization process is that $E(u)$ have a unique global minimum if $f''(x) \geq 0$ for all $x \geq 0$.

To summarize, we have three conditions to meet for a well-posed anisotropic diffusion:

1. $f'(0) = 0$.
2. $f'(\infty) \neq 0$.
3. $f''(x) \geq 0$ for all $x \geq 0$.   (5.46)

Given these conditions, it is straightforward to find out if diffusivity functions proposed in the literature lead to well-posed diffusion processes. It can be shown that the first two functions given in Table 5.1, which were proposed by Perona and Malik, do not meet the second condition given in Equation (5.46), so PM diffusion is an ill-posed process.

5.13   Total Variational-Based Diffusion

Total variation (TV)-based filtering, suggested by Rudin, Osher, and Fatemi [21], is based on the minimization of the energy functional

$$E(u) = \int_{\Omega} |\nabla u| d\Omega$$ (5.47)

subject to the two constraints $\int_{\Omega} u d\Omega = \int_{\Omega} u_o d\Omega$ and $|u - u_o| = \sigma^2$, where u, u_0 and σ^2 are the true image, the observed image, and the variance of the noise. Equation (5.47) is called the total variation of the image $u(x, y)$. It is equal to the L-1 norm of the image derivative, so it is a measure of the amount of discontinuities in the image. The first constraint signifies that the noise is zero mean. Because this constraint is automatically enforced by the evolution process during the solution of this equation, this constraint will later be dropped. The second constraint states that the standard deviation of the noise σ is known. The minimization of this energy functional subject to the constraints leads to the following Euler–Lagrange equation:

$$0 = \frac{\partial}{\partial x}\left(\frac{u_x}{\sqrt{u_x^2 + u_y^2}}\right) + \frac{\partial}{\partial y}\left(\frac{u_y}{\sqrt{u_x^2 + u_y^2}}\right) - \lambda(u - u_0) \tag{5.48}$$

Using calculus leads to

$$0 = \frac{u_{xx}u_y^2 - 2u_x u_y u_{xy} + u_{yy}u_x^2}{\left(u_x^2 + u_y^2\right)^{3/2}} - \lambda(u - u_0) \tag{5.49}$$

The first term on the right-hand side is the curvature function κ. The iterative solution of this equation can be obtained through the method of gradient descent as

$$u_t = \frac{u_{xx}u_y^2 - 2u_x u_y u_{xy} + u_{yy}u_x^2}{\left(u_x^2 + u_y^2\right)^{3/2}} - \lambda(u - u_0) \tag{5.50}$$

where Δt is our stability factor and λ is the Lagrange multiplier. The second term is to ensure that the steady-state solution is close to the original image. This is similar to the reaction term in Equation (5.9). See Rudin et al. [21] for details of the discretization of Equation (5.50). As they suggest, multiplying Equation (5.50) by $(u - u_0)$ and assuming that at steady state the left side of Equation (5.50) vanishes, leads to

$$\lambda = \frac{1}{\sigma^2} \int \frac{u_{xx}u_y^2 - 2u_x u_y u_{xy} + u_{yy}u_x^2}{\left(u_x^2 + u_y^2\right)^{3/2}}(u - u_0)dxdy \tag{5.51}$$

where the integration is performed over the image space. This equation allows the computation of λ dynamically at every iteration step. Note that we need to know σ a priori or somehow estimate it from the image. In addition to its assurance for a solution close to the original, λ plays a similar role to the scale parameter as the time parameter in our diffusion equations. To see its effect on the smallest structures preserved in the image, one can also try different λ values. λ helps improve the blotchy look that may occur in images denoised using the first term on the right-hand side of Equation (5.50). In Rudin, Osher, and Fatemi [21], a numerical procedure is provided to calculate λ. We will leave the implementation of Equation (5.51) to the reader (see Problems).

If we ignore the constraint, this is an energy functional in which the potential function is equal to $f(x) = x$. Then it is equivalent to a PM diffusion where $g(x) = 1/x$. Note also that $f'(0) = 1$ and $f''(0) \geq 0$, so this diffusion is well-posed.

The following function implements the TV-based nonlinear diffusion algorithm of Rudin, Osher, and Fatemi:

```
function dimg = miptvdiffusion(img,NofI,deltat);
% MIPTVDISSUSION PDE based image diffusion
%
% k = MIPTVDIFFUSION(IMG, NOFI, DELTAT)
%
% Diffuses images using total variation based diffusion of
% Rudin, Osher and Fatami
% img : input image
% dimg : output image
% deltat: (diffusion speed) assumes values in [0, 0.25]
%
%
% See also MIPISODIFFUSION2D

epsilon = 1;
for i=1:NofI
     dimgx  = mipcentraldiff(img,'dx');
     dimgy  = mipcentraldiff(img,'dy');
     dimgxx = mipsecondderiv(img,'dx');
     dimgyy = mipsecondderiv(img,'dy');
     dimgxy = mipsecondpartialderiv(img);
     dimgt1 = (dimgxx.*(eps + dimgy.^2) -
              2*dimgx.*dimgy.*dimgxy
                + dimgyy.*(eps + dimgx.^2));
     dimgt2 = (eps + dimgx.^2 + dimgy.^2).^(3/2);
     img    = img + deltat*dimgt1./dimgt2;
end
dimg = img;
```

Note that our implementation does not include the second term on the right-hand side in Equation (5.50). It is also straightforward to extend the implementation to the 3-D domain. Figure 5.11 shows the part of a MR brain image (sagittal view) before (left) and after (after) TV diffusion. The two images are separated by a solid line. In TV diffusion, λ was calculated adaptively at each iteration step. The original image on the left was flipped using fliplr of MATLAB for display purposes.

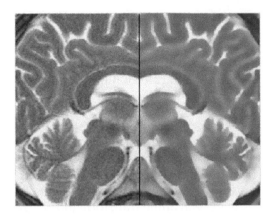

FIGURE 5.11
The part of an MR brain image (sagittal view) before (left) and after (right) TV diffusion filtering. The two images are separated by the solid line. The left image was flipped left-right before the display for display purposes.

5.14 Mean Curvature Diffusion

If we consider images as topographic surfaces defined in 3-D Euclidean space, the mean curvature diffusion (MCD) is the evolution of this surface at a rate proportional to its mean curvature [22]. In fact, Al-Fallah and Ford [22] showed that the surface evolves at a rate twice the mean curvature of the image. They also showed that the MCD removes the image noise via steepest descent surface area minimization. Considering g as the function of the surface defined in 3-D Euclidean space, the mean curvature diffusion equation can be written as

$$\partial_t I = \frac{1}{|\nabla g|}(\nabla^2 I) \tag{5.52}$$

where I is the intensity of the image. This equation is equivalent to the scalar heat equation

$$\partial_t I = c(\nabla^2 I) \tag{5.53}$$

where c is constant.

In the MCD, the image is being diffused by two factors, the inverse of the gradient magnitude and the Laplacian of the position. In other words, the diffusion is being switched from nonhomogeneous (nonlinear) to homogeneous (linear), depending on the magnitude of the surface normal (gradient). At edges where the gradient magnitude reaches the maximum, the diffusion is nonhomogeneous, whereas in flat regions, the diffusion turns into a homogeneous one.

5.15 Afine Invariant Curvature Motion

An affine transformation maps disks into ellipses and rectangles into parallelograms. A general affine transformation in a plane is written as

$$\vec{x} = Ax + B \tag{5.54}$$

where $\vec{x}$ is a vector, $A \in \mathbb{R}^{2\times2}$ is an invertible matrix with a positive determinant, and $B \in \mathbb{R}^2$ is a translation matrix. In affine transformations, colinearity is preserved. In other words, affine transformation maps the straight lines to straight lines and preserves parallelism. Translation, scaling, and shear are examples of general affine transformations. The Euclidean curvature κ based on the Euclidean arc length (see Chapter 10) is not invariant under general affine transformation as the Euclidean arc length is not invariant with respect to scaling. Intuitively, we see that the scaling will change the arc length.

A method to construct an affine invariant scale-space for planar curves has been suggested by Shapiro and Tannenbaum [23]. They define a new arc-length, instead of the Euclidean arc-length, which is invariant under affine transformations. Shapiro and Tannenbaum show that the curves evolving through the evolution equation of the form

$$\frac{\partial I}{\partial t} = \kappa^{1/3} \, \| \nabla I \| \tag{5.55}$$

based on the new arc length definition are affine invariant. Here, I is the image whose level set curve has the curvature given by

$$\kappa = \frac{I_{yy}I_x^2 - 2I_xI_yI_{xy} + I_{xx}I_y^2}{\left(I_x^2 + I_y^2\right)^{3/2}} \tag{5.56}$$

Thus, the scale-space formed by this curve evolution provides an affine multiresolution representation of planar curves.

Note that if we regard the curve as the level sets of the image I, and $\| \nabla I \|$ is the gradient magnitude, then using Equation (5.55), the images, which are defined as surfaces in 3-D Euclidean space, can also be evolved (i.e., diffused) for the purpose of removing noise.

For images, if the gradient magnitude is given by $\| \nabla I \| = \left(I_x^2 + I_y^2\right)^{1/2}$, then Equation (5.55) becomes

$$\frac{\partial I(x,y)}{\partial t} = \left(I_{yy}I_x^2 - 2I_xI_yI_{xy} + I_{xx}I_y^2\right)^{1/3} \tag{5.57}$$

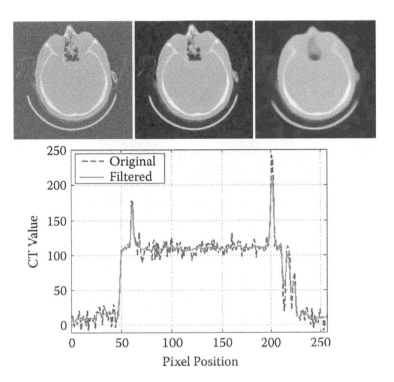

FIGURE 5.12
Top left: Noisy CT image of a brain. Top middle: Image filtered by AICM (30 iterations). Top right: Image filtered by AICM (300 iterations). Bottom: The profiles across the original and the filtered (30 iterations) images.

The evolution of an image via affine invariant curvature motion (AICM) given by Equation (5.57) is very similar to the mean curvature motion discussed in the previous section.

We already know how to discretize Equation (5.57). The discrete version of this image evolution is implemented in the function mipaffinecurvaturemove. Figure 5.12 demonstrates the performance of AICM filtering on a transaxial slice of a brain CT. The profiles across the noisy and filtered images are also illustrated.

5.16 Anisotropic Diffusion of Color Images

Anisotropic diffusion filtering has also been applied to color images [24]. Diffusion filtering of color images can be performed in many different ways. A first approach is to filter each spectrum (band) separately and recombine the filtered images. A second approach is to transform the original image in the RGB color space to another color space. Transforming

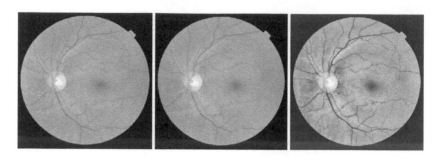

FIGURE 5.13
Images of retina acquired by a fundus camera. Left: Original image. Middle: Diffusion filtered version of the left image. Right: Image filtered after adaptive histogram equalization

images from one color space to another is commonly done to facilitate processing and analysis of images. This topic has been discussed in detail in the Applications chapter.

The L*a*b color space consists of a luminosity layer (dimension) L, and chromaticity layers a and b. Transforming images to L*a*b space also reduces the dimension of the problem from 3 (RGB colors) to 2 (colors *a* and *b*) for color analysis purposes, making color analysis easy. However, here we will remove the noise from the L layer, which carries luminosity and more structural information. As an alternative, we can enhance, for this particular application, the L layer to have better contrast using the adaptive histogram equalization technique provided in the Image Processing Toolbox. This tends to enhance the noise as well as structures, but the diffusion filtering that will ensues can easily remove the enhanced noise. The image is then retransformed back to RGB space after filtration.

Fundus cameras are optical imaging systems used in ophthalmology clinics to image the interior surface (fundus) of the eye, including the retina, optic disk, and macula, for the diagnosis of pathologic conditions. It consists of a low-power microscope and a CCD camera. Figure 5.13 shows the original images of the retina (left) acquired by a fundus camera. The middle image indicates the effect of filtering each spectrum separately. The right image was obtained by adaptive histogram equalization and diffusion filtration of the L layer. The following code can be used to implement this last approach. The original RGB image is stored in the array csub.

```
Clab    = makecform('srgb2lab');
Crgb    = makecform('lab2srgb');

Labimg  = applycform(csub,Clab);
L       = Labimg(:,:,1);
abimg   = Labimg(:,:,2:3);
Laheq   = adapthisteq(L);
```

```
dimg     = mipisodiffusion2d(double(Laheq),...
           'hgrad',30,0.1,0.5,3,'g',5);
nlabimg  = cat(3,dimg, abimg);
rimgfilt = applycform(nlabimg,Crgb);
```

It should be noted that we used a constant contrast threshold in this case. We have observed that this approach requires a different contrast threshold and a larger number of iterations owing to the enhancement performed; the enhancement process also increases the noise significantly. However, it is worth the effort as the right image shows more detail.

While filtering each band separately, we computed the gradient of each image separately as well. In Chapter 2, we discussed (with examples) how to compute the gradients of multispectral images. The disadvantages of filtering each channel separately are discussed in the same chapter. The interested reader can apply the vector-gradient methods for color images suggested there to the diffusion of color images.

5.16.1 Orthogonal Decomposition of Perona–Malik Diffusion

In this section, we will look at anisotropic diffusion from a different perspective. This will aid our understanding of the topic.

Our diffusion equation given by Equation (5.8) can be decomposed [25] into its orthogonal components as

$$\frac{\partial I}{\partial t} = g_{\xi\xi}I_{\xi\xi} + g_{\eta\eta}I_{\eta\eta} \tag{5.58}$$

where $g_{\xi\xi} = g(\|\nabla I\|)$ and $g_{\eta\eta} = \phi'(\|\nabla I\|) = g'(\|\nabla I\|)\|\nabla I\| + g(\|\nabla I\|)$.

$I_{\xi\xi}$ and $I_{\eta\eta}$ are the second derivatives of I in the orthogonal directions ξ and η (see Figure 5.14). The first term on the right-hand side of Equation (5.58) explains the smoothing across the edge or along the gradient direction, whereas the second term describes the smoothing along the edge, or the isophotes. Isophotes, level-set curves, or isolines all refer to the lines of a constant gray-level value in an image. Anisotropic diffusion can be viewed as two 1-D evolutions moving perpendicular to each other.

As seen in Figure 5.14, the unit vectors η and ξ are parallel ($\|$) and perpendicular ($\perp$) to the gradient vector ∇I. Hence, the unit vectors in the orthogonal directions can be expressed in terms of the image gradient as follows:

$$\eta = \frac{\nabla I}{\|\nabla I\|} \text{ and } \xi = \eta^{\perp}$$

The second derivatives orthogonal and parallel to the gradient direction can be written as [25]

$$I_{\xi\xi} = \frac{\left(I_{yy}I_x^2 - 2I_xI_yI_{xy} + I_{xx}I_y^2\right)}{I_x^2 + I_y^2} \tag{5.59}$$

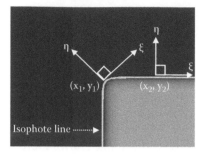

FIGURE 5.14

The curve illustrates the isophote line pointed to by the dotted arrow. The orthogonal directions on the isophote are at two different image locations $(x_{1,2}, y_{1,2})$. The unit vectors η and ξ are parallel and perpendicular, respectively, to the gradient.

and

$$I_{\eta\eta} = \frac{\left(I_{xx}I_x^2 + 2I_xI_yI_{xy} + I_{yy}I_y^2\right)}{I_x^2 + I_y^2} \tag{5.60}$$

respectively.

This decomposition helps us understand the anisotropic diffusion of Perona and Malik. The type of the diffusion in both directions depends on the signs of the diffusion coefficients $g_{\xi\xi}$ and $g_{\eta\eta}$. The (−) sign shows a backward diffusion (ill posed) and the (+) sign indicates a forward diffusion (well-posed). Diffusion along the isophotes is a forward diffusion owing to the nonnegative sign of $g_{\xi\xi}$, whereas diffusion parallel to the gradient may be forward or backward depending on the sign of $g_{\eta\eta}$ (see Problems). Thus, the whole diffusion process may be ill-posed, depending on the weights of the two components.

To shed further light on the nature of the anisotropic diffusion, we can rewrite our diffusion equation in the following form [4]:

$$\frac{\partial I}{\partial t} = g_{\xi\xi}\kappa \,\|\nabla I\| + g_{\eta\eta}\kappa_{\perp} \,\|\nabla I\| \tag{5.61}$$

where

$$\kappa = \frac{\left(I_{yy}I_x^2 - 2I_xI_yI_{xy} + I_{xx}I_y^2\right)}{\left(I_x^2 + I_y^2\right)^{3/2}} \, div\!\left(\frac{\nabla I}{\|\nabla I\|}\right) \tag{5.62}$$

and

$$\kappa_{\perp} = \frac{\left(I_{xx}I_x^2 + 2I_xI_yI_{xy} + I_{yy}I_y^2\right)}{\left(I_x^2 + I_y^2\right)^{3/2}} \tag{5.63}$$

Recall that κ is the mean curvature. The PDE evolution of the form

$$\frac{\partial I}{\partial t} = \kappa \, \|\nabla I\| \tag{5.64}$$

is the level-set version of Euclidean curve shortening in the plane and has been studied extensively [23]. Therefore, the first term on the right-hand side of Equation (5.61) is proportional to the mean curvature of the level-set of the image I, where the coefficient is our diffusivity function. You et al. [4] calls Equation (5.62) the dual of Equation (5.61) and discusses the geometric interpretation of this decomposition.

Problems

1. Show that the Gaussian function is a solution of the heat equation.
2. Find the relation between the diffusion time and the width of the Gaussian, assuming that the heat distribution initially follows a Gaussian function.
3. Experiment with the `pdetool` in MATLAB using the heat transfer demo.
4. Find the value of C_m so that the flux of the diffusivity function given by Equation (5.17) will have a maximum at the noise threshold.
5. For the C_m value found in Problem 4, plot Weickert's diffusivity and flux functions for $m = 2, 4, 10$ and, say, $\delta = 15$, and observe the effect of m on the diffusivity and flux functions.
6. Investigate if the first two diffusivity functions in Table 5.1 meet the conditions given in Equation (5.46).
7. Show that the diffusivity function $g(x) = 1/x$ leads to a well-posed diffusion.
8. To calculate λ dynamically, implement Equation (5.51) in MATLAB.
9. Observe the effect of λ in Equation (5.50) by using different values in the range $[0.015–0.05]$.
10. Show the condition for which the second part of Equation (5.61) exhibits forward diffusion if the diffusivity function is given by $g(x) = \exp(-x^2/k^2)$.

References

1. A. P. Witkin, Scale-space filtering, presented at 8th Int. Joint Conf. Art. Intell., Karlsruhe, Germany, 1983.
2. J. Koenderink, The structure of images, *Biol. Cybern* 50: 363–370, 1984.

3. P. Perona and J. Malik, Scale-space and edge detection using anisotropic diffusion. *IEEE Trans. on Pattern Anal. Machine Intelligence* 12: 629–639, 1990.
4. Y. You, W. Xu, A. Tannenbaum, and M. Kaveh, Behavioral analysis of anisotropic diffusion in image processing. *IEEE Trans. on Image Process* 5: 1539–1552, 1996.
5. K. N. Nordstrom, Biased anisotropic diffusion: a unified regularization and diffusion approach to edge detection. *Image and Vision Computing* 8: 318–327, 1990.
6. J. Weickert, *Anisotropic Diffusion in Image Processing*. Stuttgart: BG: Teubner Stuttgart, 1998.
7. B. Fischl and E. L. Schwartz, Learning an integral equation approximation to nonlinear anisotropic diffusion in image processing. *IEEE Trans. on Pattern Anal. Machine Intelligence* 19: 342–352, 1997.
8. M. J. Black, G. Sapiro, D. H. Marimont, and D. Heeger, Robust anisotropic diffusion. *IEEE Trans. on Image Process* 7: 421–432, 1998.
9. W. H. Press, B. P. Flannery, S. A. Teukolsky, and W. T. Vetterling, *Numerical Recipes In C: The Art of Scientific Computing*, 2nd ed. Cambridge: Cambridge University Press, 1993.
10. G. Gerig, O. Kubler, R. Kikinis, and F. A. Jolesz, Nonlinear anisotropic filtering of MRI data. *IEEE Trans Med. Imaging.* 11: 221–232, 1992.
11. C. Moller, *Numerical Computing with MATLAB*. Philadelphia, PA: SIAM, 2004.
12. J. Weickert, B. M. T. H. Romeny, and M. A. Viergever, Efficient and reliable schemes for nonlinear diffusion filtering. *IEEE Trans. on Image Process* 7: 398–410, 1998.
13. J. Canny, A computational approach to edge detection. *IEEE Trans. on Pattern Anal. Machine Intelligence.* PAMI-8: 679–698, 1986.
14. N. M. Alpert, D. A. Chesler, J. A. Correia, R. H. Ackerman, J. Y. Chang, S. Finklestein, S. M. Davis, G. L. Brownell, and J. M. Taveras, Estimation of the local statistical noise in emission computed tomography. *IEEE Trans. Med. Imaging* 1: 142–136, 1982.
15. Y. Yongjian and S. T. Acton, Speckle reducing anisotropic diffusion. *IEEE Trans. Image Process* 11: 1260–1270, 2002.
16. F. Catte, P. L. Lions, J. M. Morel, and T. Coll, Image selective smoothing and edge detection by nonlinear diffusion. *SIAM J. Numer. Anal.* 29: 182–193, 1992.
17. O. Demirkaya, Smoothing Impulsive Noise Using Nonlinear Diffusion Filtering, presented at CVAMIA-MMBIA 2004, 2004.
18. A. K. Jain, *Fundamentals of Digital Image Processing*. Englewood Cliffs, NJ: Prentice-Hall, 1989.
19. D. Collett, *Modeling Survival Data in Medical Research*, 1st ed. London: Chapman and Hall, 1994.
20. D. Geman and G. Reynolds, Constrained restoration and the recovery of discontinuities. *IEEE Trans. on Pattern Anal Machine Intelligence* 14: 367–383, 1992.
21. L. I. Rudin, S. Osher, and E. Fatemi, Nonlinear total variation based noise removal algorithm. *Physica* 60: 259–268, 1992.

22. A. I. El-Fallah and G. E. Ford, On mean curvature diffusion in nonlinear image filtering. *Pattern Recogn Lett.* 19: 433–437, 1998.
23. G. S. A. A. Tannenbaum, Affine invariant scale-space. *Int. J. Comp. Vision* 11: 25–44, 1993.
24. D. Tschumperlé and R. Deriche, Diffusion PDE's on vector-valued images. *IEEE Signal Processing Magazine* 19: 16–25, 2002.
25. L. Alvarez, F. Guichard, P.-L. Lions, and J.-M. Morel, Axioms and fundamental equations of image processing. *Arch. for Rational Mechanics* 123: 199–257, 1993.

6

Intensity-Based Image Segmentation

CONTENTS

6.1 Introduction

Image segmentation using histogram-based thresholding is probably the most common approach, since it is easy to implement and requires less CPU resources to run. These methods generally employ the maximization or minimization of a criterion function based on the image histogram. The optimal threshold is the gray-level intensity at which the criterion function attains its extremum (maximum or minimum). Thresholding methods are called global if a single threshold is calculated for the entire image. If the image is divided into sub-blocks and a threshold is calculated for each sub-block, then this method of thresholding is called local thresholding.

One can interpolate the threshold values for each pixel by placing the local threshold in the center pixel of each block. This is known as parametric thresholding. The major disadvantage of histogram-based thresholding methods is their disregard of the spatial context within which the intensity value occurs. In other words, they do not consider the intensity values of the surrounding pixels. Methods based on 2-D histograms consider, to some degree, contextual information. Thresholding methods are also frequently used for the initial segmentation of images prior to the application of a more sophisticated segmentation method for the purpose of reducing the convergence time [1]. A comprehensive review of the thresholding methods can be found in Mardia and Hainsworth [2] and Pal and Pal [3].

In this chapter we will discuss histogram-based thresholding methods that are ubiquitously used in image segmentation. We will also discuss the mixture modeling and K-means and fuzzy C-means clustering algorithms applied to image segmentation.

6.2 Between-Class Variance

Between-class variance was introduced first by Otsu [4] as a discriminant function to determine an optimal threshold from the image histogram to segment an image into nearly uniform regions. This criterion function does not make any assumption about underlying mixture distributions.

In this section, we will derive and discuss between-class variance and other relevant criterion functions that are used to compute optimal thresholds.

Let us first consider the normalized gray-level histogram as a discrete probability distribution function $p(i)$ of a mixture, that is,

$$p(i) = \frac{n_i}{M}, \quad p(i) \geq 0 \quad \text{and} \quad \sum_{i=0}^{N-1} p(i) = 1 \tag{6.1}$$

where n_i is the frequency of the gray level i and M is the total number of pixels in the image. Each pixel in the image assumes a gray-level value from the set $\{0, \ldots N - 1\}$, where $N - 1$ is the maximum gray-level intensity. If the histogram is divided into two classes by the gray-level intensity t (see Figure 6.1), then the probabilities of the respective classes can be expressed as

$$p_1(t) = \sum_{i=0}^{t} p(i)$$

$$p_2(t) = \sum_{i=t+1}^{N-1} p(i) \tag{6.2}$$

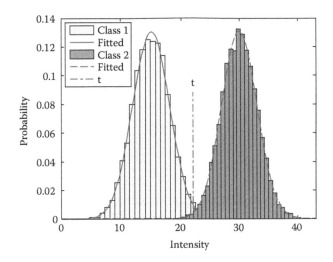

FIGURE 6.1

Histogram of an image with two normally distributed regions. The solid and dashed lines show the fitted Gaussian functions. The threshold t separates the two classes.

Similarly, the class means m_1 and m_2 are given by

$$m_1(t) = \sum_{i=0}^{t} i \cdot p(i)/p_1(t)$$

$$m_2(t) = \sum_{i=t+1}^{N-1} i \cdot p(i)/p_2(t)$$

(6.3)

Given an image, its normalized intensity histogram p can be computed using MATLAB function hist as follows:

```
[p,cbin] = hist(Img(:), nbins);
p = p/sum(p);
```

nbins is the desired number of bins for the intensity range existing in the image. p is the set of probabilities normalized by the total probability computed for the bins, whose centers are saved into the variable cbin.

The following function computes the mean of the class, which has the intensities in the range [I1, I2] given the histogram h:

```
function cm = mipcmean(h, I1, I2)
p = 0; sm = 0;
for i = I1:I2
```

```
   sm = sm + i*h(i);
    p = p + h(i);
end;
if p == 0, cm = 0;
else, cm = sm/p; end;
```

Now, the class variances are expressed as

$$\sigma_1^2(t) = \sum_{i=0}^{t} (i - m_1)^2 \cdot \frac{p(i)}{p_1(t)} \text{ and } \sigma_2^2(t) = \sum_{i=t+1}^{N-1} (i - m_2)^2 \cdot \frac{p(i)}{p_2(t)} \tag{6.4}$$

The following function computes the variance of a class whose intensities lie within the range [I1,I2] and whose mean is mu, which can be calculated using the preceding function:

```
function cv = mipcvar(h,mu,I1,I2)
p = 0;
sm = 0;
for i = I1:I2
   temp = (i-mu);
   sm = sm + h(i)*temp*temp;
   p = p+h(i);
end;
if p == 0
   cv = 0;
else
   cv = sm/p;
end;
```

Then, the total variance $\sigma_T^2 = \sigma_W^2 + \sigma_B^2$ can be divided into components, where σ_W^2 is called the within-class variance (WCV) and is expressed as

$$\sigma_W^2(t) = p_1(t) \cdot \sigma_1^2(t) + p_2(t) \cdot \sigma_2^2(t) \tag{6.5}$$

The within-class variance is the sum of the individual class variances weighted by their respective class probabilities. The σ_B^2 is referred to as the between-class variance (BCV) and is expressed as

$$\sigma_B^2(t) = p_1(t) \cdot [m_1(t) - m_T]^2 + p_2(t) \cdot [m_2(t) - m_T]^2 \tag{6.6}$$

where $m_T = \sum_{i=0}^{N-1} i \cdot p(i)$ is the total mean. The BCV provides valuable information as to how close the two classes are to each other. We will also refer to the BCV as a measure of image bimodality, which will be discussed in Section 6.2.2.

The optimal threshold t^*, which segments an image into two nearly homogenous regions, may be the gray-level value at which the between-class variance peaks or reaches maximum, that is,

$$\sigma_B^2(t^*) = \max_{0 \le t < N-1} \sigma_B^2(t) \qquad (6.7)$$

This criterion function can be easily extended to multimodal cases in which there are more than two regions. For k classes or regions, for instance,

$$\sigma_B^2 = p_1 \cdot (m_1 - m_T)^2 + p_2 \cdot (m_2 - m_T)^2 + \cdots + p_k \cdot (m_k - m_T)^2 \qquad (6.8)$$

where we have dropped the argument t for brevity.

The same optimum threshold can be obtained by minimizing the within-class variance, because its sum is equal to the total variance, a constant. However, Equation (6.6) is computationally less expensive than Equation (6.5), as the former does not require the calculation of the class variances. In a sequential search for the optimal threshold, the class probabilities and the means can be progressively computed to reduce computation time. For example, the means of the classes, when $i = t$, can be computed progressively using the following equations:

$$m_1(t) = [p_1(t-1) \cdot m(t-1) + p(t) \cdot t] / p_1(t-1) \qquad (6.9)$$

$$p_1(i+1) = p_1(i) + p(i+1) \qquad (6.10)$$

$$m_1(i+1) = \frac{m_1(i) \cdot p_1(i) + (i+1) \cdot p(i+1)}{p_1(i+1)}$$

$$m_2(i+1) = \frac{m_T - p_1(i+1) \cdot m_1(i+1)}{1 - p_1(i+1)} \qquad (6.11)$$

The function mipbcv computes the optimal threshold on the basis of the maximization of the BCV:

```
function [th,bmax,bcvf]  = mipbcv(x,nbins)
warning off all
if nargin == 1
   nbins = 64;
end
% compute histogram
[h,cbin] = mipimhist(x,nbins);
% find the indices for max & min gray levels
max_indx = max(find(h));
min_indx = min(find(h));
```

```
% initilize variables
totalMean = mipcmean(h,1,max_indx);
prevProb1 = 0;
mean1 = 0;
cf=zeros(1,nbins);
for i = min_indx:max_indx
    prob1 = prevProb1 + h(i);
    prob2 = 1-prob1;
    mean1 = (prevProb1*mean1 + h(i)*i)/prob1;
    mean2 = mipcmean(h,i+1,max_indx);
    t1 = mean1-mean2;
    bcvf(i) = prob1*prob2*t1*t1;
    prevProb1 = prob1;
end;
totalvar= mipcvar(h,totalMean,min_indx,max_indx);
if totalvar > 0
    bcvf = bcvf/totalvar;
end;
[bmax,cmax_indx] = max(bcvf);
th = cbin(cmax_indx);
```

This function will compute the threshold on the basis of the BCV criterion for the image x entered as the input variable. The variable nbins specifies the number of bins that the histogram function uses. The default value of nbins is 64. It returns the threshold th, the maximum of the criterion function bmax and the criterion function itself. Note how the probabilities and means of the classes are computed progressively in the function. The computed threshold can be used to segment the input image into two regions.

6.2.1 Criterion Functions Equivalent to BCV

An equivalent (to the BCV) criterion function was proposed by Kurita [5]. This function maximizes the likelihood of the conditional distribution of a population mixture model consisting of two normal distributions with different means and a common variance. In the case of the BCV, although we said that no explicit assumption is made earlier, this equivalency, proved in [5], shows that the BCV will perform best if the regions of the image have intensity distributions with equal variances.

Another related criterion function was suggested in the same reference [5] based on the likelihood of the joint distribution of a population mixture model consisting of two normal distributions with different means and a common variance:

$$Q(t) = \log(\sigma_W(t)) - \sum_{j=1}^{2} p_j \log(p_j) \qquad (6.12)$$

where p_j is the probability of the jth class.

Note that the first term on the right-hand side is equivalent to the within-class variance. We have an additional second term. This criterion function can be regarded as the modified version of the between-class variance for the unbalanced populations because the second term in a way corrects for the case in which populations are unbalanced.

Imaging scientists working with medical or biomedical images are likely to stumble upon both situations. In other words, they may come across images with regions of equal or unequal variances or with unbalanced populations. Therefore, one may choose an appropriate criterion function accordingly. Usually, image histograms provide adequate hints as to which situation is more likely.

The function mipkurita computes the optimal threshold using the criterion function given by Equation (6.12).

```
function [th,cf,cbin] = mipkurita(x,nbins)
warning off all
% compute histogram, pdf
[h,cbin] = mipimhist(x,nbins);
% find the indices for max&min gray levels
max_indx = max(find(h));
min_indx = min(find(h));
% initilize variables
totalMean = mipcmean(h,min_indx,max_indx);
totalvar = mipcvar(h,totalMean,min_indx,max_indx);
prevProb1 = 0;
mean1 = 0;
cf = zeros(1,nbins);
for i = min_indx:max_indx
  prob1 = prevProb1 + h(i);
  prob2 = 1-prob1;
  mean1 = (prevProb1*mean1 + h(i)*i)/prob1;
  mean2 = mipcmean(h,i+1,max_indx);
  t1 = mean1-mean2;
  cf(i) = log(totalvar-prob1*prob2*t1*t1)-...
     prob1*log(prob1)+prob2*log(prob2);
  prevProb1 = prob1;
end;
cf = cf/totalvar;
[tm,thindx] = min(cf(1:end-1));
th = cbin(thindx);
```

Note that the implementation of this function is very similar to that of the BCV function. This function also requires two input variables—the image and the number of bins—and returns the threshold, the criterion function, and the bin centers.

We will demonstrate these functions on two example images. The first one is the image of a uniform region from a SPECT image quality phantom

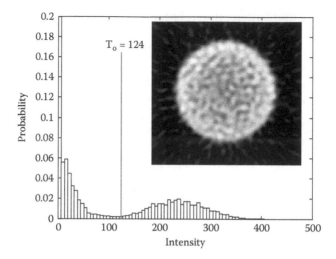

FIGURE 6.2
Image of a uniform region of a SPECT image quality phantom and its histogram. T_o is the optimum threshold computed by the BCV function.

acquired by a SPECT system, shown in Figure 6.2. The second image is the CT image of a vertebral bone, shown in Figure 6.3.

The images are shown with their histograms and the optimal thresholds computed by the criterion functions. In Figure 6.2, the threshold computed only by the BCV function is shown as the other one was the same. Figure 6.4 shows the binary images of the vertebral bone (shown in Figure 6.3), obtained by the thresholds, which illustrate that the difference between the two criterion functions is very small in this case. The computed thresholds are 109 and 118, as displayed in Figure 6.3.

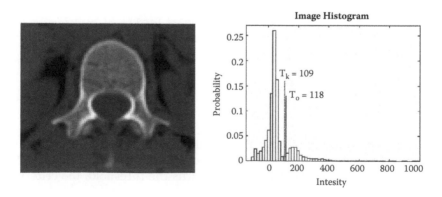

FIGURE 6.3
CT image of a vertebral bone and its histogram, with the computed thresholds.

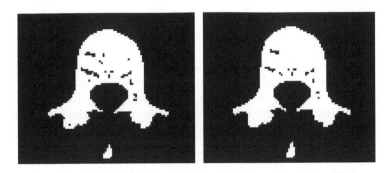

FIGURE 6.4
The binary images of the vertebral bone shown in Figure 6.3 segmented by the BCV (left) and Kurita's method (right).

6.2.2 BCV as an Image Bimodality Measure

In image segmentation, the detection of image bimodality may be required to make intelligent decisions as to the validity of the computed threshold prior to segmentation. The BCV was studied as a bimodality measure [6]. We will summarize the findings of this study here. For a more detailed discussion, the reader may refer to the aforementioned reference. The BCV function will always compute a threshold, even for a unimodal distribution, regardless of the validity of the computed threshold. In order not to unnecessarily segment a homogenous region, one should check if the computed threshold is valid.

We will demonstrate how one can use the normalized BCV expressed as

$$B(t) = \frac{\sigma_B^2}{\sigma_T^2} \tag{6.13}$$

to detect image bimodality. We will use the maximum of the $B(t)$

$$B_{\max} = \max_{0 \le t < N-1} B(t) \tag{6.14}$$

as a measure of image bimodality.

Similarly, we can normalize the WCV by the total variance and obtain

$$W(t) = \frac{\sigma_W^2}{\sigma_T^2} \tag{6.15}$$

As we mentioned earlier, $B(t)$ is equivalent to $W(t)$ as their sum is equal to one, a constant.

$B(t)$ takes on values in the interval [0,1]. For balanced uniform distributions, the theoretical value of $B_{\max}$ is easy to derive. However, for other distributions, even for the well-known normal distribution, the analytical derivation of B_{max} is quite challenging. With the help of the MATLAB Symbolic Math Toolbox, one can compute the value of B_{max} for normal distributions. For other distributions, because of the complexity of the derivation, one could easily use a simulation-based approach.

Let us show how the analytical approach can be utilized to find the bimodality thresholds for various distributions. The discussion of the simulation approach can be found in Demirkaya and Asyali [6].

6.2.2.1 Bimodality Threshold for Uniform Distribution

For a uniform distribution with a range R, the probabilities and the means of the classes that are separated by the threshold t are given by

$$
\begin{aligned}
p_1(t) &= t/R \\
p_2(t) &= (R-t)/R \\
m_1(t) &= t/2 \\
m_2(t) &= (R-t)/2
\end{aligned}
\tag{6.16}
$$

The total mean and the variance can be shown to be

$$
m_T = R/2 \text{ and } \sigma_T^2 = R^2/12
\tag{6.17}
$$

respectively.

To find B_{max} using the analytical approach, first, the class probabilities, the class means, total mean, and total variance are substituted in Equations (6.6) and (6.13). Then the value of t that maximizes $B(t)$ can be derived by differentiating $B(t)$ with respect to t, and setting the derivative equal to zero, that is,

$$
\frac{\partial B(t)}{\partial t} = 0
$$

It can be shown that B_{max} for uniform distributions is 0.75. We will leave its derivation to the reader (see Problems).

6.2.2.2 Bimodality Threshold for Normal Distribution

For a normal distribution, the probability distribution function is given by

$$
g(x) = \frac{1}{\sqrt{2\pi}\sigma} \exp\left(-\frac{(x-\mu)^2}{2\sigma^2}\right)
\tag{6.18}
$$

where μ and σ are the mean and the standard deviation, respectively. The probabilities of the classes separated by the threshold t can be computed by

$$p_1(t) = \int_0^t g(x)dx$$

$$p_2(t) = 1 - p_1(t),$$

(6.19)

and the means of the two classes by

$$m_1(t) = \int_0^t xg(x)dx$$

$$m_2(t) = \left(m_1(t)p_2(t) + \mu\right)/p_2(t).$$

(6.20)

After substituting the probabilities and the means in Equations (6.6) and (6.13), $B(t)$ can be obtained as (see Problems)

$$B(t) = \frac{\exp\left(-\dfrac{(t-\mu)^2}{2\sigma^2}\right) - \exp\left(-\dfrac{\mu^2}{2\sigma^2}\right)}{\dfrac{\pi}{2}\left(-\dfrac{5.0133}{\sqrt{2\pi}} + L(t)\right)L(t)}$$

(6.21)

where $L(t) = erf\left(\frac{(t-\mu)}{\sqrt{2}\sigma}\right) + erf\left(\frac{\mu}{\sqrt{2}\sigma}\right)$, with $erf(x) = \frac{2}{\sqrt{\pi}}\int_0^x \exp(-u^2)du$.

Again, it can be shown that $B_{\max}$ for normal distributions is equal to 0.6366. It can also be shown that $B(t)$ is a unimodal function; it has only one peak.

6.2.3 An Iterative Implementation of BCV for Trimodal Images

An iterative algorithm based on the maximization of the BCV was proposed in Reddi, Rudin, and Keshavan [7] for images with three regions. We will call these images *trimodal* images. To segment the regions in these images, we need two thresholds.

In this section we discuss and demonstrate one possible implementation of this approach. This iterative algorithm can be summarized as follows. First, we initialize the thresholds t_1 and t_2 as $R/3$ and $2R/3$, respectively. Here, R is the intensity range in the image. Then, the error functions

$$\varepsilon_1(t_1, t_2) = [m(0, t_1) + m(t_1, t_2)]/2 - t_1$$

(6.22)

and

$$\varepsilon_2(t_1, t_2) = [m(t_1, t_2) + m(t_2, \infty)]/2 - t_2 \tag{6.23}$$

where

$$m(t_i, t_j) = \frac{1}{t_i + t_j + 1} \sum_{l=t_i}^{t_j} p(l) \cdot l \tag{6.24}$$

and $p(l)$ is the image histogram, are computed.

In the next step, the thresholds t_1 and t_2 are updated to force the errors ε_1 and ε_2 toward zero.

$$\begin{aligned} t_1' &= t_1 + \varepsilon_1 \\ t_2' &= t_2 + \varepsilon_2 \end{aligned} \tag{6.25}$$

This iterative procedure continues until the errors are very small or the thresholds are no longer changing. The following function implements the iterative procedure described above.

```
function [t1,t2] = mipbcviterative(x,nbins)
warning off all
if nargin == 1
   nbins = 64;
end
[h,cbin] = mipimhist(x,nbins);
% find the indices for max&min gray levels
max_indx = max(find(h));
min_indx = min(find(h));
hstep = median(diff(cbin));
kmax = max_indx - min_indx;
t1 = fix(min_indx + kmax/3.0);
t2 = fix(min_indx + kmax*2.0/3.0);
pe1 = 0;
pe2 = 0;
FLAG = 1;
min_indx = fix(min_indx);
while (FLAG)
   e1 = (mipcmean(h,min_indx,t1) +...
      mipcmean(h,t1 + 1,t2))/2.0 - t1;
   e2 = (mipcmean(h,t1 + 1, t2) +...
      mipcmean(h,t2 + 1, max_indx))/2.0 - t2;
   if pe1 == e1 & pe2 == e2
      FLAG = 0;
   end;
   pe1 = e1;
   pe2 = e2;
```

```
    t1 = t1 + fix(e1);
    t2 = t2 + fix(e2);
end;
t1 = cbin(t1);
t2 = cbin(t2);
```

This function computes the thresholds iteratively for the input image x and returns the two optimal thresholds. Note that we can also implement Equation (6.8) to compute the optimal thresholds for multiregion images, but the aforementioned algorithm applicable to trimodal images is an iterative one and will run faster than the sequential implementation of Equation (6.8).

Figure 6.5 shows the CT image of a human head at the top left and its histogram at the bottom. As seen in the histogram as well as in the image, the image has three regions. The thresholds denoted by the vertical lines on the histogram were computed by the preceding iterative algorithm.

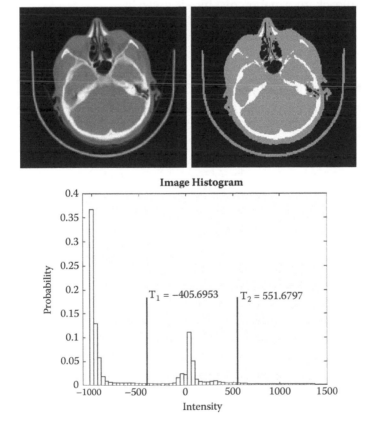

FIGURE 6.5
Top left: A CT slice of a human head. Top right: Trilevel image segmented using the iterative BCV implemented for trimodal images. Bottom: Histogram and the computed thresholds.

On the top right of Figure 6.5 is the multilevel image obtained using the two thresholds with the following MATLAB statement:

```
mimg = mipgray2multilevel(gimg,[t1,t2]);
```

where gimg is the CT image and mimg is the output. For the description of our function that converts a gray-level image to a multiple-level one, see Chapter 2.

6.3   Minimum Error Thresholding

This criterion function suggested by Kittler and Illingworth [8] is based on the minimization of the Kullback information distance. Here, we will follow Haralick's treatment [9].

The Kullback information distance is given by

$$J = \sum_{i=1}^{N} p(i) \log \left[\frac{p(i)}{f(i)} \right] \tag{6.26}$$

where f is the unknown mixture distribution and $p(i)$ is the probability of i. A mixture of two Gaussian distributions separated by threshold t can be expressed as

$$f(i) = \begin{cases} \dfrac{p_1}{\sqrt{2\pi}\sigma_1} e^{-1/2\left(\frac{i-\mu_1}{\sigma_1}\right)} & i \le t \\[4mm] \dfrac{p_2}{\sqrt{2\pi}\sigma_2} e^{-1/2\left(\frac{i-\mu_2}{\sigma_2}\right)} & i > t \end{cases} \tag{6.27}$$

where p_1 and p_2 are the mixing proportions.

We can rewrite Equation (6.26) as

$$J = \sum_{i=1}^{N} p(i) \log p(i) - \sum_{i=1}^{N} p(i) \log f(i) \tag{6.28}$$

The first term in Equation (6.28) does not depend on the unknown parameters; therefore, minimizing the second term,

$$H = -\sum_{i=1}^{N} p(i) \log f(i) \tag{6.29}$$

will be sufficient. If we substitute Equation (6.27) into Equation (6.29) and carry out the simplifications, we obtain

$$H(t) = 1 + \log 2\pi/2 + p_1(t)\log(\sigma_1/p_1(t)) + p_2(t)\log(\sigma_2/p_2(t)) \quad (6.30)$$

We will leave the complete derivation of Equation (6.30) to the reader (see Problems). We can again ignore the constant terms on the right-hand side and minimize the remaining part of the equation. In this case, the optimal threshold t^* is the gray level at which $H(t)$ is minimum.

$$H(t^*) = \min_{0 \leq t \leq N-1} H(t) \quad (6.31)$$

Kittler and Illingworth called Equation (6.31) the *minimum error function* because this is approximately equivalent to the minimization of the error due to the overlap between the two distributions that comprise the mixture. An equivalent criterion function can be obtained from the maximization of the likelihood of the joint distribution of the population mixture model consisting of two normal distributions with different variances [5].

We should note that the truncation of distributions due to the partitioning of the histogram by a threshold t biases the estimates of the distribution parameters. This is true for all the methods that estimate the distribution parameters by dividing the histogram with threshold t. Kittler and Illingworth assume that the effect of truncation is small. However, unlike the images in computer vision applications, medical and biological images do not have well-separated distributions. Chu et al. [10] have modified Kittler and Illingworth's minimum error method. They have suggested a new set of formulas for the mean and variance of the distribution, whose tail is not truncated; that is, the unbiased estimates of the parameters of the truncated distribution.

We have already discussed how to compute the probabilities and variances of the distributions from a histogram in earlier sections. The following MATLAB function computes the minimum-error criterion function and the optimal threshold:

```
function [th,cf,cbin] = mipminerror(x,nbins)
if nargin < 2
   nbins = 64;
end
% compute histogram, pdf
[h,cbin] = hist(single(x(:)),nbins);
h = h/sum(h);
% find the indices for max&min gray levels
max_indx = max(find(h));
min_indx = min(find(h));
% initilize variables
```

```
prevProb1 = 0;
mean1 = 0;
cf = zeros(1,nbins);
for i = min_indx:max_indx
  prob1 = prevProb1 + h(i);
  prob2 = 1 - prob1;
  if (prob1 ~= 0)
    mean1 = (prevProb1*mean1 + h(i)*i)/prob1;
    mean2 = mmean(h, i+1, max_indx);
    sd1 = sqrt(mvar(h, mean1, min_indx, i));
    sd2 = sqrt(mvar(h, mean2, i+1,max_indx));
    t1 = sd1/prob1;
    t2 = sd2/prob2;
    cf(i) = prob1*log(t1) + prob2*log(t2);
  else
    cf(i) = 0;
  end
  prevProb1 = prob1;
end
[tm, thindx] = min(cf);
th = cbin(thindx);
```

The input and output variables of this function are identical to their counterparts discussed in the previous sections.

Our functions `mipbcv`, `mipkurita`, and `mipminerror` assume that the images consist of two regions. The computed thresholds will not be valid or the algorithms will not perform as desired if the number of regions is greater than two.

Here, we compare these three methods of thresholding on the image of a spot that was cropped from a cDNA microarray image having, typically, about 6000 spots. The image of the original spot is shown in Figure 6.6 (left). Figure 6.7 shows the histogram of the spot image along with the

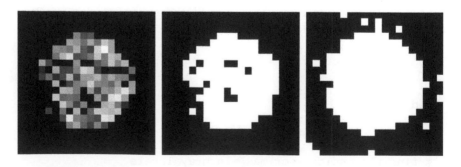

FIGURE 6.6
Images of a spot region from a cDNA microarray image. Left: Original image. Middle: Thresholded by the between-class variance. Right: Thresholded by the minimum-error thresholding method.

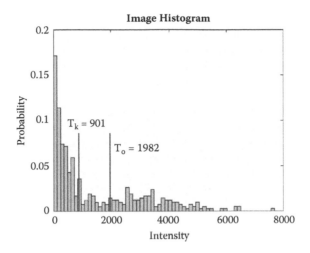

FIGURE 6.7
Histogram of the spot image shown in Figure 6.6 (left).

two thresholds computed by the minimum-error (T_k) and the BCV (T_0) criterion functions.

Kurita's criterion function computed the same threshold as the BCV and therefore is not included in the plot. The image histogram appears bimodal. Each distribution looks fairly normal, but the distributions seem to have different means and variances because one mode looks wider than the other. Again, based on visual assessment, the minimum-error thresholding appears to be providing a better threshold with a little over-segmentation, whereas the BCV appears to be undersegmenting.

Figure 6.8 shows the computed criterion functions as a function of the intensity. The criterion functions appear to be smooth and uni-modal. As seen in this figure, the intensity at which the functions have minimum or maximum differ. We know that these three criterion functions are derived with different initial assumptions. Both the BCV and Kurita's criterion assume that the two distributions have the same variances and different means, whereas the minimum-error criterion assumes that the distributions may have different means and variances. Kurita's criterion may improve the BCV in the case of unbalanced populations.

Thus, one should study the characteristics of the distributions before deciding which criterion function should be preferred. The between-class variance will compute a threshold regardless of its validity.

To study the behavior of the minimum-error function further, we have created a synthetic hexagon image. Figure 6.9 shows the synthetic hexagon image and its histogram. The minimum-error criterion function computed from this histogram is shown in Figure 6.10, denoted by the solid line. We have also created an image with one region (i.e., unimodal) only.

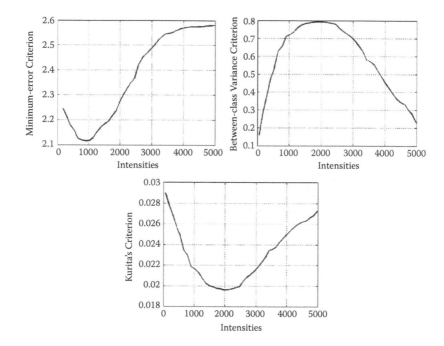

FIGURE 6.8
Criterion functions computed from the spot image plotted as a function of the intensity. Top left: Minimum-error criterion function. Top right: Between-class variance function. Bottom: Kurita's criteria function.

The dashed plot in Figure 6.10 denotes the minimum error function of the unimodal image with a mean intensity of 10.

These results illustrate that the minimum error function does not have a minimum if the image is unimodal. Hence, in using the minimum error function as part of an automated process, one may have to devise a way to

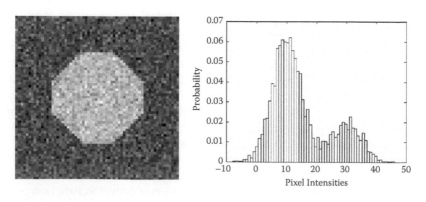

FIGURE 6.9
A synthetic hexagon image and its histogram.

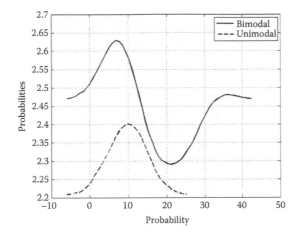

FIGURE 6.10
Minimum-error functions for the bimodal image shown in Figure 6.9 (solid line) and uni-modal image (dashed line).

find whether the criterion function has a minimum or not. The existence of a minimum in the criterion function is, in a way, also an indication of the image bimodality.

6.4 Extention to Multithresholding

Medical as well as biological images (e.g., images of tissue samples) may contain multiple regions with different intensity distribution characteristics. In such cases, the bimodality assumption cannot be met and the extension of the previously mentioned techniques to multithresholding problems would be necessary. Although the extension is fairly straightforward, the performance of these algorithms is a concern in the case of multimodal images. The distance between the modes of the distributions and the number of distributions are the key factors for the performance of these methods in multithresholding problems. Wider separation between the modes will result in better performance. If the modes are not well separated, a higher number of modes will worsen the performance. So, it is desirable to have a small number of modes that are well separated.

6.5 Entropy-Based Thresholding

In this section, we introduce some entropy-based thresholding methods for the segmentation of gray-level images. First we treat 1-D methods and then we introduce 2-D methods. The 1-D entropy-based methods only use the global information derived from the gray-level histogram, and they are effective only for certain types of segmentation. Originally, the first entropy-based method was proposed by Pun [11]. However, while deriving a lower bound for the a posteriori entropy of the gray-level histogram, Pun made a few errors in algebraic manipulations. These errors were pointed out by Kapur, Sahoo, and Wong [12] and also in the survey paper [13] due to Sahoo, Solitani, Wong, and Chen. Kapur, Sahoo, and Wong [12] proposed a new thresholding method based on the entropy of the gray-level histogram for the segmentation of gray-level images.

6.5.1 One-Dimensional Entropy-Based Method

Let $f_1, f_2, ..., f_n$ be the observed gray-level frequencies and let

$$p_i = \frac{f_i}{N}, \qquad \sum_{i=1}^{n} f_i = N, \qquad i = 1, 2, ..., n, \qquad (6.32)$$

where N is the total number of pixels in the image and n is the number of gray levels. The total entropy H_T of the image based on the distribution $(p_1, p_2, ..., p_n)$ is given by

$$H_T = -\sum_{i=1}^{n} p_i \ln p_i. \qquad (6.33)$$

In the method proposed by Kapur, Sahoo, and Wong [12], two probability distributions (e.g., object distribution and background distribution) are derived from the original gray-level distribution $(p_1, p_2, ..., p_n)$ of the image as follows:

$$A: \frac{p_1}{P_s}, \frac{p_2}{P_s}, ..., \frac{p_s}{P_s} \quad \text{and} \quad B: \frac{p_{s+1}}{1-P_s}, \frac{p_{s+2}}{1-P_s}, ..., \frac{p_n}{1-P_s} \qquad (6.34)$$

where $P_s = \sum_{i=1}^{s} p_i$. Let $H_s = -\sum_{i=1}^{s} p_i \ln p_i$. Then the entropies associated with each of the distributions are given by

$$H_b(s) := H(A) = -\sum_{i=1}^{s} \frac{p_i}{P_s} \ln\left(\frac{p_i}{P_s}\right)$$

$$= -\frac{1}{P_s}\left[\sum_{i=1}^{s} p_i \ln(p_i) - P_s \ln(P_s)\right] \qquad (6.35)$$

$$= \ln(P_s) + \frac{H_s}{P_s}$$

and

$$H_w(s) := H(B) = -\sum_{i=1+s}^{n} \frac{p_i}{1-P_s} \ln\left(\frac{p_i}{1-P_s}\right)$$

$$= -\frac{1}{1-P_s}\left[\sum_{i=s+1}^{n} p_i \ln(p_i) - (1-P_s)\ln(1-P_s)\right] \qquad (6.36)$$

$$= \ln(1-P_s) + \frac{H_T - H_s}{1-P_s}.$$

The sum of $II(A)$ and $H(B)$ is denoted by $\psi(s)$. Hence

$$\psi(s) = \ln P_s(1-P_s) + \frac{H_s}{P_s} + \frac{H_T - H_s}{1-P_s}. \qquad (6.37)$$

The function $\psi(t)$ is maximized to obtain the maximum information between the object and background distributions in the image. The discrete value t^* that maximizes $\psi(t)$ is the optimal threshold value, that is,

$$t^* = \operatorname*{Arg\,Max}_{t \in G} \psi(t) = \operatorname*{Arg\,Max}_{t \in G}\{H_b(t) + H_w(t)\} \qquad (6.38)$$

where G is the set of gray levels. The thresholding of the image $[f(m, n)]$ was achieved by the formula

$$f_t(m,n) = \begin{cases} 0 & \text{if } f(m,n) \leq t^* \\ 1 & \text{if } f(m,n) > t^*. \end{cases} \qquad (6.39)$$

The following MATLAB function computes the optimal threshold value using Equation (6.38) to Kapur, Sahoo, and Wong [12]:

```
% This function computes an optimal threshold using the
% entropy-based criterion function
% FUNCTION [th,co,h]  = mipentropy_th(x,nbins)
% outputs:
% th : optimal threshold
% co : criterion function
% h : pdf of gray levels
% inputs:
% x:image
% nbins: number of bins for the histogram
% uses hist to calculate image histogram
% function [th,co,h]  = entropy_th(x,nbins)
```

```
% warning off ;
% compute histogram, pdf
[h,cbin] = hist(x(:),nbins); h = h/sum(h);
% find the indices for max&min gray levels
max_indx = max(find(h));
min_indx = min(find(h));
% initilize variables
prob1 = 0;
ht = h;
% replace 0s with 1s in the histogram to avoid log(0) problem
% They will not affect the results as log(1)=0
ht(h==0) = 1;
% calculate total entropy
Htot = sum(h.*log(ht));
H1=0;
for i= min_indx:max_indx-1
  prob1 = prob1 + h(i);
  prob2 = 1-prob1;
  H1=H1+h(i)*log(ht(i));
  co(i) = log(prob1*prob2)-H1/prob1+(H1-Htot)/prob2;
end;
co = co/(-Htot);
co(isnan(co)) = 1;
co(max_indx) = 1;
[tm,threshold] = max(co);
th = cbin(threshold);
```

The following script was used to produce the images in Figure 6.11:

```
% Matlab Script: ksw_method.m
%
% This Matlab script computes an optimal threshold value
% using the concept of Shannon's entropy and then using the
% optimal
% value binarizes an image.
% The binarized image is displayed along with the original
% image, its gray level histogram, and the plot of the
% objective function, TotalEnt.
%
% To run this script, you have to input the name of an
% image such as rice.tif or tire.tif.
%
% This script runs only for tif or gif images.
clear all
clc
NBINS = 256;
%
% Read the user supplied image file
%
```

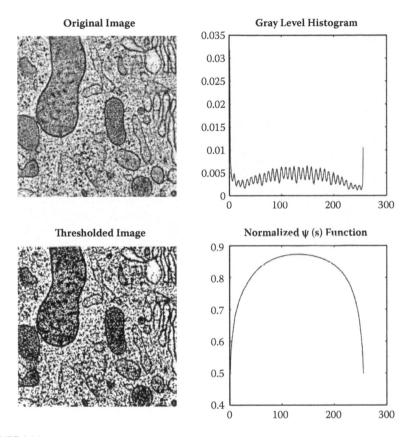

FIGURE 6.11
Top left: An original image of cells. Top right: Histogram of the original image. Bottom left: Thresholded image at the optimal threshold value 133. Bottom right: Graph of the normalized function.

```
IMAGE = input('Please enter the name of the tif image:...
    ', 's');
I = imread(IMAGE);
I3 = double(I);
numgray = NBINS;
I2 = I;
%
% Function mipentropy_th.m is used here
%
[graylevel, nco, h] = mipentropy_th(I3, NBINS);
threshold = graylevel/numgray;
BW2 = im2bw(I2, threshold);
disp(' ')
fprintf('The optimal threshold value is %3.0f \n', graylevel)
```

```
disp(' ')
%
% Display the original, binarized images and other
% information relevent to this thresholding method.
subplot(2,2,1), imshow(I2)
title('original image')
subplot(2,2,2), plot(ii,h),
title('gray level histogram')
axis('square');
subplot(2,2,3), imshow(BW2);
title('thresholded image')
subplot(2,2,4), plot(ii,0.5*nco)
title('normalized \psi (s) function');
axis('square');
%
% To print the figure into a file type from the command
% window print myfigure.ps. The figure will be save in
% postscript format in a file called "myfigure.ps"
%
print myfigure.ps
```

6.5.2 Two-Dimensional Entropy-Based Method

The advantage of the Kapur, Sahoo, and Wong method [12] is that it uses a global objective property of the histogram. Because of its general nature, this method can be used for segmentation purposes. However, one still encounters the following problems. What happens if two different pictures have the same gray-level histogram and thus the same threshold? Will it be suitable for both? A second-order statistic or some local property with the entropic concept of thresholding might give a better insight into these problems. Abutaleb [14] extended the entropy-based thresholding method of Kapur, Sahoo, and Wong [12] using 2-D entropy. The two-dimensional entropies were obtained from a two-dimensional histogram that was determined by using the gray value of the pixels. This extension due to Abutaleb was refined by Brink [15] by maximizing the smaller of the two entropies instead of maximizing the sum of the two entropies of the background class and object class. Recently, Sahoo, Slaaf, and Albert [16], and Sahoo and Arora [17,18] have considered the problem of 2-D thresholding. In this section, we present the 2-D entropy method due to Sahoo and Arora [18], where the authors have used Charvat–Havrda–Tsallis entropy. In the limiting case, this method yields the methods proposed by Brink [15] and Abutaleb [14].

Let $P = (p_1, p_2, ..., p_n) \in \Delta_n$, where

$$\Delta_n = \left\{ (p_1, p_2, ..., p_n) \mid p_i \geq 0,\ i = 1, 2, ..., n,\ n \geq 2, \sum_{i=1}^{n} p_i = 1 \right\} \qquad (6.40)$$

is the set of discrete finite n-ary probability distributions. The Havrda and Charvat entropy of degree α is defined as

$$H_n^{\alpha}(P) = \frac{1}{1 - 2^{1-\alpha}}\left[1 - \sum_{i=1}^{n} p_i^{\alpha}\right] \qquad (6.41)$$

where α is a real positive parameter not equal to one. The Tsallis entropy is a one-parameter generalization of the Shannon entropy and it is of the form

$$H_n^{\alpha}(P) = \frac{1}{\alpha - 1}\left[1 - \sum_{i=1}^{n} p_i^{\alpha}\right] \qquad (6.42)$$

where α is a real positive parameter and $\alpha \neq 1$. Both these entropies essentially have the same expression except the normalizing factor. Havrda and Charvat entropies are normalized to 1. That is, if $P = (0.5, 0.5)$, then $H_2^{\alpha}(P) = 1$, whereas Tsallis entropy is not normalized. For our application both the entropies yield the same result, and we called these entropies the Charvat–Havrda–Tsallis entropy. However, we use Equation (6.42) as the Charvat–Havrda–Tsallis entropy. Because $\lim_{\alpha \to 1} H_n^{\alpha}(P) = H_n^1(P)$, the Charvat–Havrda–Tsallis entropy $H_n^{\alpha}(P)$ is a one-parameter generalization of the Shannon entropy $H_n^1(P)$ where

$$H_n^1(P) = -\sum_{i=1}^{n} p_i \ln p_i. \qquad (6.43)$$

When $\alpha = 2$, the Charvat–Havrda–Tsallis entropy becomes the Gini–Simpson index of diversity:

$$H_n^2(P) = 1 - \sum_{i=1}^{n} p_i^2. \qquad (6.44)$$

Let $f(m, n)$ be the gray value of the pixel located at the point (m, n). A digital image of size $M \times N$ is a matrix of the form

$$[f(m,n) \mid m = 1, 2, ..., M \text{ and } n = 1, 2, ..., N] \qquad (6.45)$$

or, in short form, $[f(m, n)]$.

Let G denote the set of all gray values $\{0, 1, 2, ..., 2^l - 1\}$. Usually l is either 8 or 16. If $l = 8$ then the set $G = \{0, 1, 2, ..., 255\}$. Next we discuss (1) how to construct the 2-D histogram, (2) how to compute the probability distributions of object and background classes, and (3) the choice of the entropic criterion function.

In order to compute the two-dimensional histogram of a given image, we proceed as follows. Calculate the average gray value of the neighborhood of each pixel. Let $g(x, y)$ be the average of the neighborhood of the pixel located at the point (x, y). The average gray value for the 3×3 neighborhood of each pixel is calculated as

$$g(x,y) = \left\lfloor \frac{1}{9} \sum_{i=-1}^{1} \sum_{j=-1}^{1} f(x+i, y+j) \right\rfloor \qquad (6.46)$$

where $\lfloor r \rfloor$ denotes the integer part of the number r. While computing the average gray value, disregard the two rows from the top and bottom and two columns from the sides. The pixel's gray value, $f(x, y)$, and the average of its neighborhood, $g(x, y)$, are used to construct a two-dimensional histogram using

$$h(m,n) = \text{Prob}(f(x,y) = m \text{ and } g(x,y) = n), \qquad (6.47)$$

where $m, n \in G$. For a given image, there are several methods to estimate this density function. One of the most frequently used methods is the method of relative frequency. The normalized histogram is approximated by using the formula

$$\hat{h}(m,n) = \frac{\text{number of elements in the event } (f(x,y) = m) \,\&\, (g(x,y) = n)}{\text{number of elements in the sample space}}$$

$$(6.48)$$

$$= \frac{\text{number of pixels with gray value } m \text{ and average gray valy } n}{\text{number of pixels in the image}}.$$

The joint probability mass function, $p(m, n)$, is given by

$$p(m,n) = \hat{h}(m,n), \qquad (6.49)$$

where $m, n = 0, 1, \ldots, 255$.

The threshold is obtained through a vector (t, s), where t, for $f(x, y)$, represents the threshold of the gray level of the pixel and s, for $g(x, y)$, represents the threshold of the average gray level of the pixel's neighborhood. Using the joint probability mass function $p(m, n)$ a surface can be drawn that will have two peaks and one valley. The object and background correspond to the peaks and can be separated by selecting the vector (t, s) that maximizes a suitable criterion function $\phi_\alpha(t, s)$. Using this vector (t, s) the domain of the histogram is divided into four quadrants (see Figure 6.12).

We denote the first quadrant by $[t+1, 255] \times [0, s]$, the second quadrant by $[0, t] \times [0, s]$, the third quadrant by $[0, t] \times [s+1, 255]$, and the fourth quadrant by $[t+1, 255] \times [s+1, 255]$. Because two of the quadrants, first and

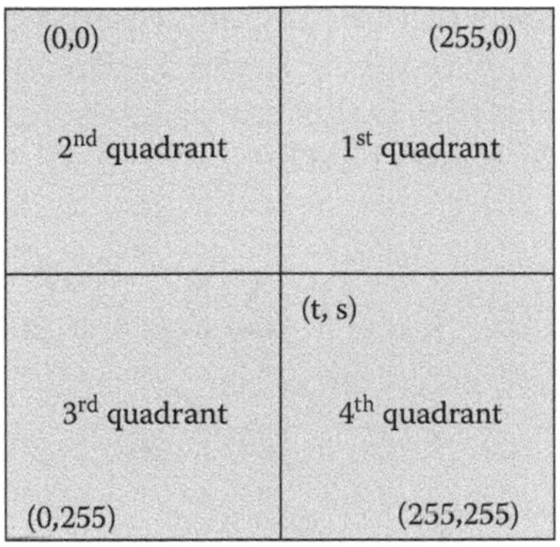

FIGURE 6.12
Quadrants in the 2-D histogram due to thresholding at (t, s).

third, contain information about edges and noise alone, they are ignored in the calculation. Because the quadrants which contain the object and the background, second and fourth, are considered to be independent distributions, the probability values in each case must be normalized for each of the quadrants to have a total probability of 1. Our normalization is accomplished by using posteriori class probabilities $P_2(t, s)$ and $P_4(t, s)$, where

$$P_2(t, s) = \sum_{i=0}^{t} \sum_{j=0}^{s} p(i, j) \quad \text{and} \quad P_4(t, s) = \sum_{i=t+1}^{255} \sum_{j=s+1}^{255} p(i, j). \qquad (6.50)$$

we assume that the contribution of the quadrants that contain the edges and noise is negligible; hence, we approximate $P_4(t, s)$ as $P_4(t, s) \approx 1 - P_2(t, s)$.

Thresholding an image at a threshold t is equivalent to partitioning the set G into two disjoint subsets:

$$G_0 = \{0, 1, 2, \ldots, t\} \quad \text{and} \quad G_1 = \{t+1, t+2, \ldots, 255\} \qquad (6.51)$$

The two probability distributions associated with these sets are

$$\left(\frac{p(0,0)}{P_2(t,s)}, \ldots, \frac{p(0,s)}{P_2(t,s)}, \frac{p(1,0)}{P_2(t,s)}, \ldots, \frac{p(t,s)}{P_2(t,s)} \right) \qquad (6.52)$$

and

$$\left(\frac{p(t+1,s+1)}{P_4(t,s)}, \ldots, \frac{p(t+1,255)}{P_4(t,s)}, \frac{p(t+2,s+1)}{P4(t,s)}, \ldots, \frac{p(255,255)}{P_4(t,s)} \right), \qquad (6.53)$$

respectively. On the basis of our previous discussion, we have approximated $P_4(t, s)$ as $1 - P_2(t, s)$, that is, $P_4(t, s) \approx 1 - P_2(t, s)$.

Thus, the Charvat–Havrda–Tsallis entropies associated with object and background distributions are given by

$$H_b^\alpha(t, s) = \frac{1}{\alpha - 1}\left[1 - \sum_{i=0}^{t}\sum_{j=0}^{s}\left(\frac{p(i, j)}{P_2(t, s)}\right)^\alpha\right]$$ (6.54)

and

$$H_w^\alpha(t, s) = \frac{1}{\alpha - 1}\left[1 - \sum_{i=t+1}^{255}\sum_{j=s+1}^{255}\left(\frac{p(i, j)}{1 - P_2(t, s)}\right)^\alpha\right].$$ (6.55)

The a priori Charvat–Havrda–Tsallis entropy of an image is given by

$$H_T^\alpha = \frac{1}{\alpha - 1}\left[1 - \sum_{i=0}^{255}\sum_{j=0}^{255} p(i, j)^\alpha\right],$$ (6.56)

where $\alpha \neq 1$ is a positive real parameter.

If one considers that a physical system can be decomposed into two statistical independent subsystems A and B the probability of the composite system is $p^{A+B} = p^A p^B$ and the Charvat–Havrda–Tsallis entropy of the system follows the nonadditivity rule:

$$H_T^\alpha(A + B) = H_T^\alpha(A) + H_T^\alpha(B) + (1 - \alpha)H_T^\alpha(A)H_T^\alpha(B).$$ (6.57)

Thus, the following equation

$$\phi_\alpha(t, s) = H_b^\alpha(t, s) + H_w^\alpha(t, s) + (1 - \alpha)H_b^\alpha(t, s)H_w^\alpha(t, s)$$ (6.58)

is used as a criterion function. The optimal threshold pair $(t^*(\alpha), s^*(\alpha))$ is obtained by maximizing the preceding criterion function $\phi_\alpha(t, s)$. Thus

$$(t^*(\alpha), s^*(\alpha)) = \underset{(t,s)\in G\times G}{\text{Arg Max}}\ \phi_\alpha(t, s).$$ (6.59)

Using the original image $[f(m, n)]$, the thresholded image $[f(m, n)]$ was computed by the formula

$$f_t(m, n) = \begin{cases} 0 & \text{if } f(m, n) \leq t^*(\alpha) \\ 1 & \text{if } f(m, n) > t^*(\alpha). \end{cases}$$ (6.60)

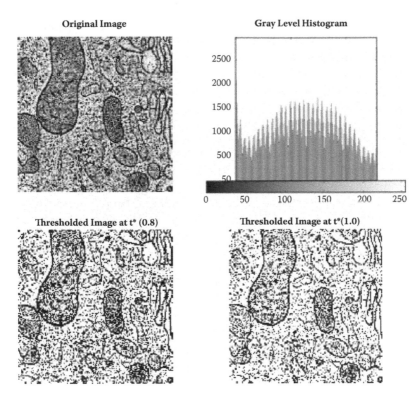

FIGURE 6.13
Top left: An original image of cells. Top right: Histogram of the original image. Bottom left: Thresholded image at the optimal threshold value 95. Bottom right: Thresholded image at the optimal threshold value 79.

The original images together with their histograms and the thresholded images obtained by using the optimal threshold value $t^*(0.8)$ and $t^*(1.0)$ are displayed side by side in Figure 6.13. Note that the thresholded image obtained by threshold value $t^*(1.0)$ is the same as the one obtained by Abutaleb's method (see Abutaleb [14]).

Our analysis is based on how much information is lost owing to thresholding. In this analysis, given two thresholded images of a same original image, we prefer the one that lost the least amount of information. Using the aforementioned ten images and also many other images, we conclude that when α is 0.8 our proposed method produced the best optimal threshold values. When α was greater than 1, this proposed method did not produce good threshold values; in fact, the threshold values produced were unacceptable. When the value of α was 1, the threshold value produced was not always a good threshold value. This method performs better than Abutaleb's method when $\alpha = 0.8$.

In this method of thresholding, we have used in addition to the original gray-level function $f(x, y)$, a function $g(x, y)$ that is the average gray-level value in a 3×3 neighborhood around the pixel (x, y). This approach can be extended to an image pyramid, where an image on the next higher level is composed of average gray-level values computed for disjoint 3×3 squares. In order to find out which pyramid level will produce an optimal threshold value, we have tested all the test images with different neighborhood sizes and different α values. In particular, we have considered neighborhood sizes of 2×2, 3×3, 4×4, 5×5, 8×8, and 16×16, respectively. Neighborhood sizes of 3×3, 4×4, 5×5, and 8×8 all produced similar optimal threshold values, giving acceptable binary images. From the point of view of computational time and image quality, a neighborhood size of 3×3 or 5×5 with α value equals to 0.8 would be ideal for thresholding with this proposed method.

The following MATLAB function computes the optimal threshold value using Equation (6.59):

```
% This function returns the optimal threshold value using
% the two-dimensional Tsallis entropy method.
%
function newmaxgray = mipsahoo_thresh(I, alpha, numgray);
[nrow, ncol] = size(I);
%
% Compute the averaged image I3 using a 3-by-3 sliding
% window This is accomplished using colfilt command.
% This command works for 'tif' and 'jpeg' images only.
% For other image formats, the command colfilt has to
% be appropriately modified.
%
% I3 = unit8(floor(colfilt(I, [3 3], 'sliding', @mean)));
%
I3 = uint8(floor(colfilt(I,[3 3],'sliding','mean')));
%
% Compute the co-occurence matrix.
I = double(I) + 1;
I3 = double(I3) + 1;
for k = 1:numgray
    for l = 1:numgray
        N(k,l) = 0;
    end
end
for i = 1:nrow
    for j = 1:ncol
        m = I(i,j);
        n = I3(i,j);
        N(m,n) = N(m,n) + 1;
    end
end
```

```
% Computation of two-dimensional cumulative sum.
% The cumsum command of the matlab has been used
% appropriately for this purpose.
%
P = N/sum(sum(N));
Pcumsum = cumsum(cumsum(P),2);
for i = 1:numgray
   for j = 1:numgray
      if Pcumsum(i,j) == 0 | Pcumsum(i,j) == 1
         Pcumsum1(i,j) = 50000;
      else
         Pcumsum1(i,j) = Pcumsum(i,j);
      end
   end
end
% Computation of AAa matrix.
%
Pcumsumal = Pcumsum1.^alpha;
Pal = P.^alpha;
PalcumsumA = cumsum(cumsum(Pal),2);
norPalcumsumA = PalcumsumA./Pcumsumal;
AAa = norPalcumsumA;
%
% Computation of BBb matrix.
%
Pnew = fliplr(flipud(Pal));
PalcumsumB = cumsum(cumsum(Pnew),2);
I4 = PalcumsumB;
I4(numgray, :) = [];
I4(:, numgray) = [];
I5 = fliplr(flipud(I4));
u = zeros(numgray-1, 1);
v = zeros(1, numgray);
I6 = [I5 u];
I7 = [I6; v];
norPalcumsumB = I7./abs((1-Pcumsum1).^alpha);
BBb = norPalcumsumB;
%
% Compute object, background and total entropies
% in the sense of Tsallis. Then compute the optimal
% threshold.
%
constant = 1/(alpha-1);
Entb = constant.*(1-AAa);
Entw = constant.*(1-BBb);
TotalEnt = Entb + Entw + (1-alpha).*Entb.*Entw;
%
% Storing the Total Entropy data in a new variable called
% TotalEntNew for later use in ploting of the entropy
% surface.
```

```
%
TotalEntNew = TotalEnt;
%
% Maximize the total entropy to calculate the optimal
% threshold value and then threshold the image in BW.
%
[maximum, rowindex] = max(TotalEnt);
[maximax, colindex] = max(maximum);
maxgray = rowindex(colindex);
newmaxgray = maxgray - 1;
newmaxgray;
```

The following function computes the optimal threshold value using Brink's method:

```
% This function returns the optimal threshold value using the
% two-dimensional Shannon entropy method.
%
function newmaxgray = mipbrink_thresh(I, numgray);
[nrow, ncol] = size(I);
%
% Compute the averaged image I3 using a 3-by-3 sliding
% window This is accomplished using colfilt command.
% This command works for 'tif' image only.
% For other format images like jpeg, this
% the command colfilt has to be appropriately modified.
%
I3 = uint8(floor(colfilt(I,[3 3],'sliding','mean')));
%
% Compute the co-occurence matrix.
%
I = double(I) + 1;
I3 = double(I3) + 1;
for k = 1:numgray
  for l = 1:numgray
    N(k,l) = 0;
  end
end
for i = 1:nrow
  for j = 1:ncol
    m = I(i,j);
    n = I3(i,j);
    N(m,n) = N(m,n) + 1;
  end
end
%
% Computation of two-dimensional cumulative sum.
% The cumsum command of the matlab has been used
% appropriately for this purpose.
```

```
%
P = N/sum(sum(N));
Pcumsum = cumsum(cumsum(P),2);
for i = 1:numgray
  for j = 1:numgray
    if Pcumsum(i,j) == 0 | Pcumsum(i,j) == 1
      Pcumsum1(i,j) = 50000;
    else
      Pcumsum1(i,j) = Pcumsum(i,j);
    end
  end
end
%
% Computation of AAa matrix.
%
Pcumsumal = Pcumsum1;
Pal = P;
PalcumsumA = cumsum(cumsum(Pal),2);
norPalcumsumA = PalcumsumA./Pcumsumal;
AAa = norPalcumsumA;
%
% Computation of BBb matrix.
%
Pnew = fliplr(flipud(Pal));
PalcumsumB = cumsum(cumsum(Pnew),2);
I4 = PalcumsumB;
I4(numgray, :) = [];
I4(:, numgray) = [];
I5 = fliplr(flipud(I4));
u = zeros(numgray-1, 1);
v = zeros(1, numgray);
I6 = [I5 u];
I7 = [I6; v];
norPalcumsumB = I7./abs((1 - Pcumsum1));
BBb = norPalcumsumB;
%
% Replace the zero or undefined entries of matrices
% AAa and BBb by one so that log(1) will be 0.
%
for i = 1:numgray
  for j = 1:numgray
    if BBb(i,j) < 0.000001
      BBb(i,j) = 1;
    end
    if AAa(i,j) < 0.000001
      AAa(i,j) = 1;
    end
  end
end
```

```
%
% Compute object, background and total entropies
% in the sense of Shannon. Then compute the optimal
% threshold.
%
Entb = - AAa.*log(AAa);
Entw = - BBb.*log(BBb);
TotalEnt = Entb + Entw;
%
% Maximize the total entropy to calculate the optimal
% threshold value and then threshold the image in BW.
%
[maximum, rowindex] = max(TotalEnt);
[maximax, colindex] = max(maximum);
maxgray = rowindex(colindex);
newmaxgray = maxgray - 1;
newmaxgray;
```

Figure 6.13 was generated using the following MATLAB script:

```
% Matlab Script: sa_method.m
%
% This Matlab script computes an optimal threshold
% value using the concept of Tsallis entropy and then
% using the optimal value binarizes an image. This
% script uses the functions mip sahoo_thresh and
% mipbrink_thresh. The thresholded images are displayed
% along with the original image and its gray level histogram.
% To run this script, you have to input the
% name of an monochrome image such as saturn.tif or
% sahoo.jpg. You need to input the alpha value used
% in the computation of Tsallis entropy. The alpha
% value should be a positive real number and it should
% not be equal to one.
%
% Read the user supplied image file
%
IMAGE = input('Enter the name of the gray-valued ...
  image:','s');
[I] = imread(IMAGE);
%
% Read the number of gray levels in the input image
%
numgray = 256;
% numgray = input('Enter the number of gray levels in
% this image:');
%
% Read the user supplied q-value for Tsallis entropy
```

```
%
alpha = input('Enter a positive q-value that is not ...
  equal to one: ');
%
% Store the input image in I2 for later use
%
I2 = I(:,:,1);
IR = I(:,:,1);
IR = double(IR);
graylevel1 = sahoo_thresh(IR, alpha, numgray);
threshold1 = graylevel1/numgray;
BW1 = im2bw(I2, threshold1);
%
graylevel2 = brink_thresh(IR, numgray);
threshold2 = graylevel2/numgray;
BW2 = im2bw(I2, threshold2);
%
disp(' ')
fprintf('The optimal threshold value with Sahoo-Arora
  method is %3.0f \n',...
  graylevel1)
disp(' ')
%
disp(' ')
fprintf('The optimal threshold value with Abutaleb-Brink
  method is %3.0f \n',...
  graylevel2)
disp(' ')
%
% Display the original, binarized images and other
% information relevent to this thresholding method.
%
figure
subplot(2,2,1), imshow(I2); title('original image')
subplot(2,2,2), imhist(I2), title('gray level histogram');...
  axis('square');
subplot(2,2,3), imshow(BW1); title(sprintf('thresholded
  at t*(%3.1f) = %3.0f',...
  alpha, graylevel1))
subplot(2,2,4), imshow(BW2); title(sprintf('thresholded
  at t*(1.0) = %3.0f',...
  graylevel2))
% To print the figure into a file type from the command
% window print myfigure.ps. The figure will be save in
% postscript format in a file called "myfigure.ps"
%
print my_sa_figure.ps
```

6.6 Image Segmentation by K-Means Clustering

Clustering, also known as unsupervised classification, looks for the natural groupings in a multidimensional data set by employing a similarity or dissimilarity measure. In clustering, classes are unknown and explored from the data themselves. Whereas clustering divides the data into similar groups, *classification* assigns an observation to one of the already-known groups. Clustering can be divided into two main categories, namely, *partitional* and *hierarchical* clustering. Given n samples, each of which may be represented by a d-dimensional feature vector, the aim of the partitional clustering method is to partition the samples into K clusters so that the features in a sample group are more similar to one another than to those features in different sample groups. Every clustering method will normally produce clusters, but they may not guarantee that the discovered clusters are always meaningful. However, clustering, in general, can be very useful as an exploratory tool.

There are two popular partitional clustering strategies: square-error and mixture modeling. The sum of the squared Euclidian distances between the samples in a cluster and the cluster center is called *within-cluster variation*. The sum of the within-cluster variations in a clustering scheme is used as a criterion in K-means clustering [19]. This clustering is also known as *minimum variance partition*.

K-means clustering is computationally very efficient and gives satisfactory results if the clusters are compact and well separated in the feature space, but the number of clusters has to be specified a priori. The K-means algorithm may or may not converge to the global minimum. It is sensitive to the initially selected cluster centers. The K-means algorithm can be run multiple times to alleviate the latter issue (see the MATLAB code in the following example).

We can view image segmentation as the partitioning of the observed intensities into similar groups. Then, a clustering method can be employed to segment images into regions or clusters.

The application of the K-means algorithm to image segmentation is reasonably straightforward. First, we will write our 2-D or 3-D image in a column-ordered vector format. This can be done by stacking each column after the previous one. Let us call our $M \cdot N \times d$ sample vector $\mathbf{v}$, each element of which comprises the gray-level intensity in the case of a gray-level image ($d = 1$) or R, G, and B values in the case of a color image ($d = 3$). Note that the column ordering results in the loss of spatial information. Hence, K-means clustering disregards the contextual or spatial information.

The K-means algorithm for image segmentation includes the following steps:

1. Initialize the number of classes K and centroids μ_j.
2. Assign each pixel or voxel to the group whose centroid is the closest.
3. After all pixels have been assigned, recalculate the centroids.
4. Repeat steps 2 and 3 until the centroids no longer change.

As we already mentioned, the K-means clustering algorithm minimizes the sum of the within-cluster variances

$$Q = \sum_{j=1}^{K} \sum_{i=1}^{n} \| v_i^j - \mu_j \|^2 \tag{6.61}$$

where v_i^j is the ith sample of jth class K_j and μ_j the center of the jth cluster defined as the mean of $v_i \in K_j$.

In calculating the centroids, different distance measures can be employed, although the Euclidian distance is probably the most common. MATLAB's kmeans algorithm offers a number of different distance measures, including the Euclidian distance. The replicate option of the algorithm allows us to repeat the algorithm a number of times and choose the solution with the lowest total sum of distances over all replicates.

We will now demonstrate the application of the K-means algorithm to image segmentation using our MRI brain image, which we assumed includes four regions or clusters. We will utilize MATLAB's kmeans algorithm. The following MATLAB script reads the image, performs K-means clustering, and finally assigns the cluster indices to the pixels. The segmented images are shown in Figure 6.14. Note

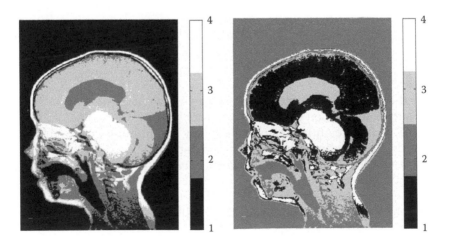

FIGURE 6.14
Left: Segmented by K-means algorithm. Right: Segmented by fuzzy C-means algorithm. In both cases, K = C = 4.

that we repeated the algorithm nRegions+1 times, as suggested by MATLAB.

```
img =imread('brain.png');
H = single(img(:));
nRegions = 4;
[ClassIndex, C] = kmeans(H,nRegions,'distance',...
    'sqEuclidean','Replicates', nRegions+1);
[r,c] = size(img);
bw = reshape(ClassIndex,r,c);
figure, imshow(bw, []);
colormap(gray(4)), colorbar('YTick',1:4)
```

6.7 Image Segmentation by Fuzzy C-Means Clustering

The fuzzy C-means (FCM) clustering algorithm was first suggested by Dunn [20] and later improved by Bezdek [21]. Unlike K-means clustering, in which each observation has a clear-cut binary membership, the FCM method proposes a fuzzy membership that assigns a degree of membership for each class. The concept of degree of membership in fuzzy clustering is similar to the posterior probability in a mixture modeling setting. By monitoring data points that have close membership values to existing classes, forming new clusters is possible; this is the major advantage of FCM clustering over K-means clustering. The FCM clustering minimizes

$$Q = \sum_{j=1}^{n}\sum_{j=1}^{C} u_{ij}^{m}\,\|v_i - \mu_j\|^2 \qquad 1 \le m < \infty \qquad (6.62)$$

where
  n is the number of samples and C is the number of clusters;
  μ_j is the d-dimension center of the cluster;
  $m \in [1,\infty]$ is a weighting exponent and any real number greater than 1;
  v_i is the ith of d-dimensional measured data; and
  $\|*\|$ is a norm expressing the similarity between any measured data and
    the cluster center.

The membership matrix **u** satisfies the condition

$$\sum_{i=1}^{C} u_{ij} = 1, \forall j = 1,...,n \qquad (6.63)$$

The memberships and the cluster centers are updated using the following relationships:

$$u_{ij}^m = \cfrac{1}{\displaystyle\sum_{k=1}^{C} \left(\cfrac{\|v_i - \mu_j\|}{\|v_i - \mu_k\|} \right)^{\frac{2}{m-1}}} \quad \text{and} \quad \mu_j = \cfrac{\displaystyle\sum_{i=1}^{n} u_{ij} \cdot v_i}{\displaystyle\sum_{i=1}^{n} u_{ij}} \tag{6.64}$$

Note that the centroids are the mean of the data weighted by their membership and normalized to the total membership. Note also that the degree of membership is inversely proportional to the distance to the cluster center.

The FCM algorithm is very similar to the K-means algorithm:

1. Choose the number of clusters or region.
2. Assign pixels their initial membership values according to equation (6.63).
3. Compute the centroid for each cluster, and the membership values using the formula in Equation (6.64).
4. Iterate until $\max_{ij}\{\|u_{ij}^{k+1} - u_{ij}^k\|\} < \varepsilon$ where k is the iteration number and ε is the error threshold; otherwise return to step 2.
5. Assign each pixel the cluster number for which its membership is maximum.

By iteratively updating the cluster centers and the membership degrees for each data point, the FCM algorithm iteratively moves toward a local minimum of Equation (6.62). Therefore, similar to the K-means algorithm, the FCM does not guarantee convergence to a global minimum. The cluster validity and impact of the parameter m have been investigated [22]. The authors conclude as follows: "Finally, our calculations suggest that the best choice for m is probably in the interval [1.5, 2.5], whose mean and midpoint, $m = 2$, have often been the preferred choice for many users of FCM." We recommend that interested readers attempt the related problems, which will also help them gather experience with different parameters' values.

We will now demonstrate the application of the FCM algorithm to image segmentation using our MRI brain image, which we again assume has four regions or clusters. We will utilize MATLAB's fcm algorithm, which performs the FCM clustering. The following MATLAB script reads the image, performs fuzzy C-means clustering for $m = 2$, and finally assigns each pixel to the cluster for which its membership is maximum. The segmented image is shown in Figure 6.14 (right).

```
img =imread('brain.png');
nRegions = 4;
H = single(img(:));
% options = [m, interations, error, info display during
% iteration];
options = [2 100 1e-5 0];
[center, U, obj_fcn] = fcm(H,nRegions,options);
maxU = max(U);
index = zeros(nRegions, length(H));
for i=1:nRegions
   tmpindx = find(U(i,:) == maxU);
   H(tmpindx) = i;
end
[r,c] = size(img);
bw = reshape(H,r,c);
figure, imshow(bw,[]);
colormap(gray(4)), colorbar('YTick',1:4)
```

This script, which is written as a function (mipfcmSegmentation), is included in the Medical Image Processing Toolbox.

As seen in Figure 6.14, both clustering algorithms provide reasonably good results on this MRI image with a multiple number of regions. These results can be used as a starting image for more sophisticated segmentation methods that utilize spatial information as well. A good initial segmentation is essential for iterative sophisticated methods (see Chapter 7) to achieve global convergence faster.

Note that we can in a similar manner apply K-means and the FCM clustering algorithms to 3-D images. One can also subsample, 2:1 for instance, a 3-D volume image to run the algorithm faster by subsampling n:1 using the following code and compute the thresholds using the sampled image to segment the original image into the same number of regions:

```
simg = img(1:n:end,1:n:end,1:n:end);
```

6.8   Mixture-Modeling–Based Segmentation

In this approach, we assume that the values of pixels forming our image come from a multimodal density. By *mode* we refer to the bumps in the image histogram. These bumps simply indicate that there are some pixel values for which the numbers of pixels attaining those values are relatively high. The modes in the histogram may correspond to certain regions or characteristics (e.g., a certain tissue type) in the image. Therefore, if we can identify or model the probability density function (pdf) of pixel values, we can then use this model to find the probabilities of any pixel value belonging to different classes/modes or regions.

Mixture modeling arose as a technique for pdf estimation [23–25] and found significant applications in various biological problems [23,26,27]. The first step in the application of this approach to an image segmentation problem would sensibly be obtaining an image histogram. The histogram gives us a rough idea about the pdf of pixel values. Even though pdf estimation is a tricky problem in itself, the histogram remains a useful/practical tool of great value. We caution the reader here because, depending on the bin selection, the appearance of the histogram may change considerably. That is, if the histogram estimate of the pdf is not obtained carefully, some modes may disappear or may appear falsely. Luckily, in the case of image data, we mostly know what the pixel values can be. For instance, while dealing with a grayscale image of 256 intensity values, it is obvious that we should set the histogram bin centers at 0, 1,..., 255.

When we look at the histogram of the MRI image of Figure 7.10, we observe that there are four modes. We will now discuss how we can model or fit normal densities to those modes and come up with an overall normal mixture model for the pdf of pixel values. In the following treatment, we will use the terms *mode*, *class*, and *mixture component* interchangeably.

Let $\mathbf{x}$ be a pixel value and $f(\mathbf{x})$ be the probability of getting that pixel value. We may also say that "$f(\mathbf{x})$ is the pdf of $\mathbf{x}$." If we have k modes or classes in the pdf of pixel values, we can argue that $\mathbf{x}$ may come from any of those k densities with different probabilities. Because these events are disjoint, we write $f(\mathbf{x})$ as the sum of those class probabilities.

$$f(\mathbf{x}) = \Pr(\mathbf{x} \text{ and } \mathbf{x} \text{ comes from Class } 1) + \ldots + \Pr(\mathbf{x} \text{ and } \mathbf{x} \text{ comes from Class } k)$$

where Pr denotes probability. $\Pr(\text{Class } i)$, $i = 1, 2, \ldots, k$ being class prior probabilities, we can then use a little mathematical trick to express the probabilities of $\mathbf{x}$ coming from different classes as

$$\Pr(\mathbf{x} \text{ and } \mathbf{x} \text{ comes from Class } i) = \Pr(\text{Class } i) \frac{\Pr(\mathbf{x} \text{ and } \mathbf{x} \text{ comes from Class } 1)}{\Pr(\text{Class } i)},$$

or, using the definition of conditional probability, as

$$\Pr(\mathbf{x} \text{ and } \mathbf{x} \text{ comes from Class } i) = \Pr(\text{Class } i) f_i(\mathbf{x} \mid \text{Class } i)$$

where $f_i(\mathbf{x} \mid \text{Class } i)$, $i = 1, 2, .., k$ represent class conditional pdfs of $\mathbf{x}$. Hence, $f(\mathbf{x})$ becomes

$$f(\mathbf{x}) = \Pr(\text{Class } 1) f_1(\mathbf{x} \mid \text{Class } 1) + \ldots + \Pr(\text{Class } k) f_k(\mathbf{x} \mid \text{Class } k) \quad (6.65)$$

In general, we assume that the pixel value $\mathbf{x}$ is of dimension d and, correspondingly, $f(\mathbf{x})$ is a multivariate pdf. That is why we have used the vector (bold) nation for **x**. For intensity images, the dimension of pixels/observations is 1, whereas for true-color images, pixels are 3-D (RGB) and d is 3.

Equation (6.65) simply states that a multimodal multivariate pdf $f(\mathbf{x})$ can be expressed as a weighted sum of k class conditional pdf's, the weights being the prior probabilities. With a little change of notation, we can rewrite equation (6.65) more elegantly as

$$f(\mathbf{x}) = \sum_{i=1}^{k} w_i f_i(\mathbf{x} \mid \boldsymbol{\theta}_i) \tag{6.66}$$

Here, we have renamed the class prior probability Pr(Class i) as w_i, representing the "weight" or "mixing coefficient" of the ith component pdf, and $f_i(\mathbf{x} \mid \text{Class } i)$ as $f_i(\mathbf{x} \mid \boldsymbol{\theta}_i)$, because each class conditional pdf is identified with a set of parameters $\boldsymbol{\theta}_i$. If we use **normal** or **Gaussian** components in our mixture model, $f_i(\mathbf{x} \mid \boldsymbol{\theta}_i)$ is a multivariate normal pdf:

$$f_i(\mathbf{x} \mid \boldsymbol{\theta}_i) = N(\mathbf{x} \mid \boldsymbol{\mu}_i, \boldsymbol{\Sigma}_i) = (2\pi)^{-d/2} \mid \boldsymbol{\Sigma}_i \mid^{-1/2} \exp\left\{-(\mathbf{x} - \boldsymbol{\mu}_i)^T \boldsymbol{\Sigma}_i^{-1}(\mathbf{x} - \boldsymbol{\mu}_i)/2\right\},$$

where $\boldsymbol{\mu}_i$ is the $d \times 1$ mean vector and $\boldsymbol{\Sigma}_i$ is the $d \times d$ covariance matrix. The corresponding length of the parameter vector $\boldsymbol{\theta}_i = (\boldsymbol{\mu}_i, \boldsymbol{\Sigma}_i^*)$, where $\boldsymbol{\Sigma}_i^*$ denotes either upper- or lower-triangular and diagonal entries of $\boldsymbol{\Sigma}_i$, is $m = d + \frac{1}{2}d(d+1)$, because of the symmetry of the covariance matrix. Depending on how the histogram looks, the choice of using normal densities in the mixture model may or may not be appropriate. We will discuss this issue in more detail later. In the rest of this discussion, we will assume that we are dealing with a normal mixture model; that is, all the components in the mixture model are normal pdfs.

One should have $\sum_{i=1}^{k} w_i = 1$ to make sure that $f(\mathbf{x})$ is a valid pdf. That is, if we know $k - 1$ weights, the last weight is determined automatically. Therefore, the total number parameters to be estimated in Equation (6.66) is $M = km + k - 1$. In order to estimate these parameters with acceptable variance/accuracy, one must make sure that $n \gg M$ where n is the number of observations. In our case, n is the total number of pixels in the image.

The joint probability of having a particular set of observations $\mathbf{x}_1, \mathbf{x}_2, \ldots, \mathbf{x}_n$, given a set of parameters $\boldsymbol{\theta} = (\boldsymbol{\theta}_1, .., \boldsymbol{\theta}_k; w_1, .., w_{k-1})$, is known as *the likelihood function* $l(\boldsymbol{\theta})$:

$$l(\boldsymbol{\theta}) = l(\mathbf{x}_1, \mathbf{x}_2, \ldots, \mathbf{x}_n \mid \boldsymbol{\theta}) = \Pr[\cap_{j=1}^{n} \mathbf{x}_j \mid \boldsymbol{\theta}] = \prod_{j=1}^{n} f(\mathbf{x}_j \mid \boldsymbol{\theta})$$

where $f(\mathbf{x}_j \mid \boldsymbol{\theta}) = \sum_{i=1}^{k} w_i f_i(\mathbf{x}_j \mid \boldsymbol{\theta}_i)$. Assuming that the observations in the data set are independent, we wrote the joint probability as a product of individual probabilities. One practical/popular way to estimate the unknown parameters of a mixture model, that is, $\boldsymbol{\theta}$, is to select it in a such way that it maximizes the likelihood function. This is called the maximum likelihood (ML) estimate of θ:

$$\theta_{ML} = \arg_\theta \max l(\theta).$$

Because maxima are unaffected by monotone transformations, we can take the logarithm of the likelihood function and convert the product into a sum:

$$L(\theta) = \log l(\theta) = \log \prod_{j=1}^n f(x_j \mid \theta) = \sum_{j=1}^n \log f(x_j \mid \theta)$$

The resultant function is called the *log-likelihood function* $L(\theta)$ and finding its maximum is usually much simpler than finding that of $l(\theta)$:

$$\theta_{ML} = \arg_\theta \max L(\theta) \tag{6.67}$$

The ML estimate of θ can be found numerically using various optimization algorithms. One particular popular optimization method that is widely used in mixture modeling is the expectation maximization (EM). The EM is an iterative method for optimizing the likelihood function when some information is missing. In our case, missing information is the class membership of the observations, that is, the pixel values. The EM algorithm was formulated by Dempster, Laird, and Rubin in their seminal paper [28] and is now a standard tool in statistics. For a good review of the application of the EM algorithm on mixture densities, we refer the reader to Redner and Walker [29]. A discussion of the convergence properties of the EM algorithm can be found in Gustafsson et al [30]. The EM algorithm for mixture modeling can be summarized as follows:

1. *Initialization:* Start with a proper initial estimate of the mixture parameters θ. Assuming that we know the number of components k, this initialization can be accomplished by using one of the available nonparametric clustering algorithms. For instance, the data can be classified into k classes using the k-means algorithm [31,32] and the initial values of the parameters can be estimated from the clustered data. Instead of using random initial parameter estimates, using this approach improves convergence of the EM algorithm significantly.

2. *Expectation step:* Compute the class conditional pdfs $f_i(x_j \mid \theta_i)$ using the current estimated value of θ and determine or estimate the posterior probability that an observation x_j belongs to class i as

$$\Pr(\theta_i \mid x_j) = \hat{h}_{ij} = \frac{w_i f_i(x_j \mid \theta_i)}{f(x_j)}; \ i = 1,2,\ldots k; \ j = 1,2,\ldots,n \tag{6.68}$$

where the dominator $f(\mathbf{x}_j)$ is given by Equation (6.66). Here, we have used the Bayes' formula, which simply states that

$$\text{posterior} = \frac{\text{prior} \times \text{likelihood}}{\text{evidence}}.$$

We then compute the new or updated w_is, i.e., class weights or prior probabilities, by averaging the posterior probabilities for each class as

$$\hat{w}_i = \frac{1}{n} \sum_{j=1}^{n} \hat{h}_{ij} \qquad (6.69)$$

3. *Maximization step:* Given the estimated weights ($\hat{w}_i$s) from the expectation step, we update the parameter vector $\boldsymbol{\theta}$ by maximizing the likelihood function, that is, by finding the ML estimate of $\boldsymbol{\theta}$. The ML estimate of $\boldsymbol{\theta}$ can be derived for different classes of pdf's using Equation (6.67). For the normal mixtures, the updates on the mean vector $\hat{\boldsymbol{\mu}}_i$ and the covariance matrix $\hat{\boldsymbol{\Sigma}}_i$ are as follows [31]:

$$\hat{\boldsymbol{\mu}}_i = \frac{1}{n} \sum_{j=1}^{n} \frac{\hat{h}_{ij} \mathbf{x}_j}{\hat{w}_i}, \quad \hat{\boldsymbol{\Sigma}}_i = \frac{1}{n} \sum_{j=1}^{n} \frac{\hat{h}_{ij}(\mathbf{x}_j - \hat{\boldsymbol{\mu}}_i)(\mathbf{x}_j - \hat{\boldsymbol{\mu}}_i)^t}{\hat{w}_i} \qquad (6.70)$$

4. Iterate (i.e., repeat the expectation and maximization steps) until the relative updates/changes in the mixture parameter estimates are smaller than a small preset tolerance level or a certain number of iterations is reached. We selected the parameter tolerance and the maximum iteration count as 0.00001 and 200, respectively.

Once a mixture model is fitted to our image's pdf, we can then assign pixels to different classes on the basis of the final estimated posterior probabilities. That is, assign the pixel $\mathbf{x}_j$ to the class that produces the highest $\Pr(\boldsymbol{\theta}_i | \mathbf{x}_j)$.

In our sample case, it was easy to determine the number of modes in the pdf of pixel values. However, sometimes we may not be quite sure about the number of modes in the pdf, as there may be some modes blocking other modes; that is, some overlapping modes may appear as a single mode. Therefore, we may try fitting several mixture models to our data's pdf with a different number of components. Then, we can check the maximum value that the likelihood or log-likelihood function attains. As we increase the number of parameters in the model, typically, the situation improves; that is, we can come up with a better model/fit and, consequently, the maximum of the likelihood function keeps increasing.

This is the well-known parsimony that one encounters in almost every modeling scheme. That is, if we use too few model parameters, the model/

fit will not be satisfactory enough in terms of explaining the composition of our pdf. On the other, if we use too many model parameters, we may produce an overfit, meaning we may be bringing in components that do not really exist. Therefore, we must determine an optimal number of model parameters (or optimal number of mixture components in our case) that will adequately explain our pdf. One popular method for evaluating/determining the quality of fit is the Bayesian information criterion (BIC) proposed by Schwartz [33]:

$$BIC = -2L(\theta) + M \log(n), \qquad (6.71)$$

where $L(\theta)$ is the maximized value of the log-likelihood function, and M and n are the numbers of model parameters and pixels, respectively. This criterion has two components acting in an opposite sense: the first one, $-2L(\theta)$, decreases as M increase, whereas the second term is directly proportional to M. Therefore, by minimization of the BIC, we can catch the balance point at which adding more parameters does not decrease the first term of the BIC much.

These ideas are implemented in the following MATLAB function named mipUnivarGMixFit_Segment. Here, Im_in is the input image to be segmented, which is a grayscale image. Im_out is the output, that is, the labeled/segmented image and K is the number of classes/segments in the image. Before proceeding with the estimation of the mixture parameters, if it is needed, the data could be preprocessed or transformed to make its distribution approximately normal. The input argument transformtype indicates the type of transform to apply to the data. Available options are 1 = no-transform (the default), 2 = log-transform (stabilizes variance), 3 = cube-root (like the log transform, stabilizes variance), and 4 = scaling by standard deviation of the data (normalizes variance).

```
function [Im_out,logL_K,bic_K] =
  mipUnivarGMixFit_Segment(Im_in,K,transformtype)
% Image segmentation via Gaussian/normal mixture modeling

if nargin==1
  K = 2; transformtype = 1;
elseif nargin==2
  transformtype = 1;
end
data = double(Im_in(:)); n = length(data); % data is nx1

switch transformtype
% case 1 data = data; No tranform, default
case 2 % log-tranform
  % avoid log of zero by shifting pixel values by 1
  data = log(1+data);
```

```
case 3 % Cube-root
  data = data.^(1/3);
case 4 % Scaling by SD
  data = data/mystd(data,n);
end

% Efficient initialization for k-means using quantiles
sorted_data = sort(data);
quantile_lims = zeros(1,K);
delta_q = 1/K; quantile_start = delta_q/2;
quantile_lims = quantile_start:delta_q:1;
mues_in = sorted_data(round(n*quantile_lims))';
% An alternative way of finding the initial means
% by using the prctile function could be as follows
% K2 = 2*K; mues_in = prctile(data,(1:2:K2)*100/K2)

% Efficient initialization for EM using k-means
pies_in = zeros(1,K); sum_k = zeros(1,K);
iter = 0; idx = zeros(n,1); idx_old = ones(n,1);
while ~isequal(idx,idx_old) & iter < 25
  idx_old = idx;
[dummy_values,idx] = min(abs(repmat(data,1,K)...
                    -repmat(mues_in,n,1)),[],2);
  for i = 1:K
    idx_k = find(idx==i);
    pies_in(i) = length(idx_k);
    mues_in(i) = sum(data(idx_k))/pies_in(i);
  end
  iter = iter+1;
end

% EM
fprintf('Mixture Model via EM\n')
pies_in = pies_in/n; vars_in = zeros(1,K);
for i = 1:K
  idx_k = find(idx==i);
  vars_in(i) = var(data(idx_k));
end
posterior_probs = zeros(n,K);
pies_up = zeros(1,K);
mues_up = zeros(1,K);
vars_up = zeros(1,K);
iter = 0; deltol = 10;
while iter < 200 & deltol > 1e-5
  for i = 1:K
    posterior_probs(:,i) = ...
      pies_in(i)*normpdfvar(data,mues_in(i),vars_in(i));
  end
  totprob = sum(posterior_probs,2);
  posterior_probs = posterior_probs./repmat(totprob,1,K);
```

```
    postsum = sum(posterior_probs);
    pies_up = postsum/n;
    mues_up = (data'*posterior_probs)./postsum;
    for i = 1:K
        xx = (data-mues_in(i)).^2; % centered data for class_k
        vars_up(i) = xx'*posterior_probs(:,i)/postsum(i);
    end
    % quit if any of the estimated component vars is close 0
    if any(vars_up<eps), break, end
    % check the relative change in weights
    deltol = abs(pies_in(1)-pies_up(1))/pies_in(1);
    % update mixture model param.s
    pies_in = pies_up;
    mues_in = mues_up;
    vars_in = vars_up;
    % finally, update the iteration count
    iter = iter+1;
end
fprintf('Mixture model converged after %d iterations...\
n',iter)
sigs_up = sqrt(vars_up);
fprintf('Weights: '), fprintf('%.4f\t',pies_up); ...
fprintf('\n')
fprintf('Means: '), fprintf('%.4f\t',mues_up); ...
fprintf('\n')
fprintf('SDs: '), fprintf('%.4f\t',sigs_up);
fprintf('\n')

% number of model parameters is K*(1+d+d*(d+1)/2)-1
% with d (data dimensionality) being 1
num_params = 3*K-1;
% log likelihood
logL_K = sum(log(totprob))
bic_K = -2*logL_K + num_params*log(n);

% % Nelder-Mead Simplex Search (uncomment to activate)
% % requires the Matlab's optimization toolbox
% theta0 = [pies_in(1:K-1) mues_in vars_in];
% fprintf('Mixture Model via Nelder-Mead Simplex
% Search\n')
% [thetamin,Lmin] = fminsearch(@myloglikelihood,theta0,
% optimset(…
% 'MaxFunEvals',3000,'TolX',1e-5,'TolF',1e-5),data,K,n);
% -Lmin
% pies = thetamin(1:K-1);
% pies_last = 1-sum(pies);
% pies_all = [pies pies_last];
% fprintf('Weights: ')
% fprintf('%.4f\t',pies_all); fprintf('\n')
% fprintf('Means: ')
```

```
% fprintf('%.4f\t',thetamin(K:2*K-1)); fprintf('\n')
% fprintf('SDs: ')
% fprintf('%.4f\t',sqrt(thetamin(2*K:end)));
% fprintf('\n')

% Generate the labeled/segmented image based on posterior
% prob.s
Im_out = Im_in;
% take the max along the second dim (rows)
[dummy_values,Im_out(:)] = max(posterior_probs,[],2);
% Produce histogram pdf and mixture pdf plots
% figure 1)
bin_centers = 0:255;
% make the hist pdf estimate plot first
myhist(data,n,bin_centers), hold on

line_colors = ['k';'b';'m';'c';'g';'y']; Lc = ...
  length(line_colors);
% colors for plotting different mixture components
fitpdf = zeros(K,256);
for i = 1:K
  fitpdf(i,:) = pies_up(i)*...
    normpdfvar(bin_centers,mues_up(i),vars_up(i));
  % cycle plot colors
  plot(bin_centers,fitpdf(i,:),line_colors(mod(i,Lc)))
end
plot(bin_centers,sum(fitpdf),'r'), hold off
xlabel('Pixel value'), ylabel('Probability')
title('Histogram estimate of pixel values pdf...
  and weighted mixture model components')
if K == 4 % this is the correct/optimal number of ...
  components
  set(gca,'ylim',[0 0.035])
  legend('Histogram','Component 1','Component 2',...
    'Component 3','Component 4','Overall mix. model fit')
end

figure
% Assess quality of mixture model's fit to data's pdf
% using qqplot
model_data = []; n_qq = 400;
for i = 1:K
  ni = round(n_qq*pies_up(i));
  % generate random data from ith component
  xi = randn(ni,1); xi = (xi-mean(xi))/std(xi);
  xi = mues_up(i) + sigs_up(i)*xi;
  % Aggragate the simulated new model data
  model_data = [model_data; xi];
end
```

```
size(model_data) % initial size (should be n_qq which ...
% is 400)
% Remove pixels with values <0 or >255 from the random
% data
model_data = model_data(model_data>=0 & model_data<=255);
size(model_data) % size of the random data after cleanup
qqplot(data,model_data)
xlabel('Quantiles of Actual Pixel Values')
ylabel('Quantiles of Random Data from Mixture Model')
axis equal, axis([0 255 0 255])
title ('QQ Plot of Random Data from Mixture Model…
  versus Actual Pixel Values')


function p = normpdfvar(x,mu,xvar)
p = exp(-(x-mu).^2/(2*xvar))/sqrt(xvar*2*pi);


function y = mystd(x,n)
if n == 1, y = NaN; return, end
y = sqrt(sum((x-mymean(x,n)).^2)/(n-1));


function y = mymean(x,n)
y = sum(x)/n;


function myhist(data,n,bin_centers)
bin_counts = hist(data,bin_centers);
ah = bar(bin_centers,bin_counts/n,1);
set(ah,'facecolor',[1 1 1],'edgecolor',[.5 .5 .5]),...
  axis tight)


function L = myloglikelihood(theta,data,K,n)
pies = theta(1:K-1); pies_last = 1-sum(pies); ...
  pies_all = [pies pies_last];
mues = theta(K:2*K-1);
vars = theta(2*K:end); % end = 3*K-1
y = zeros(n,1);
for i = 1:K
  y = y + pies_all(i)*normpdfvar(data,mues(i),vars(i));
end
L = -sum(log(y));
```

The following piece of MATLAB code first loads our sample image file, then makes several calls with different numbers of components to the UnivarGMixFit_Segment function that we discussed earlier, and finally produces figures to present the results:

```
I = imread('brain.png');
I = rgb2gray(I);
```

```
[Im_out2,logL2,bic2] = mipUnivarGMixFit_Segment(I,2);
[Im_out3,logL3,bic3] = mipUnivarGMixFit_Segment(I,3);
[Im_out4,logL4,bic4] = mipUnivarGMixFit_Segment(I,4);
[Im_out5,logL5,bic5] = mipUnivarGMixFit_Segment(I,5);

figure
subplot(211),plot(2:5,[logL2 logL3 logL4 logL5],'-o')
xlabel('K: Number of mixture components')
title('Log likelihood'), grid on
set(gca,'xtick',2:5,'xlim',[1.75 5.25])
subplot(212),plot(2:5,[bic2 bic3 bic4 bic5],'-o')
xlabel('K: Number of mixture components')
title('Bayesian Information Criterion'), grid on
set(gca,'xtick',2:5,'xlim',[1.75 5.25],'xgrid','on')


close all
figure, imshow(I,[]), colormap(gray(256)), colorbar
figure, imshow(Im_out2,[]), colormap(gray(2)),
colorbar('YTick',1:2)
figure, imshow(Im_out3,[]), colormap(gray(3)),
colorbar('YTick',1:3)
figure, imshow(Im_out4,[]), colormap(gray(4)),
colorbar('YTick',1:4)
figure, imshow(Im_out5,[]), colormap(gray(5)),
colorbar('YTick',1:5)
```

In Figure 6.15, we see the segmentation results for K (number of modes) = 2, 3, 4, and 5. Figure 6.16 shows the maximized value of the log-likelihood function (upper panel) and the BIC (lower panel) as a function of K. The BIC plot indicates that the mixture model for K = 4 is the optimal model, although in this particular case the maximized value of the log-likelihood function $L(\theta)$ peaks at K = 4 as well. However, we cannot rely on $L(\theta)$ as it is typically prone to increase indefinitely with an increasing number of model parameters or K. Figure 6.17 shows how our optimal mixture model—with 4 modes—looks compared to the histogram of pixel values.

Another powerful tool for assessing goodness-of-fit of a mixture model is the quantile–quantile (qq) plot. To verify that the normal mixture model fits the underlying distribution of the data well, we generated random data from our estimated mixture model with four components and compared their quantiles against the quantiles of the actual pixel data, and constructed the qq plot shown in Figure 6.18. Indeed, the qq plot shows that the normal mixture model with K = 4 fits the distribution of the actual data well.

Before we close this chapter, we should note that EM is not the only option/method to estimate the parameters of a mixture model. The

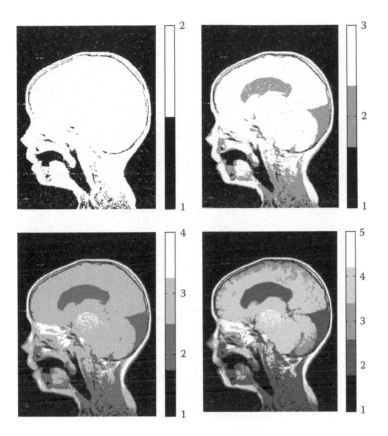

FIGURE 6.15
Mixture modeling based segmentation results. Top left, top right, bottom left, and bottom right, respectively, correspond to K = 2, 3, 4, and 5.

estimation of mixture model parameters—based on the maximization of the log-likelihood function—is a typical parameter estimation/optimization problem; as such, other optimization methods could also be utilized. For instance, we can use the simplex method of Nelder and Mead, which is a direct search algorithm that does not involve any gradient calculation. To try this out, you can uncomment the piece of code marked in red in function `mipUnivarGMixFit_Segment`. You will observe that mixture model parameter estimates that are very close to the ones obtained via the EM algorithm are obtained. However, you will also note that the maximized values of the likelihood function obtained via the EM are slightly higher, indicating that the EM is indeed doing a good parameter estimation job.

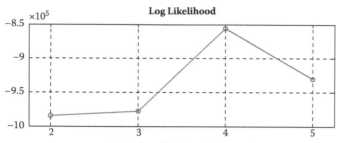

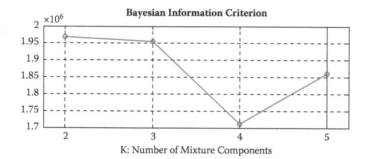

FIGURE 6.16
The maximized value of the log-likelihood function (upper panel) and the BIC (lower panel) for different values of K, the number of mixture components.

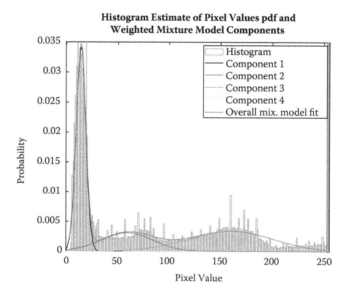

FIGURE 6.17
Histogram estimate of the pdf of pixel values and the estimated weighted normal mixture components.

QQ Plot of Random Data from Mixture Model Versus Actual Pixel Values

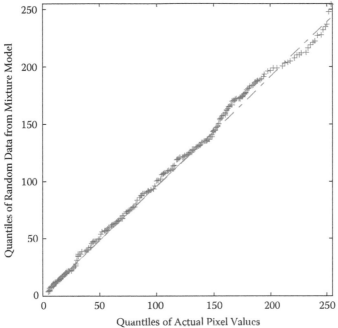

FIGURE 6.18

Analysis of the goodness-of-fit between the mixture model with four modes and the actual data. The qq plot shows quantiles of the actual data against the random data generated from the mixture model. The dashed line corresponds to the case of perfect agreement between the compared samples. If the "+" marks indicating the location of the matching quantiles roughly lie on the straight line, then the distributions of the samples have the same shape except for a possible shift and rescaling.

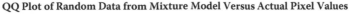

Problems

1. Show that B_{max} is 0.75 for uniform distributions.

2. For a normal distribution, show that the equation of $B(t)$ is given by Equation (6.21) using the MATLAB Symbolic Toolbox.

3. Write MATLAB code that generates images with intensities from uniform, normal, and Poisson distributions.

4. Use the code written in Problem 3 to find the B_{max} for uniform and normal distributions. Run the code a number of times to find an estimate of B_{max} and its standard deviation. Investigate the effect of the parameters of the distribution on B_{max}.

5. Repeat Problem 4 for the Poisson distribution. Investigate the impact of lambda on B_{max}.

6. Derive Equation (6.30), assuming that the mixture distribution is given by Equation (6.27).

7. Read the brain image and subsample it with a ratio n:1 (e.g., $n = 2$), and segment the subsampled image using K-means and fuzzy C-means clustering algorithms. Compute thresholds to segment the original image from the segmented image of the subsampled image.

8. Segment the brain image with different m (fuzzification) values and observe the differences.

9. Compare the segmentation results obtained via the mixture modeling approach for $k = 4$ with that of the MRF approach given in Figure 7.11 and comment on the results. Would you agree that, in contrast to the MRF methods, which also takes the neighborhood of pixel values into account, in mixture modeling, as in other thresholding—based approaches, we are losing valuable neighborhood/spatial information and this degrades the segmentation performance.

10. Devise/write a piece of MATLAB code that will perform mixture model parameter estimation using the gradient-based MATLAB optimization routines `fmincon` or `fminunc`, or both.

11. Generalize the 1-D method of Kapur, Sahoo and Wong by using the entropy given by Equation (6.42) and then write a MATLAB code to compute the threshold value for an image.

12. Extend the 1-D method of Kapur, Sahoo and Wong to include thresholding of color images. Then write a MATLAB code for your extension method.

13. Show that the entropies defined by each of the two equations, Equations (6.41) and (6.42), are a one-parameter generalization of the Shanon's entropy. That is,

14. In the 2-D entropy based method, the entropy given by Equation (6.42) was used. Show that if one uses Equation (6.41) instead of (6.42), then the value of the threshold will not change.

15. Extend the 2-D entropic method of Sahoo and Arora in Section 6.5.2 to color images and then write a MATLAB code for its implementation.

References

1. Y. Zhang, M. Brady, and S. Smith, Segmentation of brain MR images through a hidden Markov random field model and the expectation-maximization algorithm. *IEEE Trans Med Imaging* 20: 45–57, 2001.

2. K. V. Mardia and T. J. Hainsworth, A spatial thresholding method for image segmentation. *IEEE PAMI* 10: 919–927, 1988.
3. N. R. Pal and S. K. Pal, A review on image segmentation techniques, *Pattern Recogn* 26: 1277–94, 1993.
4. N. Otsu, A threshold selection method from gray-level histogram. *IEEE Trans Syst Man Cybernetics* 8: 62–66, 1979.
5. T. Kurita, N. Otsu, and N. Abdelmalek, Maximum likelihood thresholding based on population mixture models. *Pattern Recogn* 25: 1231–1240, 1992.
6. O. Demirkaya and M. Asyali, Determination of image bimodality thresholds for different intensity distributions. *Signal Process: Image Commun* 19: 507–516, 2004.
7. S. S. Reddi, S. F. Rudin, and H. R. Keshavan, An optimal multiple threshold scheme for image segmentation. *IEEE Trans Syst. Man Cybernetics* SMC-14: 661–665, 1984.
8. J. Kittler and J. Illingworth, Minimum error thresholding. *Pattern Recognition* 19: 41–47, 1986.
9. R. M. Haralick and L. G. Shapiro, *Computer and Robot Vision* 1. Reading, MA: Addison-Wesley, 1992.
10. S. Cho, R. Haralick, and S. Yi, Improvement of kittler and illingworth's minimum error thresholding. *Pattern Recogn* 22: 609–617, 1989.
11. T. Pun, A new method for gray-level picture thresholding using the entropy of the histogram. *Signal Process* 2: 223–237, 1980.
12. J. N. Kapur, P. K. Sahoo, and A. K. C. Wong, A new method for gray-level picture thresholding using the entropy of the histogram. *Computer Vision, Graphics, Image Process* 29: 273–285, 1985.
13. P. K. Sahoo, S. Sultani, A. K. C. Wong, and Y. C. Chen, A survey of thresholding techniques. *Computer Vision, Graphics Image Process* 41: 233–260, 1988.
14. A. S. Abutaleb, Automatic thresholding of gray-level pictures using two-dimensional entropies. *Computer Vision, Graphics Image Process* 47: 22–32, 1989.
15. A. D. Brink, Thresholding of digital images using two-dimensional entropies. *Pattern Recogn* 47: 803–808, 1992.
16. P. K. Sahoo, D. W. Slaaf, and T. A. Albert, Threshold selection using a minimal histogram entropy difference. *Optical Eng* 36: 1977–1981, 1997.
17. P. K. Sahoo and G. Arora, A thresholding method based on two-dimensional Renyi's entropy. *Pattern Recogn* 37: 1149–1161, 2004.
18. P. K. Sahoo and G. Arora, Image thresholding using two-dimensional Tsalllis-Havrda-Charvat entropy. *Pattern Recogn. Lett* 26: 520–528, 2006.
19. J. B. MacQueen, Some methods for classification and analysis of multivariate observations, presented at Proceedings of 5-th Berkeley Symposium on Mathematical Statistics and Probability, Berkeley, University of California, 1967.
20. J. C. Dunn, A fuzzy relative of the ISODATA process and its use in detecting compact well-separated clusters. *J. Cybernetics* 3: 32–57, 1973.
21. J. C. Bezdek, J. M. Keller, R. Krishnapuram, and N. R. Pal, *Fuzzy Models and Algorithms for Pattern Recognition and Image Processing*. New York: Springer, 1999.
22. N. R. Pal and J. C. Bezdek, On cluster validity for the fuzzy c-Means model. *IEEE Trans. on Fuzzy Syst*,3: 370–379, 1995.
23. G. J. McLachlan, R. W. Bean, and D. Peel, A mixture model-based approach to the clustering of microarray expression data. *Bioinformatics* 18: 413–422, 2002.

24. M. J. Symons, Clustering criteria and multivariate normal mixtures. *Biometrics* 37: 35–43, 1981.
25. J. H. Wolfe, Pattern clustering by multivariate mixture analysis. Multivariate Behavioral Research. *Multivariate Behav. Res* 5: 329–350, 1970.
26. M. M. Shoukri and G. J. McLachlan, Parametric estimation in a genetic mixture model with application to nuclear family data. *Biometrics* 50: 128–39, 1994.
27. I. C. McManus, Bimodality of blood pressure levels. *Stat Med* 2: 253–8, 1983.
28. A. Dempster, N. Laird, and D. Rubin, Maximum likelihood from incomplete data via the EM algorithm. *J. R. Stat. Soc* B39: 1–38, 1977.
29. R. Redner and H. Walker, Mixture densities, maximum likelihood and the EM algorithm. *SIAM Review*, Vol. 26, 195–202, 1984.
30. A. Gustafsson, B. Bake, L. Jacobsson, A. Johansson, M. Ljungberg, and M. Moonen, Evaluation of attenuation corrections using Monte Carlo simulated lung SPECT. *Phys Med Bio* 43: 2325–36, 1998.
31. W. L. Martinez and A. R. Martinez, *Computational Statistics Handbook with MATLAB*. Boca Raton, FL: CRC Press, 2001.
32. R. O. Duda, P. E. Hart, and D. G. Stork, *Pattern Classification*, 2nd ed. New York: John Wiley & Sons, 2001.
33. G. Schwartz, Estimating the dimension of a model. *Ann. Stat*, 461–464, 1978.

7

Image Segmentation by Markov Random Field Modeling

CONTENTS

7.1 From Statistical Mechanics to Image Segmentation

Markov random field (MRF) modeling of images for the purpose of segmentation or restoration was inspired by the computational techniques developed in statistical mechanics. Statistical mechanics is a discipline in physics studying the properties of atoms in condensed matter. We know that there are a large number of atoms ($\sim 10^{23}$ atoms per cubic centimeter) in a small amount of matter. Scientists in statistical mechanics have been long interested in the aggregate properties of matter, such as ensemble averages, equilibrium states, progression in time, and low-temperature behavior.

Both the intrinsic angular momentum of an electron and its rotation around the nucleus result in a magnetic dipole moment creating a magnetic field around an atom. This magnetic moment is also known as *spin*. In fact, researchers who have been working on a quantum computer exploit this unique property of electrons. The introductory articles discussing the concept and the principles of quantum computers in layman's terms can be found in references [1,2].

Each atom in a ferromagnetic material, for instance, can be viewed as a small magnet pointing in a certain direction. Under normal circumstances, the magnetic moments of these atoms may be pointing in any direction. In the presence of an external magnetic field, however, these little magnets align themselves in the same direction, resulting in a total magnetic field. The materials that exhibit spontaneous magnetization in the presence of an external magnetic field are called *ferromagnetic*. Below a certain critical temperature, which is called *Curie temperature*, the ferromagnetic materials can be antiferromagnetic, in which the magnetic moments point in directions such that the net magnetization is zero.

To be able to calculate such properties of atoms as mentioned earlier, a simpler model for ferromagnetic metals was needed. In 1924, Ernst Ising proposed a simple interaction model between atoms in a ferromagnetic metal. In this model, the interactions among the spins are constrained to the nearest neighbors of the atom, that is, to those in the directions east, west, south, and north. Figure 7.1 shows the Ising model, in which the spins are assumed to be arranged in a 2-D rectangular lattice, all pointing up. Although the Ising model may appear simple, it was by means of this simple model that the existence of the Curie temperature was discovered. Since it was published, the Ising model has become one of the most

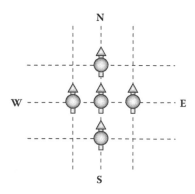

FIGURE 7.1
Interaction model proposed by Ising.

widely used models to study the properties of ferromagnetic materials by succeeding physicists/scientists.

In the Ising model shown in Figure 7.1, the energy of a particular state of the lattice is given by

$$E = -J \sum_{i,j} S_i S_j - B \sum_k S_k \tag{7.1}$$

where S_i is the value of the spin at the ith lattice site. $S_i = +1$, if the spin is pointing up, and $S_i = -1$, if the spin is pointing down. Note that the summation is carried out over the entire lattice. B is the constant energy due to the external magnetic field. J is a constant as well. However, when $J > 0$, the energy is minimized if adjacent spins point in the same direction; that is, the spin pairs have the same sign. This leads to *ferromagnetism*. When $J < 0$, the energy is minimized if the adjacent spins point in opposite directions; that is, the neighboring spins have the opposite spin values. This leads to *antiferromagnetism*.

Given the Ising model, one can compute the probability of a state or configuration using Boltzman's distribution function:

$$P(S) = \frac{e^{-E(S)/k_B T}}{\sum_A e^{-E(A)/k_B T}} \tag{7.2}$$

where $E(S)$ is the energy of the lattice in state S that can be computed using Equation (7.1). A represents all possible states or the state space of the system. T is the absolute temperature of the system measured in degrees Kelvin, and k_B is the *Boltzman's constant*, which is equal to 1.380 6505(24) × 10⁻²³ J/K.

The ensemble average μ_E, for instance, of such a system in state S_i can be calculated by subtracting the number of spins pointing up from those pointing down and weighing the difference by the probability of the state. If we denote this difference by ND_i for the ith state and the probability by $P(S_i)$, then the ensemble average can be calculated by adding the products over the state space A, that is,

$$\mu_E = \sum_A ND_i P(S_i) \tag{7.3}$$

What is the possible number of states in the state space A? For a system of N spins, for instance, there are two choices (up or down) for each site, so by the multiplication principle in probability, there are 2 × 2 × 2 × 2 × 2 × 2 × 2 × 2 ... = 2^N possible states or configurations in the state space A over which we need to perform the sum in the right-hand side of Equation (7.3). This indeed is an overwhelming task even with today's fast CPUs. Therefore, the brute force approach to calculating the ensemble average of an N-spin system considering all possible states is almost impossible within a reasonable computational time.

Metropolis et al. in 1953 introduced an algorithm to simulate such systems [3]. In their algorithm, one of the atoms in the current configuration is given a small displacement, and the change in the energy of the system ΔE is computed. If $\Delta E < 0$, the displacement, in other words, the new configuration, is accepted. If $\Delta E > 0$, the new configuration is accepted with a probability defined by the Boltzman probability $P(\Delta E) = e^{-\Delta E/kT}$. The probabilistic decision in the latter case is made by drawing a uniform random number from the interval (0, 1). Then, the new configuration is accepted, if $P(\Delta E)$ is larger than this number; otherwise the current configuration is retained. This is the essence of the well-known Metropolis algorithm, which can be used to simulate different configurations from a state space A. This algorithm is analogous to drawing samples randomly from a population, which represents, in this context, our space of all configurations, or the state space A. Instead of summing over all the configurations, which we know is not realistically feasible, one could effectively draw samples from the configuration space, of course in sufficiently large numbers, and calculate the ensemble average using only the drawn samples, which represent the entire state space.

The Metropolis algorithm was later adapted by Kirkpatric [4] to solve the minimization of NP-complete (nondeterministic polynomial)-type problems. This new class of algorithms is referred to as simulated annealing (SA) methods. We will discuss SA-based algorithms as well as the other nondeterministic types further, when we discuss the simulated annealing algorithms that have been used in the context of MRF-based image segmentation to find the maximum a priori (MAP) estimate.

7.2   Markov Random Field Modeling

We know that the pixel value in an image reflects the certain characteristics of the object in the image. Digital images consisting of pixels and defined on a bounded 2-D lattice have two important attributes. First, pixel intensities of a nearly homogenous object/region will follow a certain statistical distribution. We will call this the conditional (on the region number) intensity distribution of the pixel intensities. The pixel intensities may be scalar or a vector quantity depending on the image type (see Chapter 2). Second, the pixels close together or lying in a neighborhood will tend to have similar intensity values. The latter constraint is also known as contextual information. Intensity-based segmentation methods that we discussed in Chapter 6 disregard the latter attribute of images. In this section, we will discuss how contextual information can be modeled by means of MRF modeling. This model representing the local characteristics of the underlying image, when combined with the conditional distribution of the pixel intensities under a Bayesian

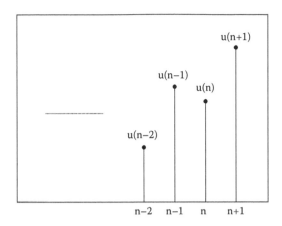

FIGURE 7.2
A discrete time sequence.

framework, will enable us to estimate the true intensities of the image much more accurately than those based on only the information derived from the image intensities.

Segmentation methods based on MRF modeling have been extensively studied and used in medical as well as nonmedical imaging applications [5–8]. They provide a convenient way to combine both the observed intensity and the contextual information under a Bayesian framework. In the following sections, we will discuss MRF modeling in detail and its application to image segmentation through a Bayesian framework.

7.2.1 Markov Random Sequence

A random sequence u is called pth-order Markov if the conditional probability of u given its entire past is equal to the conditional probability of $u(n)$ given only $u(n-1), ..., u(n-p)$ (or "present") [9], that is,

$$P(u(n)\,|\,u(n-1), u(n-2), ...) = P(u(n)\,|\,u(n-1), ..., u(n-p)) \qquad (7.4)$$

In other words, this means that if we know the recent, we can estimate the entire past. This is also known as Markovian property of sequences. For a second-order Markov sequence (see Figure 7.2), for instance, this relation can be expressed as

$$P(u(n)\,|\,u(n-1), u(n-2), ...) = P(u(n)\,|\,u(n-1), u(n-2)) \qquad (7.5)$$

7.2.2 Random Fields

If each element of a 2-D sequence is a random variable, the 2-D sequence is called a *discrete random field* [9]. In the light of this definition, we can view every image as a random field in which each pixel is regarded as a random variable. This concept of a random field can be extended to 3-D, and in the case of a 3-D image, we will regard it as a 3-D random field.

Before we start defining the MRF model, let us summarize the notation that we will be using in the remainder of the chapter. In our notation, we will primarily follow Besag's treatment [10]. Let I denote a 2-D rectangular lattice (i.e., our image) of $M_x \times M_y$ pixels. Note that a 3-D lattice (or cubic lattice) will have $M_x \times M_y \times M_z$ voxels whose center locations will lie at the lattice points. We assume that pixel or voxel i will take on values (i.e., labels) x_i from the set $L = \{1, \cdots K\}$, where K denotes the total number of regions available in the image because labels represent regions in image I. Let us assume that x^* is the true labeling of the pixels or voxels in the image. That is, our true image x^* is a realization of the random field X. The sample space Ω denotes the space of all possible realizations of our random field X. That is, $\Omega = \{1, \ldots, K\}^{M_x M_y}$ for 2-D images, and $\Omega = \{1, \ldots, K\}^{M_x \times M_y \times M_z}$ for 3-D images. Recall the multiplication principle in probability, mentioned at the beginning of the chapter, used to compute the size of the state space. Let us suppose we have three regions (i.e., $K = 3$). In this case, each pixel has three possible labels. If we suppose that we are working on a series of 512 × 512 MR images with three regions, the size of the sample space in this case would be $3^{512 \times 512} = 9.8936 \times 10^{246}$. This number illustrates clearly the magnitude of the problem that we have to deal with.

7.2.3 Neighborhood Systems

To describe or define the locally dependent MRF model, we first need to define a neighborhood system over which the MRF will be defined. Again, let I denote a $M_x \times M_y$ lattice indexing the pixels in a given target region. Also let s be the lattice point or pixel, also called site, and N_s denote the neighborhood of s. In this case, the neighborhood system N_s must satisfy the following two conditions:

1. $s \notin N_s$
2. $r \in N_s$ iff $r \in N_r$

The first condition states that a site should not be a neighbor of itself. The second condition, however, implies the symmetry requirement, which states that if r is a neighbor of s, then s is a neighbor of r. Figure 7.3 (left) shows the neighborhood systems for the center pixel s that may be defined in a 2-D image. You may recall that we have also discussed these neighborhood systems in Chapter 2, in which we have suggested a standard way to vectorize any image processing procedure that manipulates the intensity values in a neighborhood. In Figure 7.3, the neighborhood

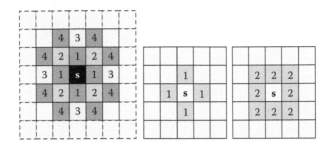

FIGURE 7.3
Neighborhood definitions (left). The middle and right show the first- and second-order neighborhood systems, respectively, whose pixels are denoted by the darker gray color.

systems are shown with different numbers. The pixels labeled by the number 1 denote the first-order neighborhood N_s^1; the pixels labeled 2 together with the pixels of the N_s^1 form the second-order neighborhood N_s^2. Note that $N^i \subset N^j$, for $i < j$, for example, in $N^1 \subset N^2$. These two neighborhood systems are also known as 4-pixel or 8-pixel neighborhood systems, respectively. As seen in the figure, this neighborhood system around the center pixel could further be extended as 3rd, 4th, ..., nth order. Note also that the neighborhood of the edge pixels will have smaller neighborhood because the lattice (image) is finite or bounded. In practice, we address this issue by symmetrical padding, which will be seen later when we discuss the implementations. Figure 7.3 shows the two neighborhood systems (middle and right) that suffice to represent contextual information in almost all real-world image processing problems.

In Figure 7.4, we see the 3-, 6-, 18-, and 26-neighborhood systems, defined over a 3-D lattice. Again, these are the systems that are widely used in 3-D image processing problems and suffice to model the contextual information in 3-D.

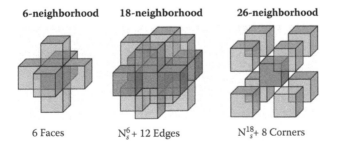

FIGURE 7.4
Three neighborhood systems for 3-D volume images.

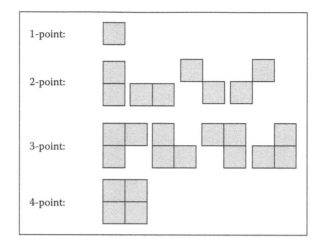

FIGURE 7.5
Clique patterns associated with the 2-D neighborhood systems shown in Figure 7.3.

7.2.4 Cliques

We now need to explain the definition of a clique, which will also be needed in defining the distribution of locally dependent MRFs. A clique is a subset of points $c \in C$, which are all neighbors of each other; $\forall \ sr \in c, r \in N_s$.

A single site s can be a clique, whereas more than one site whose pairs of sites are neighbors of each other is also a clique. Figure 7.5 shows the cliques associated with the neighborhood systems defined for 2-D images in Figure 7.3 (left). Note that one has to move, without rotation, these clique patterns around over the neighborhood system to find all cliques of the same form. For all practical purposes, the 1- or 2-pixel clique patterns are generally sufficient to define the distribution of the MRF. In this section, we will use only two-point clique patterns.

7.2.5 Gibbs Distribution

A Gibbs distribution with respect to N_s is a probability measure given by

$$P(X = x) = \frac{1}{Z} \exp\left\{-\beta U(x)\right\} \tag{7.6}$$

where the β is a positive constant that controls the size of clustering or interaction between the sites; Z is a normalizing constant, also known as the *partitioning function* and is given by

$$Z = \sum_{x \in \Omega} \exp\left\{U(x)\right\} \tag{7.7}$$

where the sum runs over all possible configurations. We know it is infeasible to calculate Z in practice. Hence, Z is said to be computationally intractable. The energy function $U(x)$, which we will also be referring to as Gibbs energy, has the following form

$$U(x) = \sum_{c \in C} V_c(x_c) \tag{7.8}$$

where C denotes the set of cliques for N_s. Note that the sum runs over all clique configurations. V_c is the potential function associated with a clique. It is a function that maps a clique configuration to a real number, that is, $V_c: I \to \mathbb{R}$. The potential function is applicable to all the neighborhoods over the image space. A widely used two-point clique potential can be given by

$$V_c(x) = \begin{cases} -1 & x_s = x_r, s, r \in C \\ 1 & x_s \neq x_r, s, r \in C \end{cases} \tag{7.9}$$

In this formulation, the potential function will be equal to −1 the pair have the same intensities and +1 otherwise. If you recall, this is equivalent to the Ising model that we discussed at the beginning of the chapter.

7.2.6 Markov Random Field

In the preceding sections, we discussed all the ingredients that we need to define the MRF. We are now ready to define the MRF model.

A random field X of I labeling the sites of I with respect to the N_s is an MRF if

- $P(X = x) > 0$ for all $x \in \Omega$
- $P(X = x_i \mid X = x_k, k \neq i) = P(X = x_i \mid X = x_k, k \in N_i$

The first property states that the labeling process assigns a positive probability to all the images in the configuration space. The second property, however, is the same Markovian property as mentioned earlier in the discussion of Markov sequences. To express the latter condition in words, the probability of labeling a pixel given all the labels in the entire image is equal to the probability of the label given the labels of its neighbors only. In other words, it is a conditional distribution that depends on the labels of the pixels in the near neighborhood. It is for this reason that MRF models are also called *locally dependent MRF models*.

The Hammersley–Clifford theorem [11] asserts that a random field is a MRF if and only if the corresponding probability distribution $P(X)$ is a Gibbs distribution. This theorem provides a means of defining conditional (or locally dependent) probability of MRFs in terms of clique potentials. We will not discuss the proof of this theorem here, but interested readers can refer to the references [7,12,13] in which the equivalence of the MRF and Gibbs distribution has been proved.

7.3 Combining the Gibbs Distribution and Conditional under a Bayesian Framework

After modeling the second source of information using MRF models, we would like to combine the two sources of information, namely, intensity distribution and contextual information, together to come up with a more powerful decision rule regarding the true label of a pixel or voxel.

We will do this by means of the Bayesian theorem, which states that one can combine prior belief together with likelihood to obtain the posterior belief about an event, that is,

$$\text{Posterior} = \frac{\text{Likelihood} \times \text{Prior}}{\text{Evidence}} \tag{7.10}$$

Let us assume that the observed image y is a realization of a random field Y, x^* is the true unknown label of the observed pixels, and $\hat{x}$ indicates the estimate of x^*. In image segmentation, the main objective is to find $\hat{x}$ given the observed image y.

Now, let us assume that $P(X)$ is our prior knowledge, and $P(Y \mid X)$ is our likelihood. In other words, $P(Y \mid X)$ is the probability of realizing the observed image given the distribution of regions in the image. Then, by Bayes' theorem,

$$P(X \mid Y) = \frac{P(Y \mid X)P(X)}{P(Y)} \tag{7.11}$$

where $P(X \mid Y)$ is our posterior. Because the evidence $P(Y)$ is a factor to ensure that total probability is one, we will disregard it in our calculations. Thus, we rewrite Equation (7.11) as

$$P(X \mid Y) \propto P(Y \mid X)P(X) \tag{7.12}$$

Our prior knowledge $P(X)$ will be described by the MRF model given by Equation (7.6). The conditional density $P(Y \mid X)$ is the intensity distribution of individual regions in the image. The most widely used conditional density that models the observed image intensity distribution is the Gaussian distribution, whose function, given the class x_s, is given by

$$p(Y = y \mid X = x_s) = \frac{1}{\sqrt{2\pi\sigma_s^2}} \exp\left(-\frac{(y - \mu_s)}{\sigma_s^2}\right) \tag{7.13}$$

where μ_s and σ_s are the parameters of the distribution of the class x_s.

Then $\hat{x}$ can be obtained by computing the maximum a posteriori (MAP) estimate, that is, the mode of the posterior given by Equation (7.12). That is,

$$\hat{x} = \arg \max_x (P(X \mid Y)) \qquad (7.14)$$

Equivalently, we can maximize the natural logarithm of the posterior:

$$\hat{x} = \arg \max_x \{ \log p(y \mid x) + \log p(x) \} \qquad (7.15)$$

If we substitute Equations (7.6) and Equation (7.13) into Equation (7.15), we obtain

$$\hat{x} = \arg \max_\lambda \left\{ -\frac{y - \mu_s}{\sigma_s} - \frac{1}{2}\log(2\pi\sigma_s^2) - \beta U(x) \right\} \qquad (7.16)$$

The first two terms inside the brackets are known as the natural log of the likelihood, and they are altogether called *log-likelihood*. We can further simplify this optimization problem by taking the negative and minimizing the resultant:

$$\hat{x} = \arg \min_{x_s \in L} \left\{ \frac{y - \mu_s}{\sigma_s} + \frac{1}{2}\log(2\pi\sigma_s^2) + \beta U(x_s) \right\} \qquad (7.17)$$

Note that the MAP estimate can easily be derived for some other conditional density distributions (see Problems).

This optimization is computationally an enormous task, as we have already discussed in Section 7.1, for the number of possible configurations for pixel labels may be too many. A number of approaches has been proposed to solve this difficult optimization problem. The solutions can, in general, be viewed under two categories: deterministic or stochastic. In the following sections, we will discuss Besag's deterministic approach known as the *iterated conditional modes (ICM algorithm)* and the two stochastic approaches; namely, Metropolis algorithm and Gibbs sampling.

7.4 Iterated Conditional Modes: A Deterministic Approach

The iterated conditional modes (ICM) algorithm, which is an approximate solution to the MAP estimate, was proposed by Besag [10]. The ICM solves the minimization problem by sequentially updating (i.e., raster scanning the image) labels by minimizing the following equation at each pixel s:

$$\hat{x} = \arg \min_{x_s \in L} \left\{ \frac{y - \mu_s}{\sigma_s} + \frac{1}{2}\log(2\pi\sigma_s^2) + \beta U(x_s) \right\} \qquad (7.18)$$

$U(x_s)$ here is simply the number of pixels in the neighborhood that have the color x_s [10]. In our MATLAB implementations, we will refer to the expression inside the brackets as total energy, which is the sum of the negative log-likelihood and the Gibbs energy.

We can look at the pairwise interactions by redefining the conditional distribution of the MRF as suggested by Besag [10]:

$$P(X = x_s) \infty \exp\left(\sum_{s,r \in C} \beta_{sr} \delta(x_s, x_r) \right) \qquad (7.19)$$

where $\delta(x_s, x_r) = \begin{cases} 1 & x_s = x_r \\ 0 & x_s \neq x_r \end{cases}$

In the aforementioned formulation, the exponential term is simply the weighted sum of the number of pairs carrying the same label as the pixel s. This formulation allows us to have different interaction parameters between the pairs of pixels in the neighborhood. For example, the β_{rs} for the diagonal pixel pairs can be factored by $\sqrt{2}$, whereas those of the horizontal and vertical pixel pairs are factored by 1 because of the Euclidian distance between the centers of the pairs of pixels.

The performance of the ICM algorithm depends heavily on the initial labeling. If a good initial labeling is possible, the ICM algorithm can quickly converge to a desired solution. If a reasonably good initial labeling is not possible, the stochastic algorithms, which will be discussed in the following sections, may be a better choice. Of course, if they can be executed in a reasonable time.

Let us demonstrate how we can implement the ICM algorithm with MATLAB. We will calculate the Gibbs energy $U(x)$ using the potential function given in Equation (7.8) as follows:

```
function energy = GibbsEnergy(img,i,j,label,beta);
% img is the labeled image
energy = 0;
% North, south, east and west neighbors
if (label == img(i-1,j)) energy = energy-beta;
else energy = energy+beta;end
if (label == img(i,j+1)) energy = energy-beta;
else energy = energy+beta;end
if (label == img(i+1,j)) energy = energy-beta;
else energy = energy+beta;end
if (label == img(i,j-1)) energy = energy-beta;
else energy = energy+beta;end
% diagonal pixels
if (label == img(i-1,j-1)) energy = energy-beta;
else energy = energy+beta;end
if (label == img(i-1,j+1)) energy = energy-beta;
else energy = energy+beta;end
if (label == img(i+1,j+1)) energy = energy-beta;
else energy = energy+beta;end
if (label == img(i+1,j-1)) energy = energy-beta;
else energy = energy+beta;end
```

Note that in the previous implementation, the 8-neighborhood system is used. Note also that this function is called at every pixel defined at pixels locations (i, j). One can use the 4-neighborhood system by simply commenting out the lines for the diagonal pixels. The previous function can easily be changed to calculate the energy of a pairwise MRF distribution (see Problem 6).

The function code in the following calculates the log-likelihood function given in Equation (7.13).

```
function LoL = LogLikelihood(img,mu,vars,i,j,label)
LoL = log((2.0*pi*vars(label)^0.5)) + ...
      (img(i,j)-mu(label))^2/(2.0*vars(label));
```

We will call the sum of log-likelihood and the Gibbs energy as the total energy, which is computed by the following function:

```
function energyTotal =
mipTotalEnergy(gimg,simg,mu,vars,i,j,label,beta)
energyTotal = LogLikelihood(gimg,mu,vars,i,j,label) + ...
              GibbsEnergy(simg,i,j,label,beta);
```

The input parameters given by gimg and simg denote the gray-level and initially labeled images, respectively. Now we can write the ICM function code that can segment 2-D images. The following function mipicm2d2r implements the ICM algorithm for images with two regions only.

```
function simg = mipicm2d2r(gimg,simg,beta,numOfIteration);
% Replicate the image edges
gimg = padarray(gimg,[1 1],'replicate','both');
simg = padarray(simg,[1 1],'replicate','both');
%initialize the variables
[row,col] = size(gimg); k = 1;
while k <= numOfIteration
  [mus,sigs] = mipregionstats(gimg,simg,2);
  vars = sigs.^2 + 0.01;
  for ii = 2:row-1
    for jj = 2:col-1
      s = simg(ii,jj);
      r = 3 - s;
      e1 = mipTotalEnergy(gimg,simg,mus,vars,ii,jj,s,beta);
      e2 = mipTotalEnergy(gimg,simg,mus,vars,ii,jj,r,beta);
      if ( e2 < e1)
         simg(ii,jj)= r;
      end
```

```
      end
    end
    k = k + 1;
  end;
  simg = simg(2:end-1,2:end-1);
```

We can extend the ICM algorithm to multiregion images. This requires calculating the total energy for every possible label and choosing the one for which Equation (7.18) is minimum. The preceding function code implements the ICM algorithm for multiregion images.

```
function simg = mipicm2dmr(gimg,simg,nClass,beta,...
  numOfIteration);
% Replicate the images edges
gimg = padarray(gimg,[1 1],'replicate','both');
simg = padarray(simg,[1 1],'replicate','both');
%initialize the variables
[row,col] = size(gimg);
k = 1;
while k <= numOfIteration
  [mus,sigs] = mipregionstats(gimg,simg,nClass);
  sigs = sigs + 0.01;
  vars = sigs.^2;
  for ii = 2:row-1
    for jj = 2:col-1
      for L = 1:nClass
        TEng(k) = mipTotalEnergyInteraction...
        (gimg,simg,mus,vars,ii,jj,L,beta);
      end
      [mn,label] = min(TEng);
      simg(ii,jj) = label;
    end
  end
  k = k + 1;
end;
simg = simg(2:end-1,2:end-1);
```

Let us experiment with the ICM algorithms on simulated images of hexagons of different intensity distributions. The following MATLAB code simulates a noisy hexagon image and does the initial labeling by simple thresholding. The function `mipgray2multilevel(img,[t1,...,tn])` converts the gray-level image into a multilevel image where the pixels with the intensity ranges $0 \le y < t_1, t_1 \le y < t_2, \cdots, t_{n-1} \le y < t_n$ are labeled as $x_s = 1, 2, \cdots, n-1$, respectively.

```
ImSize = 64;
hex1 = miphexagon(10,15,ImSize) +...
   mipimgauss([ImSize,ImSize],0,15);
hex2 = miphexagon(10,20,ImSize) + ...
   mipimgauss([ImSize,ImSize],0,15);
nimg = [hex1 hex2];
isimg = mipgray2multilevel(nimg,[12 19]);
```

As seen in the previous code, after the simulation of the noisy hexagon image, we perform initial labeling using the thresholds 12 and 19. The ICM code was iterated 15 times with a β value of 1.5.

The original hexagon image and its histogram are shown in Figure 7.6, whereas segmented hexagons are shown in Figure 7.7. As seen in the histogram, the overlap between the intensity distributions is significant.

The right hexagon appears to be segmented better around the edges than the left one, because of its better contrast with respect to its surrounding

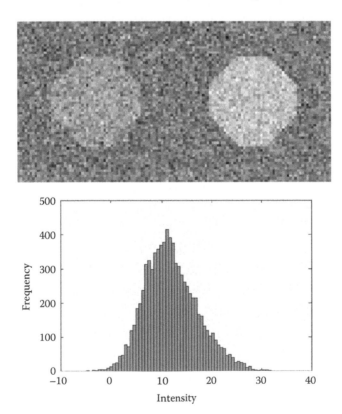

FIGURE 7.6
A simulated hexagon image with three regions and its histogram.

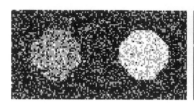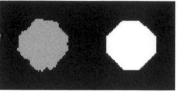

FIGURE 7.7
Segmented hexagons. Left: Initial labeling. Right: Final segmentation with the ICM algorithm.

background. Note that a histogram-based method would not give us a result as good as the ICM algorithm provided.

The impact of initial segmentation can be explored by using different threshold values during initial segmentation, which is performed using mipgray2multilevel function. We will leave it up to the reader to experiment with the impact of the initial segmentation.

As is apparent from the MATLAB code, the ICM visits each pixel (i.e., raster scan) in the image and relabels it. This code runs very slowly in the MATLAB environment, because it is carried out in two nested loops. The following function code provides a vectorized version of the multiregion ICM algorithm for 2-D images:

```
function simg = mipicmvectorized2dmr(gimg,simg,nClass,...
  nhood,beta,numOfIteration);
% Replicate the images edges
gimg = padarray(gimg,[1 1],'replicate','both');
simg = padarray(simg,[1 1],'replicate','both');
%initialize the variables
[row,col] = size(gimg); k = 1;
while k <= numOfIteration
  [mus,sigs] = mipregionstats(gimg(2:end-1,2:end-1),...
    simg(2:end-1,2:end-1),nClass);
  sigs = sigs + 0.001;
  vars = sigs.^2;
  Nimg = mipneighborhood2d(simg,nhood);
  Himg = histc(Nimg,1:nClass,3);
  for L=1:nClass
    likeimg(:,:,L) = (0.5./vars(L)).*(gimg(:,:) - ...
      mus(L)).^2 + log(sigs(L)) - beta*Himg(:,:,L);
  end
  [MN,simg] = min(likeimg,[],3);
  k = k + 1;
end;
simg = simg(2:end-1,2:end-1);
```

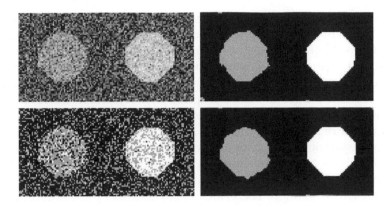

FIGURE 7.8

Comparison of the vectorized version with the sequential one. Top and bottom left images show the original and initial segmentations, respectively, whereas the top and bottom right images show the results of the vectorized and sequential implementations, respectively.

Note that in vectorization, the pixels are not labeled sequentially but rather in parallel. In addition to the vectorization or parallelization of the code, there are some other differences in this particular implementation. First, the mipneighborhood2d function, which was discussed in Chapter 2, is used to extract the labels of the neighboring pixels. Using histc function of MATLAB, the frequency of the labels in the neighborhood has been calculated. Then the Gibbs energy was computed (as suggested by Besag [10]) as beta* (frequency of the label in the neighborhood). Finally, the label for which the energy is minimum is assigned to the pixel. This vectorized code runs about eight orders of magnitude faster than that of the sequential version. Although the vectorized version violates the sequential updating requirement, it performs as well as the sequential version on the hexagon images. Figure 7.8 shows the comparison of the parallel and sequential implementations on the simulated hexagon images similar to the one shown in Figure 7.7. The top and bottom images on the right are the images segmented using the vectorized and sequential versions, respectively. These results point out that the performances of both implementations are very similar.

7.5 Simulated Annealing Algorithms

Earlier, we formulated the segmentation problem as an optimization problem. In other words, we are trying to find the MAP estimate, which is a maximization of the posterior. In the previous section, we discussed the deterministic solution, the ICM algorithm, suggested by Besag. In this section, we will discuss two simulated annealing-(SA)-based algorithms that solve the MAP estimate in a manner similar to the physical annealing process that occurs in matters. In a physical annealing process, the matter is heated at a very high temperature and then gradually and very slowly cooled to reach the ground state. Inspired by the physical annealing, the SA-based solutions introduce a temperature variable, similar to the physical temperature in concept, into our energy functions. This variable will allow us to start our optimization process from a state in which all the configurations have equal probability, in other words, from a very hot state. Then, by gradually decreasing the temperature variable, we will be reaching to the global solution. The principal advantage of these approaches is that the performance of the optimization is no longer dependent on initial labeling.

There are two well-known algorithms that fall under this category. These are Metropolis algorithm that we briefly discussed earlier and the Gibbs sampler. Now, we will discuss these two algorithms in detail and apply them to synthetic and MR images of a human brain.

7.5.1 Metropolis Algorithm

Let us first present the pseudocode for 2-D images with two regions to demonstrate how the algorithm works. We will label images with two regions with labels x_i, where $i = 1, 2$.

1. for k = 1:K
2. Select an initial temperature T_k
3. for $s = 1:N$

    Go to pixel s

    Calculate the total energies $E(x_1)$ and $E(x_2)$ for labels x_1 and x_2

    Calculate $\Delta E = E(x_2) - E(x_1)$

    Draw a random uniform number u in the range (0, 1)

    If $\Delta E/T_k < 0$

       Assign the label x_2 to the pixel s

    else if $\Delta E/T_k > u$

       Assign the label x_2 to the pixel s

    else

       do not change the label
4. Go to step # 3
5. $k \leftarrow k + 1$ and $T_{k+1} \leftarrow C \cdot T_k$
6. Go to step # 3

Note that the previous algorithm is in fact trying to minimize

$$(\log \sigma_s + (y_s - \mu_s)/\sigma_s + \beta U(x_s))/T \tag{7.20}$$

where T is the temperature parameter. Similar to the physical annealing process, we need to start with a high temperature and cool it down by decreasing the temperature very slowly. The most commonly used cooling schedule is $T_{k+1} = C \cdot T_k$, where C takes on values in the range [0.97, 1). A value of 0.97 seems to give acceptable results. In our experiments here, we will use $T_0 = 4$ as the initial temperature. Note that this temperature has no physical relevance in terms of absolute value. The following function implements the Metropolis algorithm for 2-D images with two regions:

```
function simg = mipmetropolis2d2r(gimg,simg,beta,...
  numOfIteration)
% Replicate the images edges
gimg = padarray(gimg,[1 1],'replicate','both');
simg = padarray(simg,[1 1],'replicate','both');
[row, col] = size(gimg);
% Initialize the parameters
T = 4; C = 0.97; k = 0;
% Calculate region statistics
[mus, sigs] = mipregionstats(gimg(2:end-1,2:end-1),...
  simg(2:end-1,2:end-1),2);
vars = (sigs + 0.01).^2;
while (k <= numOfIteration)
% Random numbers from uniform distribution and take the log
  aprob = log(random('Uniform',0,1,row,col));
  % raster scan the image
  for i = 2:row-1
    for j = 2:col-1
      s = simg(i,j);
      r = 3 - s;
      % Region labels start from 1,..., numRegions
    e1 = mipTotalEnergy(gimg,simg,mus,vars,i,j,s,beta);
    e2 = mipTotalEnergy(gimg,simg,mus,vars,i,j,r,beta);
      if (e2 - e1) <= 0
        simg(i,j) = r;
      elseif ( aprob(i,j) <= (e1 - e2)/T)
        simg(i,j) = r;
      end
    end
  end
  T = T*C; k = k + 1;
  [mus, sigs] = mipregionstats(gimg(2:end-1,2:end-1),...
```

```
       simg(2:end-1,2:end-1),2);
    vars = (sigs + 0.01).^2;
 end
 simg = simg(2:end-1,2:end-1);
```

We can extend our algorithm to 2-D images with multiple regions. The following function displays 2-D images with more than two regions:

```
function [simg, simgV] = mipmetropolis2dmr(gimg,simg,...
   beta, numRegions,numOfIteration)
% Replicate the images edges
gimg = padarray(gimg,[1 1],'replicate','both');
simg = padarray(simg,[1 1],'replicate','both');
[row, col]=size(gimg);
% Initilize the parameters
T = 4; C = 0.97; K = 1;
% Calculate region statistics
[mus, sigs] = mipregionstats(gimg(2:end-1,2:end-1),...
   simg(2:end-1,2:end-1),numRegions);
vars = (sigs + 0.01).^2;
% Create a matrix which will be used to draw a random
% label that is not equal to current label
regionLabels = 1:numRegions;
Lmatrix = zeros(numRegions-1);
for kk = 1:numRegions
   Lmatrix(kk,:) = regionLabels(regionLabels ~= kk);
end
while (K <= numOfIteration)
   % Random numbers from uniform distribution and take the log
   aprob = log(random('Uniform',0,1,row,col));
   % raster scan the image
   for i = 2:row-1
     for j = 2:col-1
        s = simg(i,j);
        e1 = mipTotalEnergy(gimg,simg,mus,vars,i,j,s,beta);
        rL = randomLabel(Lmatrix,s,numRegions);
        e2 = mipTotalEnergy(gimg,simg,mus,vars,i,j,rL,beta);
        if (e2 - e1) <= 0
           simg(i,j) = rL;
        elseif ( aprob(i,j) <= (e1 - e2)/T)
           simg(i,j) = rL;
        end
     end
   end
```

```
T = T*C; K = K + 1;
[mus, sigs] = mipregionstats(gimg(2:end-1,2:end-1),...
   simg(2:end-1,2:end-1),numRegions);
vars = (sigs + 0.01).^2;
simgV(:,:,K) = simg;
end
simg = simg(2:end-1,2:end-1);
```

As you see in the previous function in our main loop, we randomly select a label from the list [1, 2, ..., L] excluding the current label of the pixel. Then we execute our Metropolis algorithm to see if this randomly selected label can be accepted as a label. The following function randomLabel performs this random selection of a label that is not equal to the current label:

```
function rL = randomLabel(M,currentlabel,numRegions);
indx = ceil((numRegions-1).*rand(1,1));
rL = M(currentlabel,indx);
```

We first create a label matrix Lmatrix with rows equal to the number of regions. The *i*th row of the label matrix has all the labels except the label *i*. For the pixel label *i*, we randomly draw a label from the *i*th row.

One way to observe the progress of the Metropolis algorithm or any other iterative algorithm is to create a movie whose frames will consisted of the images obtained after every iteration step. The first part of the following script runs the Metropolis algorithm, one iteration at a time, and saves the result into a 3-D matrix. The second part of the script displays the images on a figure window, grabs the frame, and saves it into an avi movie file that is arbitrarily labeled as metropolis.avi. We suggest that the reader run the algorithm, because observing the progress of labeling may help one to understand the behavior of the algorithm in process.

```
numIterations = 100;
simgMovie = zeros([size(simg),numIterations]);
simg = isimg;
[simg, simgMovie] = mipmetropolis2dmr(nimg,simg,1.5,3,1);

mov = avifile('metropolis.avi','compression','Indeo5','fps',5)
hf = figure;
for i=1:54
   imagesc(simgMovie(:,:,i));axis image;colormap(gray)
   F = getframe(gcf);
   mov = addframe(mov,F);
end
mov = close(mov);
```

7.5.2 Gibbs Sampling

Gibbs sampling was first suggested by Geman and Geman [7] to be used in image restoration or segmentation. Similar to the Metropolis algorithm, Gibbs sampling provides a stochastic solution to the maximization problem, namely, calculation of the MAP estimate. Let us illustrate how the Gibbs sampler works by using the following pseudocode:

1. Initialize the temperature $T \leftarrow T_0$ (should be sufficiently high) and the iteration number $k \leftarrow 0$.

2. Assign initial labels to the pixels (different approaches can be chosen here). One can chose arbitrary labels for all the pixels.

3. For each pixel in the image

4. A sample is drawn such that x_s is accepted with the probability
$$\frac{\exp(-U(x_s))}{\sum_{r \in N_s} \exp(-U(r))}.$$

5. Decrease the temperature $T \leftarrow T_{k+1}$ and increase the iteration number.

As we saw earlier, the Gibbs sampler requires that we sample from a known discrete distribution. We need to know first how we can sample from a discrete distribution. This can be done by using a method known as the *inverse transform method* [14]. Let us bear in mind that our main aim is to solve the MAP estimation problem using the Gibbs sampler. Therefore, in the previous pseudocode, in Gibbs distribution, we will replace the Gibbs energy with the logarithm of the posterior. Thus, we will be sampling the posterior. Let us first discuss how we can sample from a discrete distribution.

7.5.3 Sampling from a Discrete Distribution

A random variable $Z = F(x)$, where $F(x)$ is the cumulative distribution function of the random variable X with a density function f, has a uniform distribution [15]. Hence, if U is a uniform random variable on $[0, 1]$, and $X = F^{-1}(U)$, then the cumulative distribution of X is given by F. This fact has been used to generate pseudorandom numbers from a discrete distribution whose cumulative distribution function is given by F [14]. The following pseudocode [14] summarizes a simple procedure to draw random samples from a discrete distribution whose probability mass function (pmf) is given by P:

1. Define the probability mass function

2. $P(X = x_i) = p_i \qquad x_0 < x_1 < x_2 \ldots \qquad \sum_i p_i = 1$

3. Calculate the cumulative distribution function

4. $F(X \leq x_i) = \sum_{k=0}^{i} p_k$

5. Generate a uniform number U

6. Draw the random number $X = x_i$ if

7. $F(x_{i-1}) < U \leq F(x_i)$

The example given in the following is taken from [14] and demonstrates in a simple way how we can draw samples from a known distribution whose probability distribution function is given by P. The following function implements the preceding pseudocode:

```
function x = mipsample_discretedist(P, n)
F = cumsum(P);
for i = 1:n
  U = rand(1,1);
  for k = 1:length(P)
    if U <= F(k)
      x(i) = k;
      break;
    end
  end
end
```

To demonstrate further how the method works, we will use the Poisson distribution as an example. We first compute the pmf P of a Poisson distribution with $\lambda = 2$. Then we can utilize our preceding function to generate, let us say, $n = 1000$ samples from this particular distribution, whose pmf is given by P. The following script implements this and plots the graphs of the original and sampled distributions that are shown in Figure 7.9.

```
% generate probability mass function
P = poisspdf(0:5,2)
% Draw samples from this discrete distribution
n = 1000;
X = mipsample_discretedist(P,n)
% plot the probability mass functions original and sampled
[h,cbins] = hist(X,1:6);
figure;plot(0:5,P); hold on;
plot(cbins-1,h/sum(h));
```

Now we can return to our main problem that is to find the MAP estimate using the Gibbs sampler. We will perform this by drawing samples from the posterior distribution computed at every pixel or voxel. The following

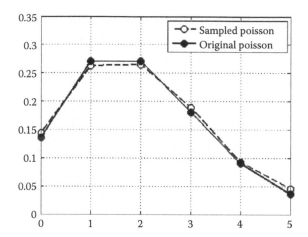

FIGURE 7.9

Sampling from a discrete distribution. Black dots show the original Poisson distribution, whereas the circles show the new distribution obtained by sampling from the original one.

pseudocode summarizes the procedure to calculate the MAP estimate using the Gibbs sampler:

1. Initialize the temperature $T \leftarrow T_0$ (should be sufficiently high) and the iteration number $k = 0$.
2. Assign initial labels to the pixels (various approaches can be taken here). One can chose arbitrary labels for all the pixels or one can use maximum likelihood estimator.
3. For each pixel in the image
4. A sample is drawn from such that x_s is accepted with the probability

$$\frac{\exp(-E(x_s)/T)}{\sum_{r \in N_s} \exp(-E(r)/T)}$$

where $E(x_s) = \dfrac{y - \mu_s}{\sigma_s} + \log(\sigma_s) + \beta U(x_s)$

5. Decrease the temperature $T \leftarrow T_{k+1}$ and the iteration number k.

As seen in the preceding pseudocode, the concept of simulated annealing is also utilized here by introducing the temperature variable. We are sampling from the Gibbs distribution whose energy is equal to the total energy, that is, the Gibbs energy and the negative log-likelihood.

For a two-region image, an object and the background, the segmentation by the Gibbs sampler can be implemented as seen in the following function code:

```
function simg = mipgibbs2d2r(gimg,simg,beta,numOfIteration)
% Replicate the images edges
gimg = padarray(gimg,[1 1],'replicate','both');
simg = padarray(simg,[1 1],'replicate','both');
[row, col] = size(gimg);
% Initialize the parameters
T = 4; C = 0.97; k = 0;
% Calculate region statistics
[mus, sigs] = mipregionstats(gimg(2:end-1,2:end-1),...
  simg(2:end-1,2:end-1),2);
vars = (sigs + 0.01).^2;
while (k <= numOfIteration)
% Random numbers from uniform distribution and take the log
  U = random('Uniform', 0, 1, row,col);
  % raster scan the image
  for i = 2:row-1
    for j = 2:col-1
      s = simg(i,j);
      r = 3 - s;
      e1 = mipTotalEnergy(gimg,simg,mus,vars,i,j,s,beta);
      e2 = mipTotalEnergy(gimg,simg,mus,vars,i,j,r,beta);
      if U(i,j) <= exp(-e2)/(exp(-e1/T) + exp(-e1/T))
         simg(i,j) = r;
      end
    end
  end
  T = T*C; k = k + 1;
  [mus, sigs] = mipregionstats(gimg(2:end-1,2:end-1),...
  simg(2:end-1,2:end-1),2);
    vars = (sigs + 0.01).^2;
end
simg = simg(2:end-1,2:end-1);
```

Note that the Metropolis algorithm and the Gibbs sampler are equivalent when the number of regions is equal to two, thereby no sampling is need. The following code implements the Gibbs sampler extended to images with multiple regions:

```
function simg = mipgibbs2dmr(gimg,simg,beta,...
  numRegions, numOfIteration)
% Replicate the images edges
gimg = padarray(gimg,[1 1],'replicate','both');
simg = padarray(simg,[1 1],'replicate','both');
[row, col] = size(gimg);
```

```
% Initialize the parameters
T = 4; C = 0.97; k = 0;
% Calculate region statistics
[mus, sigs] = mipregionstats(gimg(2:end-1,2:end-1),...
   simg(2:end-1,2:end-1),numRegions);
vars = (sigs + 0.01).^2;
while (k <= numOfIteration)
   % Random numbers from uniform distribution and take the log
   U = random('Uniform',0,1,row,col);
   % raster scan the image
   for i = 2:row-1
     for j = 2:col-1
       s = simg(i,j);
       sumE = 0;
       for s = 1:numRegions
          e(s) = exp(-mipTotalEnergy(gimg,simg,mus,vars,...
          i,j,s,beta))/T;
          sumE = sumE + e(s);
       end
       % Sampling from the posterior
       % ----------------------------
       F = 0;
       for s = 1:numRegions
           F = F + e(s)/sumE;
           if F >= U(i,j)
              simg(i,j) = s;
              break;
           end
         end
         %-----------------------------
       end
     end
     T = T*C; k = k + 1;
   [mus, sigs] = mipregionstats(gimg(2:end-1,2:end-1),...
      simg(2:end-1,2:end-1),numRegions);
    vars = (sigs + 0.01).^2;
end
simg = simg(2:end-1,2:end-1);
```

The part of the function that performs sampling the posterior is denoted by the two dashed lines. Figures 7.10 through 7.13 show the performance of the three algorithms on two MRI images. In the first example, we have a sagittal slice from an MRI image of a brain. The first image, whose histogram is shown in Figure 7.10 (right), is assumed to have 4 regions, therefore, was labeled initially using the function with the thresholds [50,100,190].

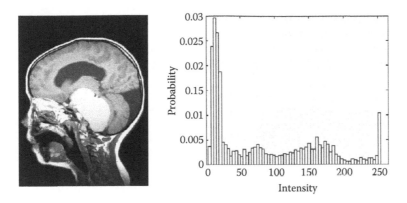

FIGURE 7.10
MRI image of brain presented in sagittal view (left) and its histogram (right).

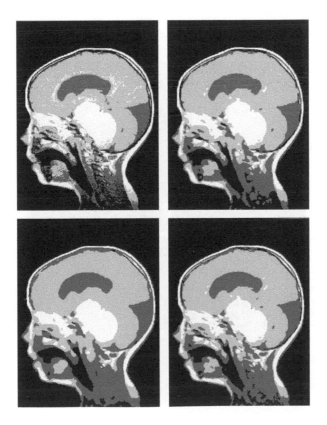

FIGURE 7.11
Segmented brain images. Top left: Initial labeling. Top right: ICM. Bottom left: Gibbs sampler. Bottom right: Metropolis algorithm.

```
isimg = mipgray2multilevel(img,[50 100 190]);
simgicm = mipicm2dmr(img,isimg,4,1.5,10);
simgmetro = mipmetropolis2dmr(img,isimg,1.5,4,30);
simggibbs = mipgibbs2dmr(img,isimg,1.5,4,30);
```

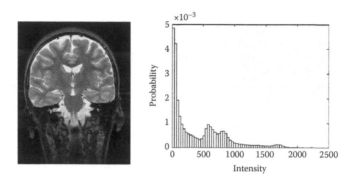

FIGURE 7.12
A coronal slice from an MRI image of brain (left) and its histogram (right).

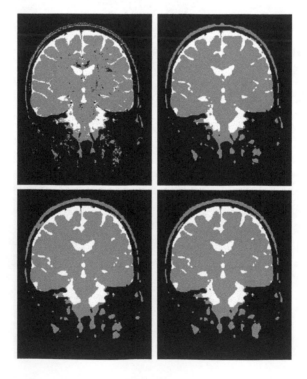

FIGURE 7.13
Segmented brain images. Top left: Initial labeling. Top right: ICM. Bottom left: Gibbs sampler. Bottom right: Metropolis algorithm.

The result of initial labeling is shown in Figure 7.11 (top left). The results of the three algorithms are presented in the same figure: top-right: ICM; bottom-left: Gibbs sampler; and bottom right: Metropolis algorithm. The parameter β was set to 1.5. The ICM was iterated 10 times, whereas the other algorithms were iterated 30 times.

The second example is a coronal view of a brain acquired by MRI. The original image and its histogram are shown in Figure 7.12. The images segmented by the three algorithms are shown in Figure 7.13.

7.6 Extension to 3-D Images

Because of the computational complexity, the 3-D simulated annealing-based algorithms are difficult to run in a reasonable time period. As the extension of these algorithms to 3-D is fairly straightforward, we leave it to the reader as an exercise. However, the 3-D version of the ICM algorithm can be run within a reasonable time period on medical images of reasonable sizes with today's CPUs.

Thus, we decided to provide you with the function for the 3-D version of the ICM algorithm. The function is named mipicm3d.m and can be found in Medical Image Processing Toolbox. This function does not label pixels in a sequential mode. It rather does it in parallel using our function mipneighborhood3d.m for speed and efficiency. The sequential version of the ICM will run slow in 3-D in MATLAB environment unless it is implemented in C or C++.

Figure 7.14 shows the coronal slices from a whole-body positron emission tomography (PET) image segmented with the 3-D version of the ICM

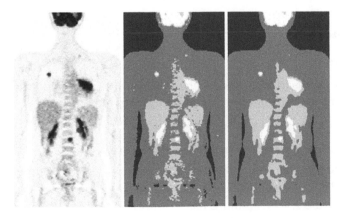

FIGURE 7.14
Coronal slices from a whole-body PET image of a patient. Left: Gray-level PET image. Middle: Initial labeling. Right: Final segmentation. The segmented image was obtained using the 3-D version of the ICM algorithm.

algorithm. The middle image shows the initial labeling, whereas the right image is the final segmented image. To avoid out-of-memory problems, we have divided the whole body PET image into several subvolumes and segments, each separately. So for large volumetric images, one can divide the image into subvolumes and segments, each separately and if possible simultaneously. This will solve both the memory and speed problems in the case of large 3-D images.

7.7 Parameter Estimation

The parameter β is perhaps the most critical parameter in all the afore-mentioned algorithms. As previously discussed, this parameter controls the interaction between the pixels or sites. In previous examples, we used a fixed value of 1.5. The question of what is the best β value to use, or can we estimate its value adaptively for each image has been considered by the researchers in this field. There are several investigations dealing with the parameter estimation issue. The methods proposed in the literature include the pseudo-likelihood, the least square estimation, and the coding method [16–19]. The readers interested in the parameter estimation issue will find the said references useful.

A fixed β value is the most common approach in practice because the algorithms behave fairly robust for a wide range of β values. If needed, task-based optimization of the β may be a reasonable approach to find the optimal value [20]. This can be done using a gold standard for the task at hand. In medical imaging, phantom or simulated images provide a means to test or validate image processing algorithms.

Problems

1. Derive the MAP estimate when the conditional follows the exponential distribution whose function is given by
   $$p(y\,|\,x_s) = \frac{1}{b_s}\exp\left(-\frac{(y-a_s)}{b_s}\right) \quad a \leq y \leq \infty, \text{ where } a_s \text{ and } b_s \text{ are the}$$
   parameters of the distribution of the class x_s.

2. Find the maximum likelihood estimators of these parameters a_s and b_s.

3. Assume $Z = F(X)$, and Z has a uniform distribution on the interval [0,1]. Then show that f, which is the probability distribution of F, is a uniform probability distribution function.

4. Assume that U is uniform on the interval [0, 1], and $X = F^{-1}(U)$. Show that the cumulative distribution of X is F.

5. Write a function that calculates the pseudo-log-likelihood function defined by $\log(\prod_{s \in I} P(X = x) = \frac{1}{Z}\exp\{-\beta U(x)\})$, where $Z = \sum_{x \in \Omega} \exp\{U(x)\}$. Compute the pseudo-log-likelihood after every iteration of the ICM algorithm to observe how pseudo-log-likelihood changes as the algorithm converges.

6. Use the pseudo-log-likelihood to optimize the parameter β simultaneously, while segmenting an image, using the following steps:

   1. Start with a β value and iterate the ICM algorithm.
   2. Try a range of β to find the optimal β that maximizes pseudo-log-likelihood.
   3. Then use this value during the next iteration of the ICM.
   4. Go to step #2.

This parameter estimation approach has been suggested by Besag [17].

References

1. L. Vaderspypen, Dot-to-dot design, *IEEE Spectrum*, 34–39, 2007.
2. D. Stick, J. D. Strek, and C. Manroe, The trap technique, *IEEE Spectrum*, 2007.
3. N. Metropolis, A. Rosenbluth, M. Rosenbluth, A. Teller, and E. Teller, Equation of state calculations by fast computing machines, *J Chem Phys* 21: 1087–1092, 1953.
4. S. Kirkpatrick, C. D. G. Jr., and M. P. Vecchi, Optimization by simulated annealing, *Science* 220: 671–680, 1983.
5. Y. Zhang, M. Brady, and S. Smith, Segmentation of brain MR images through a hidden Markov random field model and the expectation-maximization algorithm, *IEEE Trans Med Imaging* 20: 45–57, 2001.
6. K. Held, E. R. Kops, B. J. Krause, W. M. Wells, 3rd, R. Kikinis, and H. W. Muller-Gartner, Markov random field segmentation of brain MR images, *IEEE Trans Med Imaging* 16: 878–86, 1997.
7. S. Geman and D. Geman, Stochastic Relaxation, Gibbs distribution, and the Bayesian restoration of images, *IEEE Trans. Pattern Anal Machine Intelligence* 6: 721–741, 1984.
8. T. N. Pappas, An adaptive clustering algorithm for image segmentation, *IEEE Trans Signal Processing* 40: 901–914, 1992.
9. A. K. Jain, *Fundamentals of Digital Image Processing*. Englewood Cliffs, NJ: Prentice-Hall, 1989.
10. J. Besag, On the statistical analysis of dirty images, *J R Stat Soc B* 48: 259–302, 1986.
11. J. M. Hammersley and P. Clifford, Markov field on finite graphs and lattices, unpublished, 1971.

12. G. R. Grimmett., A theorem about random fields., *Bull London Math Soc* 5: 81–84, 1973.
13. J. Besag, Spatial interaction and the statistical analysis of lattice systems, *J Roy Stat Soc* 26: 192–236, 1974.
14. W. L. Martinez and A. R. Martinez, *Computational Statistics Handbook with MATLAB*. Boca Raton, FL: CRC Press, 2001.
15. M. H. Degroot and M. J. Schervish, *Probability and Statistics*, 3rd ed., Boston: Addison-Wesley, 2001.
16. D. Pickard, Asymptotic inference for an ising lattice iii. non-zero field and ferromagnetic states, *J Appl Prob* 16: 12–24, 1979.
17. J. Besag, Efficiency of pseudolikelihood estimation for simple Gaussian fields, *Biometrica* 64: 616–618, 1977.
18. H. Derin, H. Elliott, Modeling and segmentation of noisy and textured images using Gibbs random fields, *IEEE Trans Pattern Anal. Machine Intelligence* 9: 39–55, 1987.
19. D. Pickard, Inference for discrete Markov fields: The simplest nontrivial case. *J Am Sta Asso* 82: 90–96, 1987.
20. O. Demirkaya, M. H. Asyali, and M. M. Shoukri, Segmentation of cDNA microarray spots using Markov random field modeling, *Bioinformatics* 21: 2994–3000, 2005.

8

Deformable Models

CONTENTS

8.1 Introduction

General-purpose segmentation methods are difficult to apply to medical images due to the complex nature of medical images. Complexities arise from fuzzy boundaries, missing edge features, complicated backgrounds, and inconsistent image contrast. Approaches that solely depend on the low level information, local features, will most likely fail at borders with fuzzy boundaries and/or missing edge features. Figure 8.1 demonstrates this problem on an MR image of the ascending aorta and its edges detected by the Canny operator [1]. The Canny edge detector depends on the local features of the image and is very popular in imaging field; however, it has failed to fully detect the aorta boundaries due to poor contrast and fuzzy borders, giving spurious edges within the vessel due to turbulent flow. It will be difficult to automatically eliminate the spurious edges or to link the missing boundaries within such a complicated background where there are too many other edge features in close proximity.

Manual delineation is considered to be the gold standard; however it is an extremely time consuming process considering the size of the medical image datasets, and is highly observer-dependent. The pursuit for robust

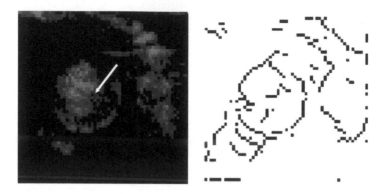

FIGURE 8.1
Ascending aorta MR image (left) and Canny edge detector segmentation result (right).

methods with minimal user intervention propelled deformable models to become one of the most popular medical image analysis methods as they utilize high-level a-priori information about the object shape and fit naturally to extract smooth and closed boundaries. Although the term deformable model has been associated with 3-D implementation in literature, this chapter generically refers to them as deformable models regardless of dimensionality. Other popular terms include active contours, active surfaces, deformable templates and snakes. In order to provide in depth information on this very exciting field, an entire chapter is dedicated rather than covering it together with the other segmentation approaches.

The strength of deformable models stems from their ability to mesh high-level information (hence the name model) with low-level local features. Since most object boundaries are smooth, closed contours, the set of possible shapes can be restricted to shapes satisfying these constraints. Kass et al introduced such controllable active contours simply called snakes [2]. Since Kass et al.'s seminal work, deformable models have been applied to many medical imaging tasks including segmentation, shape representation, registration and motion tracking. The rest of the chapter is devoted to basic theory and segmentation using deformable models.

8.2   Theory

Although deformable models are multi-dimensional by nature, this section will be limited to 2-D for the sake of simplicity. Principles remain the same in extension to higher dimensions. Deformable models can be grouped into two types: *parametric deformable models* [2] and *geometric deformable models* [3, 4]. Our focus will be on parametric deformable models first as it is the older of the two and is more intuitive to explain the deformable model concept.

8.1.2 Parametric Deformable Models

Parametric deformable model or snake is a curve $C(s)$ that can be represented as

$$C(s) = \{x(s), y(s)\}, \quad s \in [0, 1] \tag{8.1}$$

where x and y are the spatial coordinate functions and s is the parametric domain. This contour acts like a rubber band that changes its shape under a variety of local image features, and shape based and observer based constraints.

Deformation process can be best explained from energy minimization perspective. Local image features and user-defined constraints form the external energy of the system while shape based constraints form the internal energy. Internal energy E_{INT}, acts in a way similar to potential energy, attempting to prevent the contour from losing its shape-related properties (smoothness, curvature etc.). External energy E_{EXT}, analogous to kinetic energy forces the contour to deform and move towards edges. It is defined based on the local image edge features and their relative distance to the current contour. Certainly, edge locations (vessel boundaries) are unknown and indeed the outcome of the segmentation process. Gradient strength and/or distance from the zero crossings of the image Laplacian are generally used as image energy functional. The user defined external energy term introduces user intervention to the system. For example a constant energy term, called *balloon force* can be added to the system to avoid spurious edges (noisy regions have high gradient value). Special care has to be taken in user defined energy use, as it might also cause the deformable model to miss the edges that are not strong enough. This, more of an ad-hoc energy term, is excluded from our analysis. The contour that minimizes the total energy E, which is represented as

$$E = E_{INT} + E_{EXT} \tag{8.2}$$

provides the final solution, which is determined by starting from an initial seed contour placed by the operator or the algorithm itself.

8.2.1.1 Internal Energy

Calculating the shape energy contribution for each control point per iteration is computationally expensive. As an indirect measure of the shape energy contribution, two computationally inexpensive metrics are used.

These are the *continuity* and the *curvature* of the template. Kass et al [2] introduced these terms as the first and the second order derivatives of the spline contour C(s), respectively:

$$E_{INT} = \int_0^1 \alpha(s)\left|\frac{\partial c}{\partial s}\right|^2 + \beta(s)\left|\frac{\partial^2 c}{\partial s^2}\right|^2 ds \qquad (8.3)$$

where $\alpha(s)$ and $\beta(s)$ are the weighting parameters that control the tension and rigidity, respectively. Discrete approximations for the first and second derivatives at vertex vector $\mathbf{v}_i$ can be written as

$$\left|\frac{\partial c_i}{\partial s}\right|^2 \approx \frac{|\mathbf{v}_i - \mathbf{v}_{i-1}|^2}{ds^2} = \frac{(x_i - x_{i-1})^2 + (y_i - y_{i-1})^2}{ds^2} \qquad (8.4)$$

$$\left|\frac{\partial^2 c_i}{\partial s^2}\right|^2 \approx \frac{|\mathbf{v}_{i-1} - 2\mathbf{v}_i + \mathbf{v}_{i+1}|^2}{ds^4} = \frac{(x_{i-1} - 2x_i + x_{i+1})^2 + (y_{i-1} - 2y_i + y_{i+1})^2}{ds^2} \quad (8.5)$$

Williams and Shah [5] have pointed out some of the problems, such as instability, and suggested alternative approximations for the first and second order derivatives. The *continuity* term is approximated as

$$\left|\frac{\partial c_i}{\partial s}\right|^2 \approx \left|D - |\mathbf{v}_i - \mathbf{v}_{i-1}|\right|^2 \qquad (8.6)$$

where D is the average distance between neighboring points of the curve. The *curvature* term is approximated as the angle between the two curve vectors, $(\mathbf{v}_i - \mathbf{v}_{i-1})$ and $(\mathbf{v}_{i+1} - \mathbf{v}_i)$, that is, mathematically speaking,

$$\left|\frac{\partial^2 c_i}{\partial s^2}\right|^2 \approx \cos^{-1}\left(\frac{(\mathbf{v}_i - \mathbf{v}_{i-1}) \cdot (\mathbf{v}_{i+1} - \mathbf{v}_i)}{|\mathbf{v}_i - \mathbf{v}_{i-1}| \, |\mathbf{v}_{i+1} - \mathbf{v}_i|}\right) \qquad (8.7)$$

Figure 8.2 demonstrates how continuity and curvature metrics detect the problematic control points and nicely complement each other on an MR ascending aorta image. Vertices of contour are marked with filled circles and three vertices with the largest continuity and curvature values are labeled with × and + signs. The vertices that deform the most from a smooth contour are nicely detected indicating higher internal energy contribution from these points. Higher internal energy will force the contour to deform to another solution avoiding false segmentation.

8.3.1 External Energy

So far, we have discussed the internal energy and explained how to calculate the internal energy of a deformable model. The function of the internal

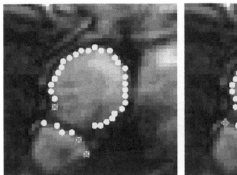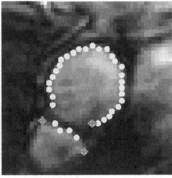

FIGURE 8.2
MR ascending aorta image. Deformable model vertices are marked with filled circle Three vertices marked with cross (×) on the left image have the largest continuity metric and three vertices marked with plus (+) on the right image have the largest curvature metric.

energy is to regularize the deformed template to shapes that are similar to the equilibrium shape of the template. The overall energy function of the model requires an external term, which will attract the template toward the image features such as edges. Because the exact locations of the features are unknown, an indirect measure of features should be employed. The magnitude of the image gradient is the most popular means of describing external energy. One can also use the distance to the zero-crossings of the Laplacian of an image; however zero crossings will likely fall on off-pixel locations, thus interpolation is needed. Once the zero-crossings are detected, the distance of every pixel in the image to the closest zero-crossing point must be calculated. Because of its simplicity and computational advantage, the gradient approach is the most popular choice.

The gradient requires a derivative calculation by definition; however, the derivative calculation is ill-posed, that is, small changes in the input can cause large deviations in the output. Looking at the Fourier Transform of the derivative operation clearly reveals this ill-posedness.

$$FT\left\{\frac{d}{ds}\right\} = i2\pi f \tag{8.8}$$

where f is the frequency. The derivative operation enhances high frequency components more than the low frequency parts when applied to images, as this term will be multiplied with the Fourier Transform of the image in Fourier domain. In the absence of noise this is a desired property; as edges are high-frequency components. Ideally, we want the external energy to attract model towards edges. However in real life, noise always exists in the form of a high frequency signal due to the imaging system. Together with the edges in the image, noise is amplified as well, reducing the signal to noise ratio of the system. To cope with this noise-enhancing problem, some sort of regularization is required prior to derivative calculations. The Gaussian filter is shown to be the optimal regularization filter before differentiation [7]. For further detail on this topic the reader may refer to Chapter 2. The gradient can be estimated using Gaussian first derivative basis filters

$$g_1^x(x,y,\sigma) = \frac{-x}{\sqrt{2\pi\sigma^3}} e^{-\frac{(x^2+y^2)}{2\sigma^2}}$$

$$g_1^y(x,y,\sigma) = \frac{-y}{\sqrt{2\pi\sigma^3}} e^{-\frac{(x^2+y^2)}{2\sigma^2}} \qquad (8.9)$$

where σ denotes the scale of the Gaussian operator. Larger scales suppress noise better and improve the capture range of the deformable model at the expense of the edge sharpness. We know that the gradient vector points in the direction of the maximum rate of change of image intensity function $I(x,y)$. The gradient of $I(x,y)$ can be approximated as:

$$\nabla I = \cos(\theta)I_1^x(x,y,\sigma) + \sin(\theta)I_1^y(x,y,\sigma) \qquad (8.10)$$

where θ is the gradient vector direction at (x, y) and

$$I_1^x(x,y,\sigma) = g_1^x(x,y,\sigma) \otimes I(x,y) \qquad (8.11)$$

$$I_1^y(x,y,\sigma) = g_1^y(x,y,\sigma) \otimes I(x,y)$$

$$\theta = \arctan(I_1^y(x,y,\sigma)/I_1^x(x,y,\sigma))$$

Based on the gradient operator, the external energy is set to

$$E_{EXT} = -\sum_{i=1}^{N} |\nabla I(v_i)|^2 \qquad (8.12)$$

where v_i corresponds to the vertices of the template. The minus sign is used to minimize the external energy when the gradient is the strongest.

Figure 8.3 shows an ascending aorta MR image, its gradient response, and the external energy in the subplots from left to right. In the gradient image, higher gradient levels are marked with a brighter color. In the image energy, the darker pixels indicate smaller image energy. The smooth closed contour of the vessel boundary is clearly visible in image energy map.

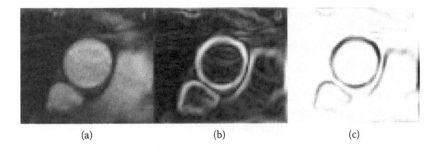

(a) (b) (c)

FIGURE 8.3
Gradient as a measure of image energy. (a) Ascending aorta MR image. (b) Gradient of the image. (c) Image energy based on the image gradient.

Tension and rigidity weighting parameters $\alpha(s)$ and $\beta(s)$ could be treated as constants or more complex monotonic functions. Ascending aorta segmentation is quite challenging as its shape, position, and blood flow profile varies significantly throughout the cardiac cycle. An asymmetric flow profile and turbulent flow degrade the ascending aorta vessel wall representation. Figure 8.4 demonstrates deformable model segmentation

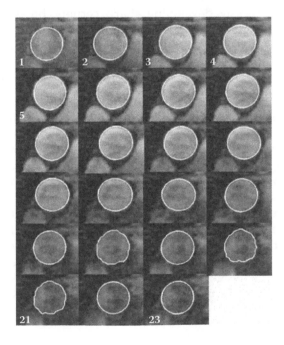

FIGURE 8.4
Ascending aorta MR segmentation results with deformable models. 23 total frames were acquired using a cardiac-gated acquisition.

results on a healthy volunteer. A total of 23 time frames are acquired with cardiac gating within each cardiac cycle. Despite the turbulent flow and frame-to-frame ascending aorta motion, the deformable model successfully extracted the boundaries of the ascending aorta. In this case, an initial seed was dropped in one of the frames and the rest were segmented automatically. Even the challenging low flow frames towards the end of the cardiac cycle demonstrating the well-suited nature of deformable models for medical image analysis tasks.

Readers are encouraged to refer to [7] for more detailed technical discussion and the literature overview.

8.3   Geometric Deformable Models

Geometric models are based on curve evolution and level set method [8]. The basic idea is to represent contours as the zero level set of an implicit function defined in a higher dimension, usually referred as the level set function, and to evolve the level set function according to a partial differential equation (PDE). This approach, albeit its complexity, presents unique advantage over the parametric deformable model. The contours represented by the level set function handles the topological changes naturally by seamlessly developing sharp corners, breaking or merging during the evolution. This becomes very useful with three or higher dimensional segmentation problems as the surfaces become inherently complex for parametric representations.

8.3.1   Level Set Representation

Level set representation provides the mathematical framework on how to track evolution of boundaries (interfaces). An intuitive explanation would be appropriate for level set representation in order to understand the adaptive capability of the geometric deformable models against topological changes. For further details on the topic, readers are encouraged to refer to [9].

Instead of tracking the contour in its original dimensionality, level set representation adds an extra dimension to the problem. Although more dimensions normally mean increased complexity, dealing with the topological changes at a higher dimension provides the much needed flexibility. For simplicity, letís again assume a 2-D contour in x–y plane. Level set representation adds dimension z to create the level set function ϕ:

$$z = \phi(x, y, t = 0) \tag{8.13}$$

Hence z becomes the height and represents the distance of (x, y) to the interface at $t = 0$. This representation builds a surface as demonstrated with

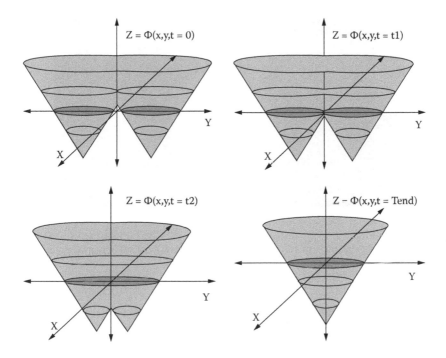

FIGURE 8.5
Level set function (surface) shown in gray color at different time frames. Zero level set is plotted in darker gray. Evolution of the interface is matched by the level set function's zero level set by adjusting the height of the level set.

gray color in Figure 5. The "zero level set" is defined as the intersection of the level set surface with x–y plane. Therefore, level set function ϕ returns distance of each (x, y) location to the zero level set at a given time t. It is called zero level set because it is collection of all points that has the zero height and it provides the deformable model contour. Mathematically, level set formulation of the geometric deformable model $C(t)$ is:

$$C(t) = \{(x, y) \mid \phi(x, y, t)\} = 0 \qquad (8.14)$$

Figure 8.5 demonstrates "zero level set" or deformable model contour with darker gray color at different time frames. Our goal is to figure out how to change the height of the level set so that it matches the evolution of the deformable model at the zero level set. If we can do this, then as the contour evolves, we can now stand at each fixed point (x,y) and adjust the height of the level set. From an implementation perspective, this means that the level set function remains a function on a fixed grid, allowing efficient numerical solution. Going back to Figure 5, initial contour is given as two elliptic shaped closed contours shown in darker gray in the first

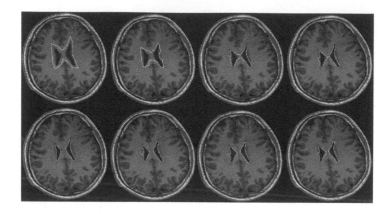

FIGURE 8.6
Geometric deformable model evolution demonstrating how a deformable model gracefully handles changes in topology.

image. At time t_1, the contours intersect and the level set function height was adjusted to move another level set to zero to reflect the topology change. At time t_2 the two contours merged into a one contour and height of the level set was adjusted again to match the zero level set. The final curve is a single elliptical contour indicating that the object of interest has elliptical shape and the zero level set at this particular time has become single curve rather than two.

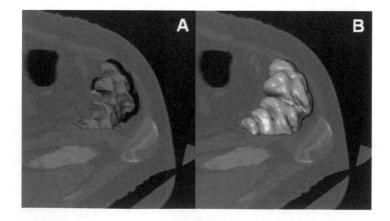

FIGURE 8.7
Fully automated 3-D segmentation of the colon using geodesic deformable model. Initial surface on the left (A) and final surface on the right (B). Images are courtesy of Dr. Christopher Wyatt from Virginia Polytechnic Institute and State University.

The beauty of level set framework becomes evident when extending it to 3-D or higher dimensions as strategy remains the same regardless of the dimensionality: extend the problem into one higher dimension; and adjust the value of this higher dimension function to compute the zero level set to find the position of the propagating interface.

Figure 8.6 demonstrates how deformable models naturally handle the changes in topology on an axial brain MR image. The top left image shows the initial contour. The deformable model starts as a single closed curve and crosses itself in the process (top right image) and automatically splits into two closed contours (bottom right) and extracts the object of interest (bottom left).

Figure 8.7 provides an example using the 3-D geodesic deformable model from Yezzi et al. [10] to segment a region of the colon in CT colonography images. The initial surface in (A) is automatically generated from threshold based segmentation and a distance map. The final surface is shown in (B) after the model converges.

Robustness against change in topology offers unique advantage to the geometric deformable models; they are widely used in medical imaging especially for 3-D segmentation tasks.

8.3.2 Level Set Evolution

Evolution of the level set function ϕ is derived by taking the time derivative of the level set function and is governed by the formula:

$$\frac{\partial \phi}{\partial t} + F|\nabla \phi| = 0 \qquad (8.15)$$

where F defines the speed at which the level set moves. F stays perpendicular to the interface as shown in Figure 8.8, and any tangential component will have no effect on the propagation. For segmentation purposes, F depends on the image data and the level set function ϕ.

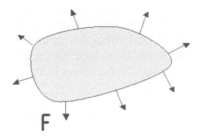

FIGURE 8.8
Speed function remains perpendicular to the interface.

In their pioneer paper, Osher and Sethian focused on motion under mean curvature flow where the speed term is expressed as the divergence (*div*) of the normalized level set:

$$F = div\left(\frac{\nabla\phi}{|\nabla\phi|}\right) \tag{8.16}$$

Caselle et al [11] improved upon this speed function by adding a constant inflation force term v and multiplying the speed by a term inversely proportional to the smooth gradient of the image as an edge indicator function

$$F = G(|\nabla\phi|)\left(div\left(\frac{\nabla\phi}{|\nabla\phi|}\right) + v\right)$$

$$G(|\nabla\phi|) = \frac{1}{1 + |\nabla g(x, y, \sigma) * I(x, y)|^2} \tag{8.17}$$

One common problem with the level set function ϕ is that it can develop shocks or sharp corners during the evolution, which jeopardizes stable curve evolution. One popular remedy is to initialize the function ϕ as a signed distance function before the evolution, and then "reinitialize" it to be a signed distance function periodically during the evolution:

$$\frac{\partial\phi}{\partial t} = sign(\phi_0)(1 - |\nabla\phi|)$$

$$sign(x) = \begin{cases} -1 & x < 0 \\ 0 & x = 0 \\ 1 & x > 0 \end{cases} \tag{8.18}$$

where ϕ_0 is the function to be re-initialized. Re-initialization period must be chosen carefully to balance the computational efficiency and risk of failure, as the function can deviate greatly from its previous value. Since its inception, many flavors of geometric deformable models using alternate evolution and speed frameworks have been proposed in order to improve robustness and convergence. However the general principles remain the same. This section is intended to provide the conceptual understanding of geometric deformable models. More in-depth coverage can be found in the mentioned references.

8.4   MATLAB and Deformable Models

The MATLAB Image Processing Toolbox can be utilized to great extent to implement deformable models. For instance, the `fspecial` function provides the 2-D Gaussian filter, which can be used to smooth images prior to gradient calculation. Below example generates a Gaussian kernel with standard deviation of 1.5 covering ±5 standard deviations.

```
sigma = 1.5;
G = fspecial('gaussian', 2*5*sigma+1, sigma);
```

The conv2 function can convolve an image with the Gaussian kernel to generate a smooth image. Since both gradient operation and Gaussian filtering are linear operations; we can exchange the order of operation; performing the filtering before the gradient calculation. The following statement filters the image.

```
smoothImg=conv2(Img,G,'same');
```

The smooth image can then be passed the gradient function, which computes the directional gradients. The gradient magnitude image sI can be computed as

```
[sIx,sIy]=gradient(smoothImg);
sI = sqrt(sIx.^2 + sIy.^2);
```

Note that element-wise square values are easily calculated using ".^" operator in MATLAB. Once the gradient term of the smoothed image is calculated, the external energy term for parametric deformable models as well as edge functional $G(|\nabla\phi|)$ for geometric deformable models can be calculated very easily. Figure 8.9 shows the mesh plot of the sample Gaussian kernel (top left), a sagittal MR brain image (top right), the geometric deformable models edge functional $G(|\nabla\phi|)$ with (bottom right) and without Gaussian filtering (bottom left). This example demonstrates the need for Gaussian filtering prior to gradient calculation, as the functional is less noisy after Gaussian filtering, which should help with level set evolution process.

The roipoly function can be utilized to define the initial contour for deformable models. The output binary mask image created by roipoly can be used to define the initial level set function (LSF). In the example below the initial LSF curve LSF0 is set to −5 for the points inside the contour and 5 for the points outside contour.

```
K0 = 5;
Imagesc(smoothImg);
BW    = roipoly;
LSF0  = 2*K0*(1-BW) ñ K0;
```

Once the initial contour is placed, the deformable model evolution can be implemented using a for loop to do time marching, and by updating the

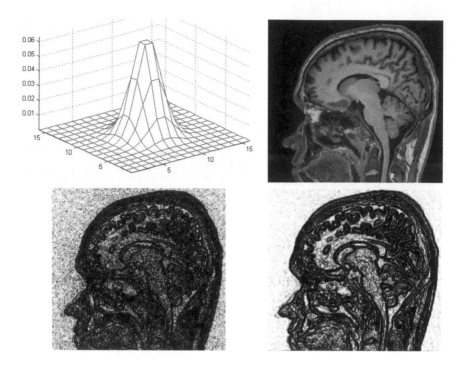

FIGURE 8.9

Top Left: Gaussian kernel with sigma = 1.5. Top Right: Noisy MR brain image. Bottom Left: Edge functional calculated without the Gaussian filtering. Bottom Right: Edge functional calculated after the Gaussian filtering.

curvature and continuity terms at each iteration for parametric deformable models and the level set propagation for geometric deformable models.

Problems

1. Implement two MATLAB functions to calculate the continuity and the curvature terms of an arbitrary contour as given in Equations (9.6) and (9.7).

2. Implement a MATLAB function based on Equation (9.3) to calculate the internal energy term (hint: can utilize "sum" function in place of integral).

3. Implement the external energy function with and without Gaussian smoothing (use the the phantom function in MATLAB to produce a 256 × 256 Modified Shepp-Logan phantom).

4. Use R = normrnd(mu,sigma, M, N) to add noise to the Shepp-Logan phantom to experiment with different levels of noise and explain how Gaussian smoothing filter impacts external energy term.

5. Explain what would happen if very large sigma values are used with the Gaussian smoothing filters. What would be the advantages and disadvantages of using large values?

References

1. J. Canny, A computational approach to edge detection, *IEEE Trans. Pattern Analysis Machine Intelligence*, vol. 8, no. 6, pp. 679–698, November 1986.
2. M. Kass. and A. Witkin, and D. Terzopolous, Snakes: Active Contour Models, International Conference on Computer Vision, vol. 1, pp. 321–331, 1987.
3. V. Caselles, F. Catte, T. Coll, and F. Dibos, A geometric model for active contours, Numer. Math., vol. 66, pp. 1–31, 1993.
4. R. Malladi, J. A. Sethian, and B. C. Vemuri, Shape modeling with front propagation: A level set approach, *IEEE Trans. Pattern Anal. Machine Intell.*, vol. 17, pp. 158–175, 1995.
5. D.J. Williams and M. Shah, A Fast Algorithm for Active Contours and Curvature Estimation, *CVGIP: Image Understanding*, vol. 55, no. 1, pp. 14–26, 1992.
6. J.J. Koenderink, *The Structure of Images, Biological Cybernetics*, vol. 50, pp. 363–370, 1984.
7. T. McInerney and D. Terzopoulos, Deformable Models in Medical Image Analysis: A Survey. *Medical Image Analysis*, 1(2): 91–108, 1996.
8. S. Osher, J. A. Sethian, Fronts Propagating with Curvature Dependent Speed: Algorithms based on Hamilton-Jacobi formulations, *J. Comp. Phys.*, vol. 79, pp. 12–49, 1988.
9. J. A. Sethian. Tracking interfaces with Level Sets, *American Scientist*, pp. 254–263 May-June 1997.
10. A. Yezzi, S. Kichenassamy, A. Kumar, P. Olver, and A. Tannenbaum, A geometric snake model for segmentation of medical imagery, *IEEE Trans. on Medical Imaging*, vol. 16, pp. 199–209, 1997.
11. V. Caselles, F. Catte, T. Coll, and F. Dibos, A geometric model for active contours in image processing, *Numer. Math.*, vol. 66, pp. 1–31, 1993.

9

Image Analysis

CONTENTS

9.1   Introduction

The image processing and analysis pipeline can be divided into three stages. Figure 9.1 depicts this pipeline. As seen in this diagram, these stages include image acquisition, preprocessing, intermediate-level processing, and image analysis. The preprocessing stage is also known as low-level processing.

Following image acquisition, the preprocessing or low-level processing may include tomographic reconstruction, noise filtering, image enhancement, and removal of image degradations, which may be due to the image formation process, such as nonuniformity in magnetic resonance imaging (MRI) and light microscopy, or the removal of the image artifacts such as streak or beam-hardening artifacts in CT. In some tomographic imaging modalities such as positron emission tomography (PET) and single photon emission tomography (SPECT), some of the innate degrading factors such

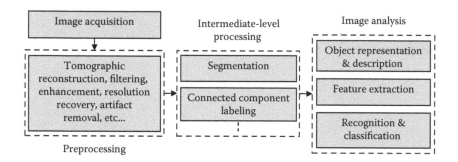

FIGURE 9.1
Image processing and analysis pipeline.

as the ones causing resolution loss are corrected during the tomographic image reconstruction process.

Image segmentation is considered part of the intermediate level processing stage. Connected component labeling and/or boundary extraction usually follow image segmentation. Connected component labeling involves labeling of the pixels of different regions in a 2-D or 3-D image identified during image segmentation. Boundaries may also be directly detected using an edge detection technique, which is often considered a segmentation method, as the edges may correspond to the boundaries between different regions.

Image analysis is the last stage of the of the image processing and analysis pipeline. It may include boundary representation/description, feature extraction, and pattern recognition or classification.

Image analysis is such a broad subject that comprehensive coverage of the whole field in a single chapter is impossible, so our treatment here is in no way comprehensive. Over the years many scientific papers have been published proposing new solutions to the problems of image analysis. Image analysis also includes topics such as feature extraction, shape representation, and object recognition and classification. Here, we will cover only some of the fundamental topics that have found widespread applications in medical image processing.

9.2 Region Properties

Following the extraction of the region representing the object of interest, it is required to quantify its properties. This is the principle aim of image processing and analysis. For instance, if we are interested in the ejection fraction of an abnormal heart, which is the percentage of the blood that is pumped out of the left ventricle during each heartbeat, the image analysis algorithm needs to quantify the blood volume during the systolic and diastolic phases of the heart from the gated SPECT images. The region properties that one may be interested in depend on the problem at hand. In general, the most common region or object (i.e., volume) properties that are needed are the area, volume, perimeter, circularity, orientation of the region, and the location, normally denoted by its centroid.

A region comprises pixels $R = \{(x_1, y_1, z_1, I_1), (x_2, y_2, z_2, I_2), ..., (x_N, y_N, z_N, I_N)\}$ that are connected together by a neighborhood relationship. Each pixel has a position defined by (x_i, y_i, z_i) and a gray-level intensity denoted by I_i. Regions in intensity images are separated using the methods of image segmentation.

Following the identification of regions, their pixels are identified from binary images using the method of connected-component labeling. This method, which we will not discuss here, is a process in which all the pixels of different regions in an image are tagged with unique labels. The MATLAB functions `bwlabel` and `bwlabeln` are the connected-component labeling functions for 2-D and N-D images, respectively, that perform connected-component labeling. Following connected-component labeling, the region properties or features of the objects can be computed, as we already know all the pixels or voxels that comprise a particular region or object.

One can compute the region properties based on the gray-level intensities. The mean intensity and the variance are typical examples. The co-occurrence matrix–based measures or Haralick textural features, named after Haralick, who suggested these measures in reference [1], may provide clues about the textural properties of a region. The MATLAB Image Processing Toolbox includes functions that calculate co-occurrence–based features. These features may be used for the purpose of identification of different regions. So, they may also be used for classification purposes. Abnormal tissue structures, for example, may be ascertained by comparing these features against that of normal tissue of the same kind. Texture identification is another interesting subject by itself that we will not delve into.

Now we will discuss some of the widely used region properties in medical and biological imaging applications.

The *area* of a region can be defined as the number of pixels in the region:

$$A = \sum_{x,y \in R} 1 \qquad (9.1)$$

To find the area in actual units, we need to multiply the area A by the area of a single pixel in actual units.

Centroid of a region R denoted by $(\bar{x}_c, \bar{y}_c)$ can be found using

$$\bar{x}_c = \frac{1}{N} \sum_{i=1}^{N} x_i \text{ and } \bar{y}_c = \frac{1}{N} \sum_{i=1}^{N} y_i \qquad (9.2)$$

where N is expressed in terms of number of pixels. If the region is an object with volume, then we add the z-coordinate of the centroid to Equation (9.2). The centroid is the point equal to the average of the coordinates of the pixels or voxels.

The *perimeter* of a region in a 2-D image can be computed after the identification of its boundary pixels. Let us suppose that the boundary of a region comprises an ordered sequence of pixels defined in the x–y coordinate system. The pixels are connected with either 4 or 8 connectivity. The distance between two consecutive pixels is 1 or $\sqrt{2}$ units if they are 4 or 8 connected, respectively. The following simple function code calculates the perimeter on the basis of the connectivity between pixels:

```
SQRT2 = sqrt(2);
plength = 0.0;
p = [p; p(1,:)];
npoints = size(p,1);
for j = 2:npoints
    if abs(p(j,1) - p(j-1,1)) > 0 & abs(p(j,2)- p(j-1,2)) > 0
        plength = plength + SQRT2;
    else
        plength = plength + 1.0;
    end
end
```

To compute the perimeter in actual units, the perimeter can be multiplied by the actual size of the pixel, assuming that the pixel dimensions are equal.

There are a number of measures suggested for *compactness* or *circularity*. Because these measures are widely accepted and used, we will not provide references. The first one is given by

$$\frac{\|Perimeter\|^2}{Area} \qquad (9.3)$$

For a circular region this ratio is equal to a constant, that is, $\frac{(2\pi r)^2}{\pi r^2} = 4\pi$.

The second measure is the ratio of the major to minor axis lengths. For a circular shape, these two should be similar. A larger ratio indicates a larger deviation from circularity. An alternate measure of circularity [2] is given by

$$\mu_R / \sigma_R \qquad (9.4)$$

This measure is based on the mean distance (Euclidean distance) μ_R from the centroid to the region boundary, and the standard deviation σ_R of the distances from the centroid to the region boundary. They are defined by

$$\mu_R = \frac{1}{N} \sum_{i=1}^{N} \| (x_i, y_i) - (\bar{x}_c, \bar{y}_c) \|$$

(9.5)

$$\sigma_R = \frac{1}{N} \sum_{i=1}^{N} [\| (x_i, y_i) - (\bar{x}_c, \bar{y}_c) \| - \mu_R]^2$$

where $(\bar{x}_c, \bar{y}_c)$ is the coordinates of the centroid, and N is the total number of boundary pixels. Haralick [2] shows that this circularity measure (1) increases monotonically, as the shape becomes more circular; (2) is similar for similar digital and continuous shapes; and (3) is orientation and area independent. The following function code calculates the circularity given in Equation (9.4):

```
function c = mipcircularity(p)
xmean = mean(p(:,1));
ymean = mean(p(:,2));
npoints = size(p,1)
for i=1:npoints
    d(i) = pdist([p(i,1) p(i,2) ;xmean ymean]);
end
mur = sum(d)/npoints;
sgmr = 0;
for i=1:npoints
    sgmr = sgmr + (d(i) - mur)^2;
end
sgmr = sgmr/npoints;
c = mur/sqrt(sgmr);
```

Assuming a circular region, the *equivalent diameter* of a circular region with the same area is given by

$$D = \sqrt{(4 * Area / \pi)}$$

(9.6)

The `regionprops` function in the Image Processing Toolbox calculates the properties of a region in a 2-D image. The input image should be labeled first using the function `bwlabel`. We use this function extensively to calculate the properties of regions. We also remove small structures, which we refer to as debris, prior to calculating region properties. Our function `miprmdebrisn` calculates the sizes of regions and excludes the regions smaller than a certain size (i.e., debris).

We will demonstrate (see Figure 9.2) the use of `regionprops` on an image of small cells using the following script. In the script, we load the cell image, segment the cell regions, remove the small fragments, detect the region boundaries, compute the region properties, and finally display

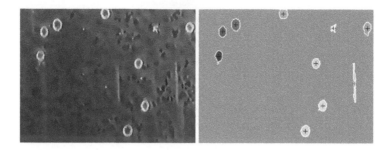

FIGURE 9.2
Filtered gray-level image of the cells (left) and the segmented cell regions (right).

both the gray level and segmented image. Note that we identify the outer boundaries of regions, that is, coordinates of the boundary pixels in the following script using the MATLAB function bwboundaries:

```
load filteredcell.mat
thw = mipbcv (double(csub),64);
bw = csub > thw;
[BW2,IDX] = bwfill(bw,'holes');
BW2 = rmdebris(BW2,50);
imshow (csub);

[B,L] = bwboundaries(BW2,'noholes');
% Labels and computes the region properties
RPROPS = regionprops(bwlabel(BW2),'all');
centroids = cat(1, RPROPS.Centroid);

imsow(label2rgb(L, @gray, [.5 .5 .5]));hold on;
plot(centroids(:,1), centroids(:,2), 'b+','Markersize',8);
for k = 1:length(B)
    boundary = Bknown;
    plot(boundary(:,2), boundary(:,1), 'w', 'LineWidth', 2)
end
```

The output structure of RPROPS is a structure array with 10 elements, each of which has the following 22 fields:

1. Area	12. Image
2. Centroid	13. FilledImage
3. BoundingBox	14. FilledArea
4. SubarrayIdx	15. EulerNumber
5. MajorAxisLength	16. Extrema
6. MinorAxisLength	17. EquivDiameter
7. Eccentricity	18. Solidity
8. Orientation	19. Extent
9. ConvexHull	20. PixelIdxList
10. ConvexImage	21. PixelList
11. ConvexArea	22. Perimeter

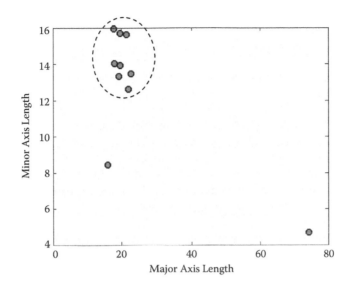

FIGURE 9.3
The graph of major and minor axis lengths of the objects.

We will leave it to the reader to explore the detailed explanation of these parameters in the MATLAB help pages.

Here we will demonstrate, in an example, how we can identify noncellular structures or cell fragments using the major and minor axis lengths of the cells. Let us place these two parameters of all the objects segmented into two different arrays and plot them against each other using the following statements:

```
majaxis = cat(1,RPROPS.MajorAxisLength);
minaxis = cat(1,RPROPS.MinorAxisLength);
plot(majaxis,minaxis,'o');
```

Figure 9.3 shows the graph of the major and minor axes of the objects against each other.

If we were to cluster segmented objects on the basis of their major and minor axis length, as seen in the graph in Figure 9.3, we would have three fairly distinct clusters. Note that the long region, which is not a cell, and the small cell-like region have distinct major and minor axis lengths when compared to those of the eight cells. We can also observe this from their ratios. We will not further discuss what else can be done with the region properties provided by regionprops; we will leave this to the imagination of the readers, and it depends very much on the problem at hand, anyway. This example suffices to shows that the region parameters calculated by regionprops gives us many options to calculate, process, and analyze the region properties of objects.

9.2.1 Surface Area and Volume of the Convex Hull

In this section, we will explain the methods to calculate the volume and surface area of the convex hull of a 3-D object of an arbitrary shape. Our objects consist of a set of voxels that are neighbors and defined by their center locations $\{(x_i, y_i, z_i)\}$ in $\mathbb{R}^3$. The convex hull is the smallest convex region or space that envelopes the entire object. For a 2-D data set, the convex hull is a polygon. For a 3-D object, however, it is a convex polyhedron that consists of small triangular planes, called facets, each of which is defined by three points in $\mathbb{R}^3$. These points are called vertices of the plane.

Again, before any feature extraction or calculation, we need to use the MATLAB bwlabeln to perform connected-component labeling to identify voxels of our object in the image. We assume that the object is already segmented from an intensity image.

The MATLAB convhulln function can then be used to find the convex hull of the object. The MATLAB convexhulln function returns the indices, denoted by K in the following script, of the points in object X that comprise the facets (triangular planes) of the convex hull of X. X is an $m \times n$ array representing m points in n-D space. If the convex hull has p facets, then K is $p \times n$. The function convhulln also returns the volume of the convex hull.

To demonstrate this on an example object, let us create a sphere (see Figure 9.4) using our mipspehereimage function using the following statement:

```
imgs = mipsphereimage([32,32,32],10,[16,16,16]);
```

The output of the function is a binary image of the shell. The binary volume image can also be visualized using our display GUI imlook3d. To compute the convex hull of the sphere, we first need to label the binary image using bwlabeln. We then get the pixel list of the sphere shell using the regionprops function of MATLAB. From the pixel list, the convhull function finds the indices of the vertices of the triangular planes that form the convex hull and also returns its volume. The following MATLAB script performs the labeling and convex hull calculations:

```
Lbw = bwlabeln(imgs);
PL = regionprops(Lbw,'PixelList');
X = PL.PixelList;
[K,v] = convhulln(X)
figure;
trisurf(K,X(:,1),X(:,2),X(:,3))
err=4/3*pi*18^3/(v-4/3*pi*18^3)
```

The surface area of the convex hull can be calculated by adding the areas of small triangles whose vertices are returned by the convhulln function.

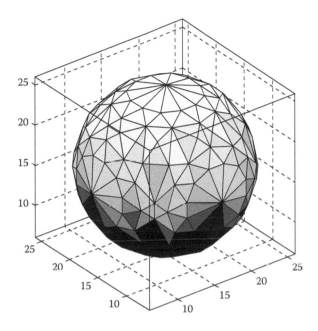

FIGURE 9.4
The surface plot of the sphere using `trisurf`.

We know, given the vertices of a triangle, its area can be calculated using the cross product operation. We know from basic calculus that the cross product of two vectors, denoted as $\mathbf{v}_1 \times \mathbf{v}_2$, is another vector whose magnitude is equal to the area of the parallelogram (see Figure 9.5) formed by these two vectors. Then the area of the triangle defined by the three points $\{p_1, p_2, p_3\}$ in $\mathbb{R}^3$ (see again Figure 9.5) is simply equal to half of the area of the parallelogram:

$$Area = \frac{1}{2} |\mathbf{v}_1 \times \mathbf{v}_2| \tag{9.7}$$

where $\mathbf{v}_1 = p_2 - p_1$ and $\mathbf{v}_2 = p_3 - p_1$.

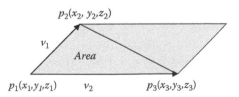

FIGURE 9.5
A parallelogram formed by the two vectors. *Area* refers to the area of the half of the parallelogram.

The surface of the polyhedron consists of *n* triangular surfaces whose vertex points are defined in $\mathbb{R}^3$. As we stated earlier, the surface area of this polyhedron can be found by adding the areas of the individual triangles forming the polyhedron. The following MATLAB code calculates the total surface area of the convex hull:

```
[C,vol] = convhulln(P);
d = [1 2 3];
nTriangle = size(C,1);
A = 0;
for i = 1:nTriangle
      j = C(i,d);
      v1 = P(j(2),:)-P(j(1),:);
      v2 = P(j(3),:)-P(j(1),:);
      A = A + 0.5*norm(cross(v1,v2));
end
```

We will demonstrate this numerically using the example given in the MATLAB help pages. We will calculate the surface area and the volume of a cube whose 8 corner points (vertices) are generated by the following script:

```
d = [-1 1];
[x,y,z] = meshgrid(d,d,d);
X = [x(:),y(:),z(:)];% 8 corner points of a cube
C = convhulln(X);
```

The following code, taken from the MATLAB, helps pages plots the convex hull by drawing the triangles as 3-D patches (see Figure 9.6):

```
figure, hold on
d = [1 2 3 1];    % Index into C column.
for i = 1:size(C,1) % Draw each triangle.
      j= C(i,d);    % Get the ith C to make a patch.
      h(i)=patch(X(j,1),X(j,2),X(j,3),i,'FaceAlpha',0.9);
end % 'FaceAlpha' is used to make it transparent.
hold off
view(3), axis equal, axis off
camorbit(90,-5); % To view it from another angle
```

Now we will compute the surface area and the volume of this cube whose sides are 2 units long. Our library function mipvolprop.m, run as shown in the following statement, computes the convex hull first, and then the volume and the surface area as 8 and 24, respectively:

```
[C,vol,A] = mipvolprop(X);
```

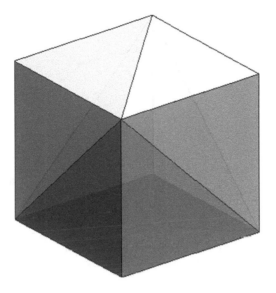

FIGURE 9.6
Plot of the cube consisting of triangular planes.

9.3 Boundary Analysis

Boundary analysis is required, for instance, to break the object boundary into homogeneous line segments or arcs for the purpose of shape analysis or recognition. Boundary analysis provides ways to identify salient points on a boundary curve. It can also help find vertices, if one wishes to find a more efficient polygonal representation of the boundary. In this section, we will discuss boundary analysis methods. It is not within the scope of this section to discuss the extraction of boundaries from a gray-level image. We assume that boundaries are identified using image segmentation or edge detection.

9.3.1 Boundary Curves and Parametric Representation

The boundary curve of an object extracted from an image is an ordered set of points connected with 8-connectivity, and whose positions are defined normally in Cartesian coordinates, $\mathbb{R}^2$, in the image space. Figure 9.7 shows the curve of the hemicircle sampled at intervals in the range [a, b]. The sampling points of the boundary curve are symbolized by $t_i \in [a, b]$. The boundary curve, which normally forms a closed contour, can be represented by the parametric vector equation $(x(t), y(t))$. In parametric representation, the

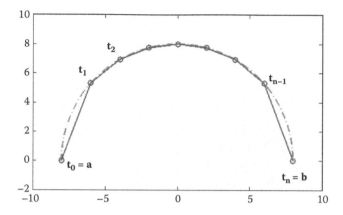

FIGURE 9.7
A hemicircle sampled at certain intervals. The dashed curve was sampled with a larger number of samples to approximate the analytic curve. The polygon formed by connecting the sampled points represents the curve.

s is the arc length that satisfies $\frac{ds}{dt} = \sqrt{\dot{x}^2 + \dot{y}^2}$, where $\dot{x} = \frac{dx}{dt}$. The total curve length S_t can be expressed as

$$S_t = \int_a^b \sqrt{\dot{x}^2 + \dot{y}^2}\, dt \qquad (9.8)$$

Note that here (.) and (') will be used to denote partial derivatives with respect to t and x, respectively. This representation is also known as the natural representation of the curve and simplifies computations performed on curves such as curvature calculations. Note that for closed curves, $x(t)$ and $y(t)$ are periodic functions.

The following code demonstrates how parametric representation makes it easy and convenient to compute 20 points $(x(t_i), y(t_i))$ along the curve where $t_i \in [0, 2\pi]$ and $i = 0, \cdots, 19$:

```
X  = linspace(0,2*pi,20);
xt = cos(X)';
yt = sin(X)';
xt = [xt ; xt(1)];
yt = [yt ; yt(1)];
```

Let us now calculate the curve length using the MATLAB function pdist. By default, pdist uses Euclidean distance unless specified otherwise.

```
P = [xt yt];
dismat = squareform(pdist(P));
St = sum(diag(dismat, 1));
```

The pdist function computes the distance between a pair of points. For this sampling rate, the total length of the curve is calculated as 6.2832. Note that the true perimeter of this curve is $2\pi = 6.2546$ as the radius is 1. If the number of samples is increased, the error between the true and estimated perimeter should decrease. We will leave the experimentation with different sampling rates to the reader as an exercise. A simpler function, which will run faster than the preceding code, can be written to calculate the curve length.

The Euclidian arc length given by Equation (9.8) is invariant with respect to rotations and translations. However, it is obviously not invariant with respect to scaling. Therefore, the curve length, or arc length, is said to be not invariant under affine transformation. An affine invariant arc length measure was proposed by Blaschke [3] in 1923. Affine invariant image evolution developed on the basis of the affine invariant arc length and has been discussed in Chapter 5 together with various partial-differential-equation-based diffusion techniques.

9.3.2 Resampling Boundary Curves

In an eight-connected boundary, the Euclidean distance between successive boundary pixels may not be equal, as they may be connected with either 4- or 8-connectivity; that is, the boundary curve is not evenly sampled (see Figure 9.8).

To obtain an evenly sampled boundary curve, the curve should be resampled in the parametric space. This is performed by first creating a continuous curve consisting of straight line segments joining successive points. The continuous curve is then resampled at a constant distance interval $\Delta s = 1/S_t$, where S_t is the total curve length obtained by adding

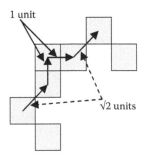

FIGURE 9.8
Boundary pixels connected with 4- or 8-connectivity. The distance between the centers of the pixels varies depending on the connectivity type. The pixels connected diagonally are $\sqrt{2}$ units apart, whereas the pixels connected vertically or horizontally are separated by 1 unit.

the Euclidean distances between successive points. This normalized (to the total length) arc length s takes on values ranging over the closed interval $[0, 1]$. Resampling has a smoothing effect in addition to an increase in the number of boundary points. This increase is a disadvantage, as the complexity of subsequent stages may be a function of the number of points. Note also that after resampling the boundary points will not lie on the image grid.

9.3.3 Circular Convolution

As we mentioned earlier, the coordinates of the closed boundary curves are periodic. If we need to smooth, for instance, our boundary curve with a Gaussian kernel, we need to perform circular convolution. Here, we will demonstrate how we can do this in a very simple manner. We will add, *circularly*, to the leading and trailing ends of the point list $m = (l - 1)/2$ number of points, where l is the length of the Gaussian kernel as seen in the following figure:

$$\overbrace{x_{n-(m-1)}, \cdots x_{n-2}, x_{n-1}, x_n}^{\text{added } m \text{ points}}, \underbrace{x_1, x_2, x_3, \cdots x_{n-2}, x_{n-1}, x_n}_{\text{actual } n \text{ boundary points}}, \overbrace{x_1, x_2, x_3, \cdots, x_m}^{\text{added } m \text{ points}}$$

This adding or padding can be done using the `padarray` function in MATLAB as seen in the following statement:

```
xnew = padarray(x,[0 m],'circular','both');
```

As can be seen, the length of the new data list is now $n + 2 * m$. In the next step, we convolve this new series with a Gaussian kernel and remove the points from both ends of the result to get the same length as that of the original point list using the following statements:

```
y = conv(xnew,h);
y = y(2*m+1:end-2*m);
```

Note the number of points we remove from both ends to obtain the same number of points as the original curve. Our library function `mipcircconv` computes the circular convolution of a signal with a kernel.

9.3.4 Curvature

Let us represent a closed object boundary by a sequence of points $C = \{(x_n, y_n)\}$, where $(x_n = x(t_n), y_n = y(t_n))$. The curvature at a point on this

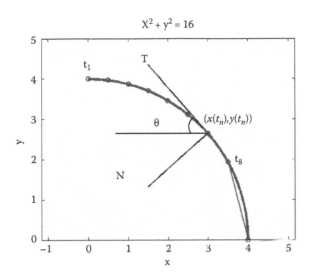

FIGURE 9.9
A quadrant of a circle ($x^2 + y^2 = 16$). The circle is sampled at certain intervals. **T** and **N** denote the tangent and normal vectors.

planar curve, defined by the sequence of boundary points, is the rate of change of the angle (see Figure 9.9) with respect to arc length; that is

$$\kappa = \frac{d\theta}{ds} \tag{9.9}$$

where s is the arch length parameter. The curvature is a local geometric property of the curve.

The tangent vector **T** shown in Figure 9.9 is defined by $T = [\dot{x} \quad \dot{y}]^T$. The normal vector **N**, which is perpendicular to the tangent vector, is given by $N = [-\dot{y} \quad \dot{x}]^T$.

The tangent of the angle θ (see Figure 9.9) at $(x(t_n), y(t_n))$ is given by

$$\tan \theta = \frac{dy}{dx} = \frac{\dot{y}}{\dot{x}} \tag{9.10}$$

Then it can be shown that the curvature κ of the parametric curve can be written as

$$\kappa = \frac{\ddot{x}\dot{y} - \dot{x}\ddot{y}}{(\dot{x}^2 + \dot{y}^2)^{3/2}} \tag{9.11}$$

It can also be shown that for a curve of the form $y = f(x)$, the curvature is given by

$$\kappa = \frac{y''}{\left[1 + \left(y'\right)^2\right]^{3/2}} \tag{9.12}$$

The reciprocal of the curvature at $(x(t_n), y(t_n))$

$$\rho = \frac{1}{\kappa} \tag{9.13}$$

is called the *radius of the curvature*. This is equal to the radius of the best-fit circle, in the least-squares sense, to the points abutting $(x(t_n), y(t_n))$. At a *point of inflection*, the curvature is equal to 0 as the second derivative at that point is zero.

The following script computes the curvature and the radius of curvature of a curve consisting of points $v = (x(t_n), y(t_n))$. Note that we use epsilon = 0.01 to avoid possible division-by-zero error.

```
x = v(:,1); y = v(:,2);
epsilon = 0.01;
dx = gradient(x); dy = gradient(y);
dxx = gradient(dx); dyy = gradient(dy) ;
grdsq = dx.*dx + dy.*dy;
grdsq(grdsq == 0) = epsilon;
cvt = (dx.*dyy - dy.*dxx)./(grdsq).^1.5;
```

The gray level and binary images of the vertebra are shown in Figure 9.10. It also shows the binary image (right) of vertebra along with the inner and outer boundaries superimposed. Figure 9.11 shows the boundaries on which the positive and negative curvatures are labeled with different

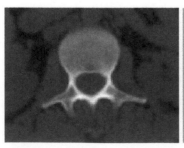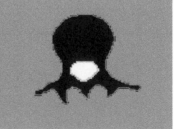

FIGURE 9.10
Left: Gray-level and binary (segmented by Otsu's method) CT images of spinal vertebral bone. Right: The boundary curves of the bone and of its internal hole are superimposed on the binary image.

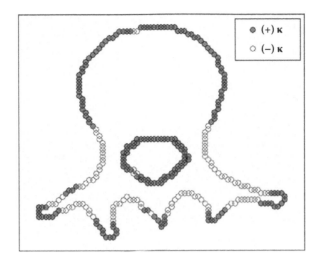

FIGURE 9.11
Inner and outer boundaries of the spinal vertebral bone. The points with positive and negative curvature values are labeled with filled and empty circles, respectively.

markers. The two graphs shown in Figure 9.12 depict the curvature functions for the inner and outer boundaries, respectively. In the curvature function for the inner boundary (of the hole), the curvature is positive everywhere except at three points. However, the curvature function of the outer boundary (bottom) exhibits peaks at five locations, which represent the processes (spinous and transverse) and facet joints of the vertebra. The negative curvature points represent the laminas of the vertebra.

We know that the transverse view of the vertebra in a CT image varies depending on the location of the individual vertebra along the vertebral column. Note also the positive and relatively smaller curvature values around the vertebral body. The curvature values are negative when the boundary curve is convex. If we compare the two curvature functions, the curvature function of the outer curve certainly has a larger variance. This feature may be used as an indicator of the boundary irregularity. Note also that the body of the vertebra has relatively smaller positive curvature values. Given the curvature of the outer curve, the vertebral body may be identified from the values and the signs of the curvature. So, the curvatures of boundary curves carry unique signatures that may be utilized for shape identification or characterization.

9.3.5 Tangential Deflection

Anderson and Bezdek [4] have proposed a method to compute the angle, the tangential deflection, between the two successive curve segments or arcs on a boundary. Tangential deflection can be defined as the angle between the least-squares-fit lines of the two data sets.

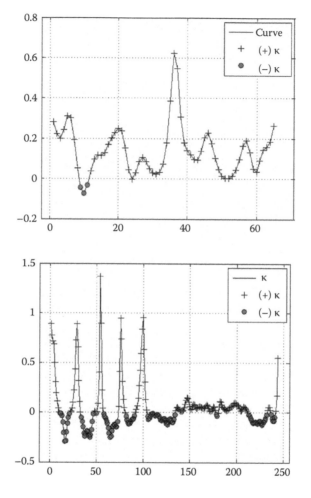

FIGURE 9.12

Top: Curvature function of the inner boundary. Bottom: Curvature function of the enclosing (outer) boundary. The negative and positive curvature values are denoted by different markers.

Let us denote the two arcs of a closed boundary curve C around a center point x_c as the data sets in $\mathbb{R}^2$ by

$$P_1 = \{(x_1, y_1), (x_2, y_2), \cdots, (x_n, y_n)\} \text{ and } P_2 = \{(x_1, y_1), (x_2, y_2), \cdots, (x_m, y_m)\}.$$

Then the normalized scatter matrices for the data sets are given, respectively, by

$$A = \frac{S_{P_1}}{trace\left(S_{P_1}\right)} = \begin{pmatrix} a_{11} & a_{12} \\ a_{21} & a_{22} \end{pmatrix}, B = \frac{S_{P_2}}{trace\left(S_{P_2}\right)} = \begin{pmatrix} b_{11} & b_{12} \\ b_{21} & b_{22} \end{pmatrix} \quad (9.14)$$

The scatter matrix here denoted by S_p is the scaled version of the covariance matrix V_p, that is, $S_p = (n-1)V_p$.

The covariance matrix V_p is expressed as

$$V_p = \begin{pmatrix} \sigma_{xx} & \sigma_{xy} \\ \sigma_{xy} & \sigma_{yy} \end{pmatrix} \tag{9.15}$$

where

$$\sigma_{xx} = \frac{1}{n-1} \sum_{i=1}^{n} (x_i - \mu_x)^2$$

$$\sigma_{yy} = \frac{1}{n-1} \sum_{i=1}^{n} (y_i - \mu_y)^2$$

$$\sigma_{xy} = \frac{1}{n-1} \sum_{i=1}^{n} (x_i - \mu_x)(y_i - \mu_y)$$

$$\mu_x = \frac{1}{n} \sum_{i=1}^{n} x_i \text{ and } \mu_y = \frac{1}{n} \sum_{i=1}^{n} y_i$$

The trace of a matrix is the sum of its diagonal elements. The trace of the scatter matrix $trace(S_p)$ is therefore equal to $\sigma_{xx} + \sigma_{yy}$. The σ_{xx} and σ_{yy} denote the variances of the variables x and y, respectively. And $\sigma_{xy} = \sigma_{yx}$ is the covariance of x and y. The scatter matrix is a 2×2 positive semi-definite matrix. The following statements calculate the scatter matrix and normalized scatter matrix:

```
scatmat = (length(x1)-1)*cov(x1,x2);
nscatmat = scatmat/trace(scatmat);
```

The eigenvalues of the normalized scatter matrices A and B can be used to obtain shape information about the boundary line segments or arcs.

The function `mipnormscattermat` in the Medical Image Processing Toolbox returns the normalized scatter matrix for a given set of points.

The characteristic equation for A is given by $\lambda^2 - \lambda + \det A = 0$, where $\lambda = (\lambda_1, \lambda_2)$ refers to the eigenvalues of the matrix A. Thus the eigenvalues are given by

$$\lambda_1 = \frac{1+d_s}{2} \text{ and } \lambda_2 = \frac{1-d_s}{2} \tag{9.16}$$

where $d_s = \sqrt{(1-(4\det A))} = \lambda_1 - \lambda_2$. Note that $\lambda_1 + \lambda_2 = 1$ due to normalization by the trace. The eigenvalues of the normalized scatter matrix can be computed by

```
lamda = eig(a);
```

There are three cases for the eigenvalues:

1. λ_1 or $\lambda_2 = 0$. In this case, all the points of P_i lie on a straight line.
2. $\lambda_1 = \lambda_2 > 0$. Then P_i is a circular bivariate normal. The covariance matrix is a constant multiple of the identity matrix. The x and y coordinates are not correlated.
3. $\lambda_1 > \lambda_2 > 0.1$. Then p_i is elliptical.

The λ values refer to the major and minor axes of the best-fit ellipse. Thus, the difference of eigenvalues d_s will tell us approximately whether the segment has a linear or an elliptical shape. The expression d_s is easy to compute and takes on values ranging over the closed interval [0, 1]. Similarly, the three corresponding cases for d_s can be given as

1. $d_s = 1$, then P_i is linear
2. $d_s = 0$, then P_i is circular
3. $0 < d_s < 1$, then P_i is elliptical

The shape index d_s can be calculated using the following MATLAB command:

```
ds = sqrt(1-4*det(a));
```

Our library function `miparcshapeindex.m` computes both the eigenvalues and the shape index of an arc.

Anderson and Bezdek [4] further proved that the principal angle between two consecutive arcs, say P_1 and P_2, denoted by $\Delta\theta$, can be expressed in terms of their normalized scatter matrices as

$$\cos 2\Delta\theta(P_1, P_2) = \frac{(a_{22} - a_{11})(b_{22} - b_{11}) + 4a_{12}b_{12}}{\sqrt{(1 - 4\det A)(1 - 4\det B)}} \tag{9.17}$$

where $\det A$ and $\det B$ are the determinants of the respective normalized scatter matrices A and B. The following script computes the tangential deflection angle θ from the scatter matrices a and b:

```
t1 = (( a(2,2) - a(1,1) )*( b(2,2) - b(1,1) ) + …
    4*a(1,2)* b(1,2));
t2 = sqrt( (1 - 4*det(a))*(1 - 4*det(b)) );
theta = acos(t1/ t2);
theta = 180*(theta/2)/pi;
```

In their paper, Anderson and Bezdek have suggested an algorithm for vertex detection. Their algorithm utilizes tangential deflection and the segment shape information d_s. These detected vertices may also be used, for instance, to represent the curve as a closed polygon with fewer vertices.

9.4 Scale-Space Analysis of Boundaries

Real-world images include structures that comprise a range of scales. A frequently cited example is the case of a tree. In the case of a tree image, we cannot talk about microscales as none of the tree structure exists in this very small scale. The braches, leaves, the trunk of a tree, and the forest that the trees belong to, all appear in different scales in an image. We quite often do not know a priori the scale at which our object of interest appears in the image. Thus, scale-space analysis may be required to find the scale at which we can identify the object that we are interested in. Noise is another factor that contaminates our scale range and makes it hard to distinguish between noise and the structure of interest. To address these problems, the theory of scale-space has been introduced. The scale-space is a mapping of our image or can also be a 1-D signal (i.e., a boundary curve of an object) into a new space where the image or the signal is represented in a range of scales varying from the original fine to coarser levels.

One way of performing this is to smooth the original signal with kernels of increasing sizes. In this case, the scale-space representation is parameterized by the size of the smoothing kernel denoted by t. The Gaussian kernel seems to be unique in satisfying the requirements of the scale-space representation, known as scale-space axioms, such as linearity, nonenhancement of local extrema or nonappearance of new structures, and invariance with respect to rotation, translation, and scaling [5–7], in other words, under affine transformations.

The concept of scale-space was first introduced into image processing by Witkin [8] and Koenderik [9]. Extensive discussions of scale-space theory can be found in references [5–7].

Mokhtarian and Mackworth [10] have rewritten a curvature function based on the parametric representation of the curve as

$$\kappa = \frac{\dot{x}\ddot{y} - \ddot{x}\dot{y}}{(\dot{x}^2 + \dot{y}^2)^{3/2}} \tag{9.18}$$

where $\dot{x} = x * g'$, $\ddot{x} = x * g''$, $\dot{y} = y * g'$, $\ddot{y} = y * g''$, and g is a Gaussian function

$$g(x, \sigma) = \left(\frac{1}{\sqrt{2\pi \cdot \sigma}}\right) \exp\left(-\frac{x^2}{2\sigma^2}\right) \tag{9.19}$$

and g' and g'' are the first and second derivative of the Gaussian function with respect to x, respectively. The $*$ sign denotes the convolution operation. Note that Equation (9.18) is the same as Equation (9.11) except the smoothing with a Gaussian kernel. This new formulation permits the computation of the curvature function at different scales or σs.

We know that convolving signals with a Gaussian kernel has a smoothing effect. Smoothing a curve causes shrinkage toward the center of the curvature. The shrinkage arises from the fact that each point on the curve is being averaged with its neighbors. The degree of shrinkage depends on the degree of smoothing, that is, σ in the case of Gaussian smoothing, as the degree of smoothing determines the size of the neighborhood along which the points are averaged. The location of the boundary features (e.g., minimum negative curvature) will change, depending on the degree of smoothing. Lowe [11] proposed a method to smooth curves without shrinkage. He formulated the magnitude of shrinkage as a function of the smoothing factor and the curvature value for a given point on the curve. He then compensated for the likely shrinkage by adding the amount of shrinkage to the point.

For instance, in a curve-partitioning process, the minimum negative curvature points on a curve can be selected from the minimum curvature points below the zero line. During the process, it may be necessary to distinguish spurious minimum negative curvature points from the salient ones to detect the candidate break points that will partition the boundary curve into segments. Multiresolution analysis of the curvature function can be utilized to determine these salient minimum negative curvature points.

Let us demonstrate how one can create the scale-space representation of a 1-D signal. Our 1-D signal is the boundary curve of our vertebral bone. The coordinates of the curve are saved into the variable pv. In the following script we compute the curvature of the boundary using Equation (9.18) implemented in the function mipcurvature for a range of σ values. Note that σ takes on values in the range [1, 20] with increments of 0.2. We saved the computed curvature function as rows of an image that we call scale-space image. In the script, the scale-space image of the curvature is saved into cvt and shown in Figure 9.13 (top). The scale σ increases at each row of the image from top toward bottom. The bottom image shows the contour lines of the scale-space image. The bright regions extending vertically in the scale-space image correspond to high curvature points (to processes and facet points of the vertebral bone). The sharper and longer processes survive longer in the scale-space, whereas smaller features eventually diminish as the scale gets larger.

```
count = 1;
for sigma = 1:0.2:20
    cvt(count,:) = mipcurvature (pv,sigma);
count = count+1;
end
[C,h] = contourf(cvt,10);
```

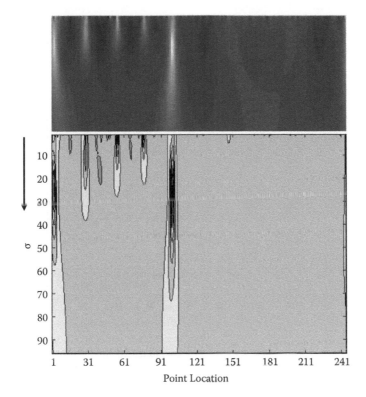

FIGURE 9.13
Top: Scale-space image of the curvature function. Bottom: The filled contour plot of the isolines of the scale-space image. The areas between isolines are filled with constant color.

The scale-space analysis process does not end here. Usually, next step is the determination of the salient features. This requires detection of the features that survive at large scales, and the tracking of these features in the scale-space to find their locations in the original fine scale.

As discussed in Chapter 5, one of the motivations for proposing the anisotropic diffusion technique of Perona and Malik was to produce the scale-space representation of an image or 1-D signal without blurring and displacing the object features. Figures 9.14 and 9.15 show the plots of the boundary curves and the curvature functions, respectively. The boundary curves seen in Figure 9.15 were smoothed (dashed) with a Gaussian kernel ($\sigma = 3$) and diffused (solid) with the 1-D version of the anisotropic diffusion filtering. Note the greater smoothing and dislocation of the curve caused by the Gaussian smoothing. Therefore, using an anisotropic diffusion-filtering technique may alleviate the difficulties of feature tracking in the scale space.

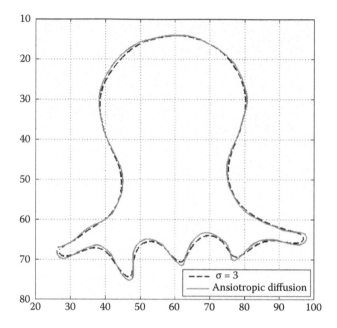

FIGURE 9.14

Boundary smoothed with a Gaussian ($\sigma = 3$) kernel (dashed) and anisotropic diffusion filtering (number of iterations = 30, noise threshold = 0.8, lambda = 0.05, Weickert's diffusivity function).

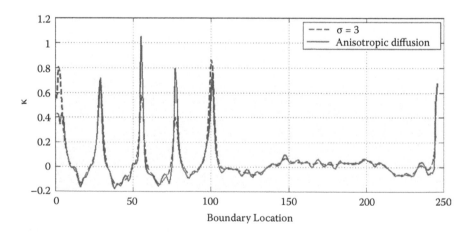

FIGURE 9.15

The curvature functions of the smoothed curves seen in Figure 9.14 using a Gaussian kernel with $\sigma = 3$ and 1-D anisotropic Perona–Malik diffusion (see Chapter 5 for details).

9.5 Direct Least-Squares Fitting of Ellipses to Boundary Curves

In medical and biological imaging, the objects that we deal with are often round or elliptical. Fitting the boundary curve of an elliptical object often facilitates subsequent shape analysis process. In fact, this may be a rather prudent approach to obtaining a smooth boundary curve if the object boundary is reasonably elliptical.

Here we will discuss the method of Fitzgibbon [12] for fitting ellipses to a sequence of N data points that may be defining a closed curve or a curve segment. The advantages of this method are its invariance to affine transformations, robustness to noise, uniqueness of the solution, and computational efficiency. In introducing the method, we will follow Fitzgibbon's notation.

Let us define a general conic by

$$F(\mathbf{a}, \mathbf{x}) = \mathbf{a}\mathbf{x} = ax^2 + bxy + cy^2 + dx + ey + f = 0 \qquad (9.20)$$

where $\mathbf{a} = \begin{bmatrix} a & b & c & d & e & f \end{bmatrix}^T$ and $\mathbf{x} = \begin{bmatrix} x^2 & xy & y^2 & x & y & 1 \end{bmatrix}^T$.
$F(\mathbf{a}, \mathbf{x})$ is the distance between a point (x, y) and the conic. Direct least-squares fitting of Fitzgibbon minimizes

$$E = \|D\mathbf{a}\|^2 \text{ subject to the constraint } \mathbf{a}^T C \mathbf{a} = 1 \qquad (9.21)$$

where C is a 6×6 constraint matrix. The minimization reduces it to the following system of equations after introducing a Lagrange multiplier and differentiation:

$$\mathbf{S}\mathbf{a} = \lambda C \mathbf{a}$$
$$\mathbf{a}^T C \mathbf{a} = 1 \qquad (9.22)$$

where S is the scatter matrix that we are familiar with.

The eigenvalue-eigenvector pairs of this system $(\lambda_i, \mu \mathbf{u}_i)$ for any μ will provide a solution to the system. We can obtain μ_i from the constraint equation as $\mu_i = \sqrt{\frac{1}{\mathbf{u}_i^T C \mathbf{u}_i}}$ then the solution is given by $\hat{\mathbf{a}}_i = \mu_i \mathbf{u}_i$. Fitzgibbon [12] also shows that the minimization of Equation (9.21) with the general ellipse constraint $4ac - b^2 = 1$ yields a unique solution, which is an ellipse. The following function code presented in their paper implements this effective method:

```
% x,y are the vectors of coordinates
function a = fit_ellipse(x,y)
% Build design matrix
```

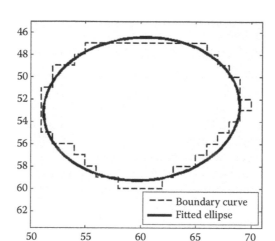

FIGURE 9.16
Boundary curve of a cell and the ellipse fitted by Fitzgibbon's [12] algorithm.

```
D = [ x.*x x.*y y.*y x y ones(size(x)) ];
% Build scatter matrix
S = D'*D;
% Build 6x6 constraint matrix
C(6,6) = 0; C(1,3) = -2; C(2,2) = 1; C(3,1) = -2;
% Solve eigensystem
[gevec, geval] = eig(S,C);
% Find the negative eigenvalue
[NegR, NegC] = find(geval < 0 & ~isinf(geval));
% Get fitted parameters
a = real(gevec(:,NegC));
```

An improved code with prior data scaling can be downloaded from Fitzgibbon's Web site. We have included the improved code in our library without any change except the function name. Figure 9.16 shows the boundary curve of a cell and the direct least-squares fit of the ellipse.

The computed parameters of this ellipse are $C_x = 52.84$, $C_y = 60.06$, $r_x = 8.91$, $r_y = 6.41$, and $\theta = -1.5$. The first two parameters are the coordinates of the center, whereas the following two are the radii in the x and y directions. The last parameter is the angle between the x-axis and the major axis of the ellipse.

9.6   Hough Transform

It is almost always desirable to locate some certain shapes in images for automated analysis and/or detection purposes. The Hough transform is a tool to find or locate some groups of pixels that lie on regular shapes such as lines or circles. Although there is also a generalized version of the Hough transform that can be applied for the detection of any (irregular) shape, we will just deal with its application on detection of lines and circles here. Once the idea behind this tool is understood in the example cases that we will study, the extension of the technique to other possibly more complicated cases will hopefully be simpler.

As we will see in a moment, while implementing the Hough transform, we use parametric equations that describe the shapes; therefore, dealing with regular shapes such as lines and circles whose parametric equation is known is relatively easy.

The first step in the application of the Hough transform is to obtain the edgemap,[*] giving the boundaries of the shapes or objects in our image. This is done through *edge detection*, which is a classical topic in image processing. In the following examples, we use Canny's method for edge detection. This method, along with many others, is implemented in the MATLAB Image Processing Toolbox's edge function. Here is an excerpt regarding the Canny method from the edge function's help documentation:

> The Canny method finds edges by looking for local maxima of the gradient of input image. The gradient is calculated using the derivative of a Gaussian filter. The method uses two thresholds, to detect strong and weak edges, and includes the weak edges in the output only if they are connected to strong edges. This method is therefore less likely than the others to be fooled by noise, and more likely to detect true weak edges.

9.6.1 Line Detection

Let (x_0, y_0) be a point on the edgemap; given this point we aim to find lines that may have given rise to this point. As we see in Figure 9.17, we can have infinitely many lines going through (x_0, y_0).

In Cartesian coordinates, a line can be described by its slope m and its y-axis intercept n as $y = mx + n$. However, this type of representation is not suitable for our line detection purposes. This is because if we calculate the slope and intercept for the possible lines going through (x_0, y_0), we observe that the range of the slope will be from $-\infty$ to ∞, whereas the intercept will luckily be limited by the vertical extent of the image area. To understand why the range of the slope is so wide, start with a horizontal line that passes through our point (x_0, y_0) and start rotating the line in the counterclockwise direction. As

---

[*] In edge detection, through various high-pass-filtering or gradient operations, a grayscale *edge image* is obtained first. The pixels with strong/high values in the edge image are assumed to correspond to the edge areas in the original image. Then, by thresholding the edge image with a suitable threshold, a binary *edgemap* is obtained, where pixels with a value of 1 correspond to possible edges.

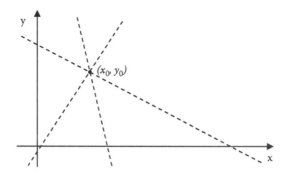

FIGURE 9.17
An infinite number of lines may pass through a point on the edgemap.

we approach a vertical line, the slope increases from 0 to ∞. As soon as we pass 90° (the vertical), the slope (simply being the change in y over the change in x) jumps down to $-\infty$, and it then starts approaching zero from the left.

One remedy to deal with this problem (i.e., to cover a wide range of slopes) could be the use of a logarithmic axis or scale for the slope. Or, instead of dealing with lines in the Cartesian domain, we can use polar coordinates to represent the lines. This is illustrated in Figure 9.18, where L is just one of the many possible lines going through (x_0, y_0) and N is the normal or perpendicular line drawn from the origin to L. The polar representation (see Figure 9.18) is based on the angle θ from the horizontal axis to N and the distance r of L from the origin.

Because the slope of the normal line N is $\tan(\theta)$, the slope of L in terms of θ should be

$$m = -\frac{1}{\tan(\theta)} = -\frac{\cos(\theta)}{\sin(\theta)}.$$

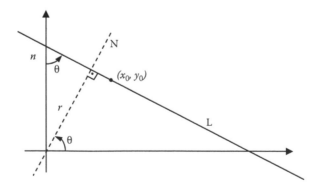

FIGURE 9.18
Polar coordinate system for representation of lines.

Using simple trigonometry, we also find that

$$\sin(\theta) = \frac{r}{n} \text{ or } n = \frac{r}{\sin(\theta)}.$$

Then, if we substitute these expressions for m and n in polar coordinates in our line equation $y = mx + n$, we obtain

$$y = mx + n = -\frac{\cos(\theta)}{\sin(\theta)} x + \frac{r}{\sin(\theta)} \qquad (9.23)$$

$$y \sin(\theta) = -\cos(\theta)x + r \text{ or } r = x\cos(\theta) + y\sin(\theta)$$

This way, we have expressed the line $y = mx + n$ in terms of r and θ. We already know that this line goes trough the point (x_0, y_0), therefore, we can substitute these values in Equation (9.23) and obtain a specific function that relates r and θ:

$$r(\theta) = x_0 \cos(\theta) + y_0 \sin(\theta) \qquad (9.24)$$

We should note here that this function is generated by a single point on the edgemap, and for each point on the edgemap we will have a similar function. That is, Equation (9.24) represents is a *point-to-curve transformation*, and we will have as many of these curves as the number of points (i.e., white pixels or pixels with a value of 1) in the edgemap.

We will now discuss how we can form the 2-D Hough transform matrix (or *accumulator array*, as it is commonly referred to in the literature) for line detection. In order to scan all the possible lines that the points on the edgemap can line on, we need to come up with r and θ arrays first.

As a refresher, we would like to remind the reader at this point that, in our view, images are just matrices with entries consisting of pixel values. In accordance with the matrix indexing scheme, the upper left corner of the image is our origin. Then, the x and y coordinates in terms of row and column indices (i, j) will be $x = j$ and $y = M - i$, where M is the number of rows.

If we go back to the issue of setting up proper arrays for r and θ, we can see that for any point on the edgemap, the distance from the origin r will vary from 0 to R, where R is the largest possible extent of the points on the edgemap from the origin. For an image I, R can be found by issuing the following MATLAB commands:

```
[M,N] = size(I)
R = sqrt(M^2+N^2)
```

The angle θ, on the other hand, will vary from 0 to 2π. Another typically used convention for covering the (r, θ) domain is obtained by letting θ vary from 0 to π and allowing negative values of r to represent the lines in

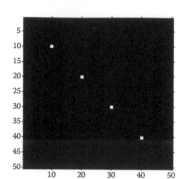

FIGURE 9.19
The test edgemap to demonstrate the sinusoidal structures in the Hough transform.

the upper- and lower-half planes, respectively. Similar to this convention, MATLAB Image Processing Toolbox's hough function uses a convention whereby r and θ, respectively, vary from $-R$ to R and from $-\pi/2$ to $\pi/2$. We leave it to the reader to confirm that all of these different ways of scanning the (r,θ) domain do indeed cover the whole domain, so the information contained in them is equivalent but with differences.

If a number of points lie on the same line, then the sinusoidal curves corresponding to these points will intersect at the (r,θ) location or pair that corresponds to that particular line. The MATLAB below code demonstrates this point nicely.

To simulate an edgemap, we first generate a synthetic image of size 50 by 50 pixels of class logical and place 4 white pixels along the $-45°$ line going through the origin (see Figure 9.19). We then take its Hough transform using the hough function with its defaults, where r and θ resolutions are, respectively, 1 pixel and 1°, and finally display the resultant transform matrix in Figure 9.20.

```
I = logical(zeros(50));
I(10,10) = 1; I(20,20) = 1;
I(30,30) = 1; I(40,40) = 1;
imshow(I,[],'InitialMagnification',100), axis on
[h,theta,radius] = hough(I);
figure
imshow(h,[],'XData',theta,'YData',radius,…
        'InitialMagnification','fit')
axis on, grid
xlabel('\theta')
ylabel('\itr')
h_max = max(h(:)); % h_max is 4
map = gray(h_max); % graylevel colormap
map = map(end:-1:1,:); % reverse the colormap
colormap(map)
```

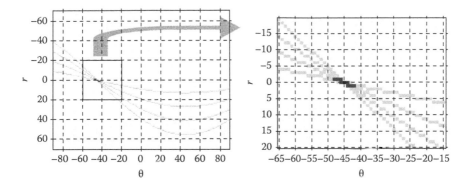

FIGURE 9.20
The Hough transform of the edgemap shown in Figure 9.19. Left panel: The whole transform domain. Right panel: Zoomed view of region around $r = 0$ and $\theta = -45$.

As we see in Figure 9.20, the four sinusoidal curves corresponding to the four points in the edgemap (which we made collinear) intersect at $r = 0$ and $\theta = -45°$ and produce a value of 4 in the Hough transform matrix.

After the Hough transform matrix is obtained, we then look for local maximums corresponding to possible lines in the transform domain. We can then find or extract lines with the desired properties by processing the peak (local maxima) information. These ideas are implemented in the MATLAB Image Processing Toolbox functions houghpeaks and houghlines. The help documentation of these functions and the demos given therein provide plenty of information about line detection applications in image processing.

As a word of caution, we should note here that a noisy edgemap (with some salt-and-pepper type of noise for instance) may confuse the Hough transform and, consequently, can make it difficult to detect lines in the Hough domain. Some morphological operators, such as the removal of isolated single pixels, could be carried out on the edgemap before proceeding with the Hough transform.

9.6.2 Circle Detection

We again obtain an edgemap of the image of interest first; then, while analyzing the points (pixels with a value of 1) in the edgemap, we imagine that those points can potentially lie on a circle. Let (x_0, y_0) be a point in the edgemap; given this point, we need to locate the centers of the circles with radius r that may have given rise to this point. The location, that is, the centers (a, b) of those circles, is given by the following equation of a circle:

$$(x_0 - a)^2 + (y_0 - b)^2 = r^2 \tag{9.25}$$

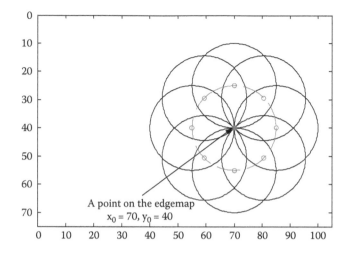

FIGURE 9.21
Several possible circles (solid line) that may have produced the white pixel at $(x_0, y_0) = (70, 40)$.
The geometric location of all possible circles (centers) is shown the by the dashed line.

Let us illustrate how several different circles can give rise to the same point on the edgemap, using MATLAB. Here, for a point on the edgemap with coordinates $(x_0, y_0) = (70, 40)$, we will draw eight circles that may have produced this point. The result is shown in Figure 9.21.

```
function demo_circle
x = 70; y = 40; r = 15;
delta_theta = pi/4;
theta = 0:delta_theta:2*pi-delta_theta;
L = length(theta);
a = x+r*cos(theta);
b = y+r*sin(theta);
hold on
for i = 1:L
    draw_circle(a(i),b(i),r,'k')
end
draw_circle(x,y,r,'r--')
axis image, axis ij, box on
axis([0 100 0 100])


function draw_circle(x,y,r,linestyle)
theta = 0:pi/100:pi/2;
xr = r*cos(theta); yr = r*sin(theta);
plot(x+[xr -yr -xr yr],y+[yr xr -yr -xr],linestyle)
plot(x,y,'ro') % mark the center
```

Using these ideas, we first set up an accumulator array for each radius value that we would like to work with. We then scan through all of the points in the edgemap, and for each point we find possible center locations using Equation (9.25). Consequently, we update or increase the accumulator values at those center locations by 1. This is demonstrated in Figure 9.22, where the point of interest in the edgemap is shown with the cross sign and all of the potential circles with centers (a,b) that may have given rise to this point are marked with circles. To make the update of the (a,b) centers in the accumulator array faster, we have employed a little programming trick that is also shown in the figure. Instead of going through all the points along the circle, we covered just 1/8th of the circle with a loop, and determined the other possible center locations using circular symmetry. We note that because we are operating on a pixel grid, the actual center locations (indicated by the solid line circle in the figure) are rounded to the closest pixel positions (i.e., small circles).

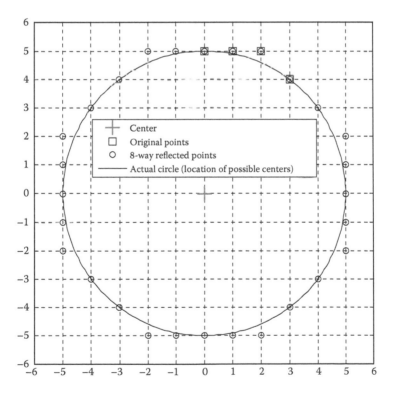

FIGURE 9.22
Given a point (white pixel) on the edgemap (the cross mark), the small circles show the centers in the (a, b) accumulator array to be incremented by 1.

The following MATLAB code processes an edgemap to locate centers of the circles with radius `rmin` to `rmax` and fills in a 3-D accumulator array:

```
function h = miphoughcircle(edgeim,rmin,rmax)
% Implements Hough transform for circle detection
% edgemap is the input binary image
% rmin and rmax are min and max radii for possible
% circles in the edgemap


% first initialize the Hough transform accumulator array h
[rows,cols] = size(edgeim);
nradii = rmax-rmin+1;% number of different radii that we
% will search
h = uint16(zeros(rows,cols,nradii));
% h is 3-dimensional, the 3rd dimension is the radius
% dimension


% Find coordinates of the edge points (white pixels)
[i,j] = find(edgeim); % i: y
npoints = length(i); % j: x


% Increment accumulator values for possible centers for
% each radii
fprintf('Doing circle search from radius %d to …
    %d\n',rmin,rmax)
for n = 1:nradii
    radius = n+rmin-1;
    h2 = zeros(rows,cols);
    for pt = 1:npoints
        h2 = mipaddcircle(h2,j(pt),i(pt),rows,cols,…
                        radius);
        end
    h(:,:,n) = h2; % n is the index in the radius dim.
    % Progress indicator
fprintf('Searching circles at radius %d (%d/%d)\n',…
  radius,n,nradii)
end


function h = mipaddcircle(h,cx,cy,hr,hc,radius)
% This function does the circle search for a given
% (single) radius
% in the Hough transform accumulator array h
% h is the 2-d accumulator array (indicating the strength of
% possible centers)
% (cx,cy) is a white pixel on the edgemap
% hr and hc are row and column size of the edgemap
```

```
% first find x and y coordinates for a circular arc
% (1/8th of a circle) with the given radius
x = 0:fix(radius/sqrt(2)); y = round(sqrt(radius^2-x.^2));

% Now fill in the 8-way symmetric points on the circle
% and shift the origin to the given white pixel
px = cx + [x x -x -x y y -y -y];
py = cy + [y -y y -y x -x x -x];

% (px,py) are the possible centers for circles that may have
% produced the white pixel (cx,cy) on the edgemap

% remove points that are outside the limits
validx = px>=1 & px<=hc;
validy = py>=1 & py<=hr;
valid = find(validx & validy);
px = px(valid); py = py(valid);

% update the accumulator array value at the correct index
ind = py+(px-1)*hr;
h(ind) = h(ind)+1;
```

Once we carry out the Hough transform and obtain the accumulator array indicating the strength of possible circle centers, we need to find the local maximums in the 3-D accumulator array. We have developed the following function to accomplish this task. This function utilizes the bwlabeln function, which labels connected components in a binary matrix of arbitrary dimensions, of the MATLAB Image Processing Toolbox. In our case, connected components correspond to possible circle centers.

```
function mipextractcircles(I,h,rmin,thres)
% This function detects the possible circles in the Hough
% transform matrix h by checking the local maxima
% I is the original image on which the detected circles
% will be overlaid
imshow(I,[]), hold on
[r,c] = size(I);
% thres is the cutoff to threshold the 3-d Hough transform
% accumulator array h
% for instance thres could be 50% of the max. value of h,
% i.e. thres = .5*max(h(:));
bwh = h > thres;
% Form labeled connected components and reduce the number of
% possible circles to a reasonable size (in this case 30) by
% increasing the thresholding level successively by 5%
[bwh,nregions] = bwlabeln(bwh); nregions
while nregions>30
```

```
        thres = 1.05*thres;
        bwh = h > thres;
        [bwh,nregions] = bwlabeln(bwh); nregions
end
% initialize the vectors for storing centers(x,y) and radii
% of the circles to be extracted/detected
% maxvec is the circular strength vector
% strength of a detected circle is calculated as the ratio
% of points on the circle, i.e. the current local maxima
% of h,
% to the radius of the circle
xvec = zeros(nregions,1);
yvec = xvec; radvec = xvec; maxvec = xvec;
for i = 1:nregions
        % Form a mask for each region
        mask = uint16(bwh==i);
        % Extract the region from the 3-d Hough transform
        region = immultiply(mask,h);
        % catch the local maximum and its location
        [maxval,z] = max(region(:));
        depth = fix(z/r/c)+1;
        [maxval,x] = max(region(:,:,depth));
        [maxval,y] = max(maxval); x = x(y);
        xvec(i) = y; yvec(i) = x;
        radius = depth+rmin-1;
        radvec(i) = radius; maxvec(i) = double(maxval)/
        radius;
        fprintf('Possible circle found at center [%d %d] with …
           radius %d\n',y,x,radius)
end
% sort the circles according to their strength
[maxsort,idx] = sort(maxvec,'descend');
xvec = xvec(idx); yvec = yvec(idx);
radvec = radvec(idx); maxvec = maxvec(idx);


% remove (filter out) circles with close centers
xthres = .04*c; ythres = .04*r;
Rlim = xthres^2+ythres^2;
jlist = cell(nregions-1,1);
for i = 1:nregions-1
        for j = i+1:nregions
            dist = (xvec(i)-xvec(j))^2+(yvec(i)-yvec(j))^2;
            if dist<Rlim
                jlist{i} = [jlist{i} j];
            end
        end
end
all_close_list = cat(2,jlist[13]);
idx_remove = unique(all_close_list)
```

```
idx_good = setdiff(1:nregions,idx_remove)
lengood = length(idx_good);
fprintf(sprintf('%d circles are detected...\n',lengood))
for i = idx_good
    fprintf('Circle detected at center [%d %d] with …
        radius %d and strength %.2f\n',yvec(i),xvec(i), …
        radvec(i),maxvec(i))
    circle([xvec(i),yvec(i)],radvec(i),'w')
end


function circle(c,r,lcolor)
nsides = 16; a = [0:pi/nsides:2*pi];
line(r*cos(a)+c(1),r*sin(a)+c(2),'color',lcolor,'linew',2)
```

Before we apply our implementation of the Hough transform for circle detection to a real-life biomedical problem such as cell counting, it is a good idea to test it on a synthetic image containing circles. We first generate a binary image with a circular ring using the following simple MATLAB function:

```
function I = generate_test_circle(S,a,b,d)
% S is size of the square test image
% (a,b) is the center and d is the radius of the ring
I = logical(zeros(S));
lim1 = (d-1)^2;
lim2 = (d+1)^2;
for x = -d:d
    for y = -d:d
        C = x^2+y^2;
        if C >=lim1 & C<=lim2
            row = b-y; col = a+x;
            I(row,col) = 1;
        end
    end
end
end
```

We can then use these functions to confirm that our circle detection method works properly as expected. (Examine the following MATLAB code whose result is shown in Figure 9.23.)

```
I = generate_test_circle(100,50,50,20);
subplot(1,2,1), imshow(I,[]), axis on
title('Test Image: A Circle with Radius 20 at center …
    [50,50]')
r1 = 10; r2 = 30;
h = miphoughcircle(I,r1,r2);
```

Test Image: A Circle with Radius
20 at Center [50,50]

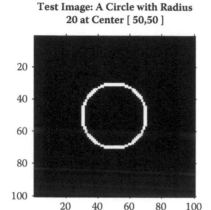

Detected Circle

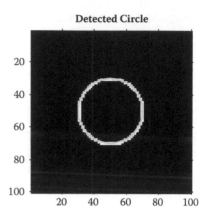

FIGURE 9.23
Left panel: A synthetic edgemap containing a circular ring. Right panel: The circle detected (gray) using our Hough transform functions/routines is overlaid on the original synthetic edgemap.

```
thres = .5*max(h(:));
subplot(1,2,2)
mipextractcircles(I,h,r1,thres), axis on
title('Detected circle')
```

To further investigate how the Hough transform of our synthetic image looks, we can generate a 3-D view of our accumulator array using the following MATLAB commands. The resultant graph is shown in Figure 9.24, where we observe that the maximum is visible at the slice taken for $r = 20$.

```
figure
h = double(h);
x = 1:100;
r = 10:30; % radius range
graph_handle = slice(x,x,r,h,[],[],10:5:30);
alpha('color')
set(graph_handle,'EdgeColor','none','FaceColor','interp',…
                 'FaceAlpha','interp')
alphamap('rampdown')
alphamap('decrease',.2)
colormap(hsv)
xlabel('Circle Center X Coordinate')
ylabel('Circle Center Y Coordinate')
zlabel('Circle Radius')
title('Slices from 3-D Hough Transform Matrix of the …
  Test Image')
```

Slices from 3-D Hough Transform Matrix of the Test Image

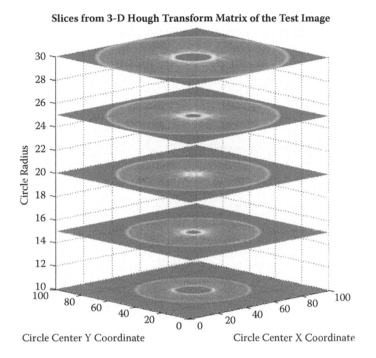

FIGURE 9.24

Three-dimensional view of the Hough transform of the synthetic edgemap consisting of a circular ring centered at (50, 50).

We will now apply our circle detection method on some embryo images, with our aim being to count the number of cells in the embryo. This can be handy for automated analysis or for processing of embryo images at an in vitro fertilization (IVF) lab, for instance. The following MATLAB function `mipcelldetect` loads the image of interest first; it then converts the input image into grayscale if necessary and performs the edge detection using Canny's method. Next, it displays the edgemap so that the user can see whether the circular structures in the edgemap are identifiable. Then, it asks the user to click on two points at the edges of the smallest and largest circular structures in the edgemap to determine the minimum and maximum radii values. (These are radii limits within which we will do the circle search.) As the final step, it calls the Hough transform functions that we have discussed previously and overlays the detected circles on the original image. Two test embryo images and the results of circle detection on these images are shown in Figures 9.25 and 9.26.

```
function mipcelldetect
% Cell detection demo on embryo images using the Hough
% transform
if nargin==0 % no input image is supplied (ask for one)
    fn = uigetfile({'*.jpg';'*.tif';'*.png';'*.*'});
    if isempty(fn)
        return
    end
    try
        [I,map] = imread(fn);
    catch
        error('Could not read the image file...')
    end
    Iinfo = imfinfo(fn);
    imtype = Iinfo.ColorType;
    if ~strcmp(imtype,'grayscale')
        disp('Input image is not grayscale, trying to …
          convert it to grayscale...')
        if imtype == 'truecolor'
          I = rgb2gray(I);
        elseif imtype == 'indexed' & ~isempty(map)
          I = ind2gray(I,map);
        else
            error('Could not convert the image into  …
                    graylevel format...')
        end
    end
end
clf, imshow(I,[]), pause
eI = edge(I,'canny',.3);
% display complemented version of the edgemap for efficient
% printing
imshow(~eI), axis on, pause
xlabel(sprintf('There are %d "on" pixels in the …
                edgemap',sum(eI(:)))), pause
title('Select small diameter by clicking on two points …
  on a potential small circle')
[x,y] = getpts; line(x,y,'color','k'), pause
r1 = floor(max(abs([diff(x) diff(y)]))/2);
title('Select large diameter by clicking on two points …
  on a potential large circle')
[x,y] = getpts; line(x,y,'color','k')
pause
r2 = ceil(max(abs([diff(x) diff(y)]))/2);
h = houghcircle(eI,r1,r2);
thres = .5*max(h(:));
mipextractcircles(I,h,r1,thres)
```

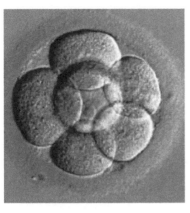

**Select Small Diameter by Clicking on Two Points
on a Potential Small Circle**

**Select Small Diameter by Clicking on Two Points
on a Potential Small Circle**

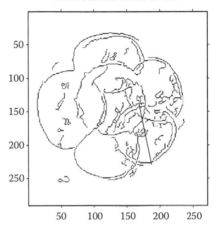

There are 2921 "on" Pixels in the Edgemap

**Select Large Diameter by Clicking on
Two Points on a Potential Large Circle**

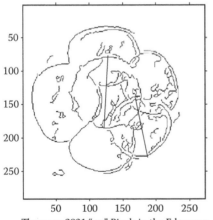

There are 2921 "on" Pixels in the Edgemap

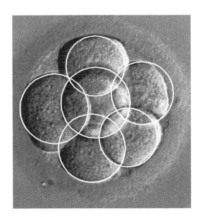

FIGURE 9.25
Upper left: Original embryo image. Upper right: Edgemap of the embryo image. Lower left:
Determination of search range for the radius. Lower right: Detected six circles overlaid on
the embryo image. (Image courtesy of Advanced Fertility Center of Chicago, http://www.
advancedfertility.com/pics/8 cell.jpg)

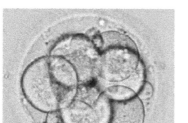

Select Small Diameter by Clicking on Two Points on a Potential Small Circle

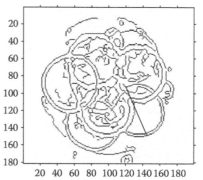

There are 2914 "on" Pixels in the Edgemap

Select Large Diameter By Clicking On Two Points On A Potential Large Circle

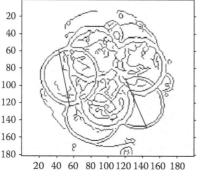

There are 2914 "on" Pixels in the Edgemap

FIGURE 9.26
Upper left: Original embryo image. Upper right: Edgemap of the embryo image. Lower left: Determination of search range for the radius. Lower right: Detected six circles overlaid on the embryo image. (Image courtesy of IVF Dallas, http://www.ivfdallas.com/images/embryo-division_lg.jpg.)

Problems

1. For a closed curve approximated by set of points, show that the relation for the curve length is given by Equation (9.8).

2. What should be the sampling rate for a boundary curve to estimate the curve length with 10% error?

3. What should be the pixel size to estimate the area enclosed by the object boundary with 10% error? Hint: Use the MATLAB function `polyarea`.

4. Explain how the rotation of the object affects curvature calculations.

5. Explain how the scaling of objects can affect curvature values.

6. Explain how flipping (left–right flip) of a sequence of boundary points can affect curvature values.

7. Load the vertebra image and detect the boundary curve and create the scale-space representation of the curvature of the boundary. Perform multiresolution analysis to identify the salient minimum curvature points on the boundary.

References

1. R. M. Haralick, K. Shanmugam, and I. H. Dinstein, Textural features for image classification, *IEEE Trans. on Systems, Man, and Cybernetics* 3: 610–621, 1973.
2. R. M. Haralick, K. Shanmugam, and I. H. Dinstein, Measure of circularity of digital figures, *IEEE Trans on Systems, Man, and Cybernetics* 4: 394–396, 1974.
3. W. Blaschke, *Vorlesungen uber Differentialgeometrie II*. Berlin: Springer, 1923.
4. I. M. Anderson and J. C. Bezdek, Curvature and deflection of discrete arcs: A theory based on the commutator of scatter matrix pairs and its application to vertex detection in planar shape data, *IEEE Trans. on Pattern Analysis and Machine Intelligence* 6: 27–40, 1984.
5. T. Lindeberg, *Scale-Space Theory in Computer Vision*: Norwell, MA: Kluwer Academic Publishers, 1994.
6. B. T. H. Romeny, *Front-End Vision and Multi-Scale Image Analysis*: Dordrecht, the Netherlands: Kluwer Academic Publishers, 2003.
7. J. Sporring, M. Nielsen, L. M. J. Florack, and P. Johansen, eds. *Gaussian Scale-Space Theory*, vol. 8 of computational imagins and vision series, 2nd ed. Dordrecht, the Netherlands: Kluwer Academic Publishers, 1997.
8. A. P. Witkin, Scale-space filtering, presented at 8th *Int. Joint Conf. Art. Intell.*, Karlsruhe, Germany, 1983.
9. J. Koenderink, The structure of images, *Biological Cybernetics* 50: 363–370, 1984.
10. F. Mokhtarian and A. Mackworth, Scale-based description and recognition of planar curves and two-dimensional shapes, *IEEE Trans. on Pattern Analysis and Machine Intelligence* 8: 34–43, 1986.
11. D. G. Lowe, Organization of smooth image curves at multiple scales, presented at ICCV, Tampa, FL, 1988.
12. A. W. Fitzgibbon, M. Pilu, and R. B. Fisher, Direct least-squares fitting of ellipses, *IEEE Trans. on Pattern Analysis and Machine Intelligence* 21: 476–480, 1999.
13. N. R. Pal, and S. K. Pal. 1993. A review on image segmentation techiniques. *Pattern Recogn* 26(9): 1277–1294.

Application 1

Quantification of Green Fluorescent Protein eXpression in Live Cells: ProXcell

CONTENTS

A.1.1 Introduction

The green fluorescent protein (GFP) is a protein produced by jellyfish, such as *Aequorea victoria*. It is a special protein that emits fluorescence when excited by UV light. When introduced into other living organisms, it makes them fluoresce.

It is possible to generate the DNA sequence or the gene that codes GFP. To introduce or express the GFP protein in various cells, the GFP-coding DNA sequence is fused downstream of a suitable promoter DNA sequence presented in a special type of DNA molecule called expression vectors. Promoters control transcription of genes, that is, the making of messenger RNA (mRNA). The mRNAs are ultimately decoded to make protein in a process called *translation*. The expression vectors having the GFP gene can be introduced into the cells by the process called *transfection* mediated by lipofectamine reagent. In this process, lipofectamine is mixed with vector DNA, resulting in the formation of lipid–DNA complexes. These complexes are easily taken up by cells through *phagocytosis* or membrane fusion. A successful transfection will result in the expression of GFP gene and, hence, green fluorescence of the cells. The entire cytoplasm or nucleus will light up green when excited with UV light, as the GFP protein is distributed throughout the cell. The amount of fluorescence produced depends on the number of active GFP molecules made. In

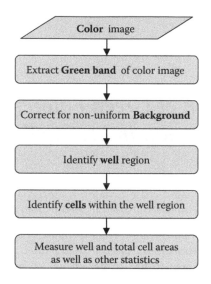

FIGURE A.1.1
The flowchart of image processing and analysis.

this case, the GFP plays a role similar to that of a reporter gene. Reporter genes are frequently used in vivo or in vitro molecular imaging to monitor the expression or repression of genes, that is, the amount of mRNA or proteins made.

In this study, the biologist was interested in quantifying the amount of green fluorescence protein expressed in live cells that are treated under different experimental conditions.

The cells grown at standard culture conditions, 3×10^4 cells per well in 96-well plates, were transected with the GFP plasmids. The GFP constructs emit light at 503 nm, which falls within the lower green portion of the visible spectrum, when excited at the optimum excitation wavelength of 488 nm. To quantify the amount of protein expression in cells, we applied a series of image processing and analysis methods. The flowchart of image processing and analysis is shown in Figure A.1.1. In the following sections, we will explain each step along with the MATLAB code. The sample images presented here are made available on our Web site (see Appendix D).

A.1.2 Image Acquisition

The images of cells consisting of ~1944 × 2592 pixels were captured in color using a Zeiss fluorescence microscope. In all cases, exposure time, zoom, and other settings were kept constant to allow fair comparison of different experimental conditions.

A.1.3 Nonuniform Background Correction

Images were captured by a high-resolution digital color camera. As we are interested only in the green fluorescence, we first extracted the green band of the color image. This may simply be done by

```
Gimg = Img(:,:2)
```

These images may suffer from serious nonuniform illumination. As seen in Figure A.1.2, the intensities are brighter in the center of the well than they are in the periphery.

To remove this nonuniformity, we first reduced the image size by about 60%. The main reason for this reduction is to decrease the processing time. As the nonuniform illumination is a low-frequency signal, that is, it gradually changes over the image space, the size reduction does not affect the background illumination pattern. Before we reduce the size, we save the number of rows and columns of the original image. Then we use a morphological opening (imopen) operation with a disk-shaped structuring element. The size of the structuring element depends on the size of the cells within the image. As the cell size will vary with magnification, disk size at one magnification may not work on images captured at another magnification. Then the opened image is filtered using a Gaussian filter to blur out sharp edges that may result from the opening operation. Finally, we resized the image to its original size before we subtract this nonuniform illumination pattern from the gray-level image. The following MATLAB code performs the operations described above. Figure A.1.2 shows, on the right, the computed nonuniform illumination pattern.

```
se = strel('disk',15);
h = fspecial('gaussian',11,2);
[rov,col = size(Gimg)
```

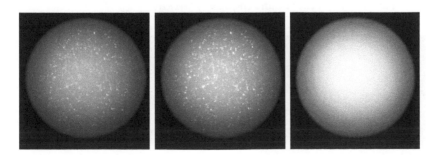

FIGURE A.1.2
Original color image (left), its green band (middle), and the computed background nonuniformity (right).

```
sImg = imresize(Gimg,0.4);
bkg = imopen(sImg,se);
blurred = imfilter(bkg,h,'replicate');
blurred = imresize(blurred,[row,col]);
nGimg = Gimg-blurred;
```

A.1.4   Segmentation of Well Region

As seen in Figure A.1.2, the well region has distinct gray-level character-istics compared to the dark background around it. To improve the cell segmentation, we segment the well region first.

This can be done using the thresholding method of Otsu (see Chapter 6) applied to the background illumination pattern. Following the closing operation, objects smaller than a certain size are removed. As we are inter-ested in a very large object, the size threshold is not difficult to choose. In this application it was chosen as 50 pixels. As we have a fairly large back-ground around the well region, we wanted to crop the well region again to save memory and speed in the ensuing processes. To do this, we label the binary image and compute the bounding box for the well region. We use this bounding box to crop the well region. In the following MATLAB code, the well region from the labeled image was identified as the region with the largest area. Figure A.1.3 shows the segmented well region (left) and the cropped well region already corrected for the nonuniform illumi-nation (middle).

```
% identify well region
thw = otsu_th(double(blurred),64);
bwdish = Gimg>round(thw);
bwdish = bwareaopen(bwdish,50);

% Extract the well region
L = bwlabel(bwdish);
s = regionprops(L,'BoundingBox','Area');
```

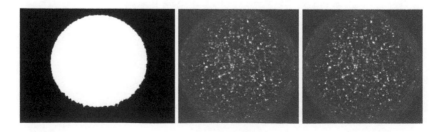

FIGURE A.1.3
The identified well region (left), cropped well region before (middle), and after (right) aniso-tropic diffusion filtering.

```
[mx,idx] = max([s.Area]);
rect = round(s(idx).BoundingBox);
csub = imcrop(nGimg,rect);
[r,c] = size(csub);
bwdish = ismember(L,idx);
```

A.1.5 Anisotropic Diffusion Filtering

The corrected and cropped well region is further processed to filter the noise in the image to improve the performance of the following cell segmentation step. Anisotropic diffusion filtering methods are discussed in Chapter 5. This code filters the cropped image csub using our function anisodifftwod with the parameters given. Figure A.1.3 shows the filtered image (right). Although it is not very visible, the filtering removes the noise and improves the segmentation.

```
% Anisotropic diffusion filtering
csub = anisodifftwod(csub,5,8,0.25);
```

A.1.6 Segmentation of Cells

Then, the cells within the well region are segmented by applying the minimum-error thresholding algorithm (see Chapter 6) twice as seen in the following code:

```
% Identify cell pixels
thc1 = kittler_th(single(csub),64);
H1 = csub(csub > thc1);
H2 = H1(H1 > thc1);
thc2 = kittler_th(single(H2),64);
bwcell = gray2multilevel(csub,[thc1 thc2]);
bwcell = bwcell>2;
```

The reason for applying the thresholding twice is that the intensity distribution of the cell population is not uniform, primarily due to the focusing of the microscope. The segmented cells are shown in Figure A.1.4 as white regions.

After the identification of cells, the total cell and well areas in pixels, and the total green intensity within the cell regions were calculated and saved into an ASCII file in tab-delimited format.

The area is computed by adding the number of pixels, whereas total green intensity is computed by adding the intensities of the pixels belonging to the cell population.

We integrated all the aforementioned steps in a graphical user interface (GUI) named *ProXcell*. The screenshot of the GUI is shown in Figure A.1.5.

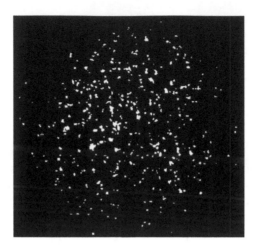

FIGURE A.1.4
Segmented cells.

The GUI allows processing a single image as well as multiple images in batch mode. The different cell cultures are placed into the wells of a 98-well plate. The new image acquisition system captures the images of the wells as one image. Then, each cropped well region is saved as a separate image and undergoes the processes shown in Figure A.1.1.

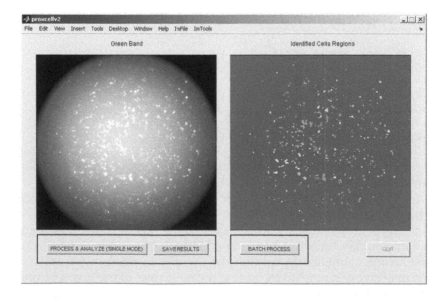

FIGURE A.1.5
The screenshot of the GUI named *ProXcell*.

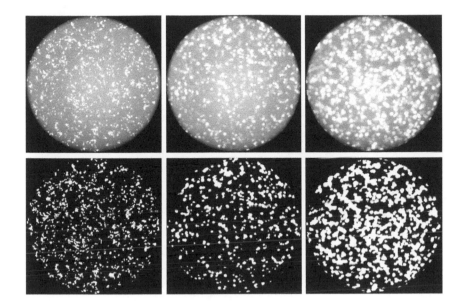

FIGURE A.1.6
A set of images in which cell populations have different levels of GFP expression: green bands of the color images (top row); identified cell regions (bottom row). The total green intensities in cell areas (left to right) are: 66,392,666; 79,220,850; 187,097,491.

Figure A.1.6 shows a set of images in which cell populations have different levels of GFP expression. The method presented previously and amalgamated into the GUI *ProXcell* was used by biologists to quantify the GFP expression and the results were published in Al-Zoghaibi et al. [1].

Reference

1. Al-Zoghaibi, F., Ashour, T., Al-Ahmadi, W., Abulleef, H., Demirkaya, O., and Khabar, K. S. A., Bioinformatics and experimental derivation of an efficient hybrid 3' untranslated region and use in expression active linear DNA with minimum poly(A) region, *Gene* **391**(1–2): 130–139, 2007.

Application 2

Calculation of Performance Parameters of Gamma Cameras and SPECT Systems

CONTENTS

A.2.1 Introduction

Medical physicists working in the field of nuclear medicine have to perform a battery of tests routinely on their gamma camera systems (GCSs), known as routine quality control (QC) testing. Such tests are essential to both measuring the performance characteristics and ensuring that the images produced by GCSs are clinically uncompromised. Among these tests, flood field uniformity is performed daily by technologists to check both image uniformity and any other significant defect that may have occurred since the last flood field verification. The technologist should also be looking for more subtle changes that may occur gradually over time.

Normally, a more rigorous testing known as *acceptance testing* is performed at installation to verify if the camera performs as published in the manufacturer's specification sheet, to establish the baseline parameters, and to identify any other problems that gamma cameras may have. Although manufacturers are supposed to test their systems at the factory before shipment, the condition of a system may deteriorate during the

379

shipment. There may even be problems that go unnoticed, if the system is not thoroughly checked during the factory testing.

Acceptance testing, similar to regular QC testing, consists of three main steps. These include (1) preparation of the test equipment, usually a phantom; (2) data acquisition; and (3) analysis or the calculation of the performance parameter. In acceptance testing, all of these steps may be rather involved and complicated. The National Electrical Manufacturers Association (NEMA) has published a guideline [1] that standardizes these steps. In this guideline, these steps are described in detail to avoid potential variations in implementations. Due to the complexity of the data acquired in some of these tests, it is very difficult to do the calculations without sophisticated software [2]. In general, the vendor provides analysis tools sufficient to analyze the QC tests performed routinely, but they may not include all the necessary tools to analyze the data acquired in an acceptance test.

In this application, we present some image analysis methods to show how to calculate some of the performance parameters of GCSs from the image data generated in an acceptance or routine QC testing. Our principle aim here is to show how advanced image processing techniques can be utilized to automate the sophisticated calculations in the acceptance testing of gamma cameras. We have developed a comprehensive software application named *GCAnalyze* [2] that performs most of the calculations required in an acceptance testing. In the following sections, we present ways to approach the problem at hand. We by no means imply that these are the best methods. Rather, our intention here is to show how one can approach an image analysis problem.

A.2.2 Resolution from Line Source

In gamma cameras, resolution is expressed in terms of full width at half maximum (FWHM) and full width at tenth maximum (FWTM) measured from a line-source profile. A typical profile looks similar to the Gaussian profile shown in Figure A.2.1. To calculate FWHM and FWTM, one approach is to fit a Gaussian function to the line-source profile and calculate the resolution parameters using the relation *full width at percent maximum* defined by

$$FWPM(p) = 2\sqrt{-2 * \ln(p)}\sigma \qquad (11.1)$$

where $0 < p \leq 1$ is the percentage of the maximum. Note that FWHM (i.e., $FWPM(0.5)$) and FWTM (i.e., $FWPM(0.1)$) are equal to $2.3548*\sigma$ and 4.2919σ, respectively.

However, the algorithm we describe in the following text, which is suggested by NEMA, first finds the peak point with maximum counts in the

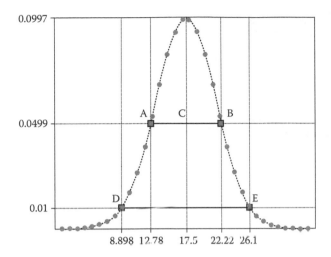

FIGURE A.2.1
A Gaussian profile in which FWHM points A and B along with the center point C and FWTM points D and E are denoted.

profile and then fits a parabola to the peak and its adjoining points, that is, a three-point parabolic fit. The maximum of the profile is then recalculated using the parameters of the fitted parabola. The actual FWHM points A and B shown in Figure A.2.1 are calculated through linear interpolation using the points just above and below the half-maximum value. Similarly, the FWTM points D and E, shown in Figure A.2.1, are also calculated using the points just above and below the tenth-maximum value. This method may be more appropriate if the line-source profile deviates from a Gaussian profile.

Let us demonstrate the calculation steps described here on a line profile extracted from an actual image of a dual-line-source acquired by a gamma camera. We need only one line source.

Let us first read our dual-line-source image (Figure A.2.2 [left]), which is in Digital Image Communication in Medicine (DICOM) format. It can be read using the MATLAB function dicomread. Next, we interactively crop a region of interest (ROI; the middle image in Figure A.2.2) including only one of the line sources. Then we average three adjacent profiles (or rows) somewhere in the middle of the ROI to obtain a single profile whose graph is shown in Figure A.2.2 (right). Averaging multiple line profiles may affect the resolution adversely if the line source is slanted and not perfectly straight. The following script reads the image, allows cropping of the ROI, and averages three profiles in the middle of the ROI image:

```
ImInfo = dicominfo('NM0001.dcm');
Img = dicomread(ImInfo);
subImg = imcrop;
```

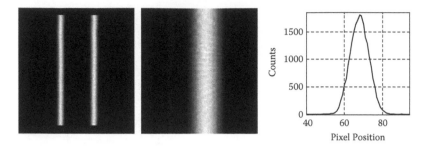

FIGURE A.2.2
Left: Image of a dual-line source acquired by a gamma camera. Middle: Image of the cropped ROI including single-line source. Right: Average of three profiles in the middle of the ROI.

```
lprof = mean(subImg(round(size(subImg,1)/2)...
  -1:round(size(subImg,1)/2)+1,:),1);
```

Now we can find the maximum of the new profile and its location to identify the maximum and its two adjoining points to fit a three-point parabola. The following script performs all these tasks:

```
pixelSize = ImInfo.PixelSpacing(1);
[my,mp] = max(lprof);
x = pixelSize*(mp-1): pixelSize(mp+1);
y = lprof(mp-1:mp+1);
p = polyfit(x, y, 2);
```

After fitting the parabola, we calculate the new peak value and its position before we proceed with the calculation of the FWHM and FWTM values. The following code carries out these tasks:

```
peakpos = -(p(2)/(p(1)*2));
calcPeak = p(1)*peakpos^2+p(2)*peakpos+p(3);
fwpmValue = calcPeak*0.5;
```

In the following script, we threshold our profile to identify the points right above and below the FWHM values. Note that this is done using the MATLAB function find. Then, using a simple linear interpolation, we estimate the location of the calculated FWHM values denoted by A and B in Figure A.2.1. We can also calculate the location of the center of the profile, which is denoted by C in Figure A.2.1, by simply using the points of the FWHM.

```
bw = lprof > fwpmValue;
[L,numR] = bwlabel(bw);
Label = L(mp);
ppf = find(L == Label,1,'first');
pps = find(L == Label,1,'last');

FWPMP(1) = ppf - (lprof(ppf) - ...
  fwpmValue )/(lprof(ppf)-lprof(ppf-1));
```

```
FWPMP(2) = pps + (lprof(pps) - ...
   fwpmValue )/(lprof(pps)-lprof(pps+1));
FWPM = FWPMP(2) - FWPMP(1);
centerPos = FWPMP(1) + (FWPMP(2) - FWPMP(1))/2;
```

We integrated this code into our function `mipresolutionlineProfile` for general use. We will be employing this function in the next section to calculate the resolution from a point source.

A.2.3   Resolution from Point Sources

In single photon emission tomography (SPECT), the x and y resolutions from the image of a point source or line source are calculated to find the resolution characteristics of a SPECT system, which are known as *radial*, *central*, and *tangential* resolutions. These parameters are defined in terms of the x and y resolutions of multiple point sources or cross sections of the line sources scanned in SPECT mode. In this section, we will describe how to calculate the x and y resolutions from a given point source.

After the selection of a rectangular ROI centered at the pixel with maximum count inside the point source, the ROI is summed along the rows (x direction) and columns (y direction). The resultant profiles are the y and x profiles of a point source, respectively. These two profiles are analyzed using the method discussed in the previous section.

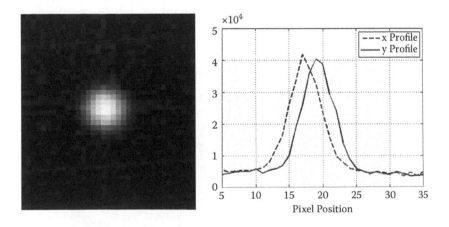

FIGURE A.2.3
Left: Transaxial slice from the tomographic image of a line source. The point source seen in the image is a cross section of a line source. Right: Profiles obtained by columnwise and rowwise summations of the left image.

We will demonstrate this process using our point source image shown in Figure A.2.3. Let us assume that our image represents the ROI centered on its maximum-count pixel and is saved into the matrix subImg. First, we sum along the two directions to produce the x and y count profiles. The following two statements calculate the x and y profiles:

```
xprof = sum(subImg,2);
yprof = sum(subImg,1);
```

To calculate the FWHM points, we will run our function on xprof and yprof as seen in the following statements:

```
P = 0.5;
[FWHMX,FWHMPX,fpeakx] = mipresolutionlineProfile(xprof, P);
[FWHMY,FWHMPY,fpeaky] = mipresolutionlineProfile(yprof',P);
```

The output parameter FWHMX holds the FWHM value for the x profile and the location of the points A and B. We can calculate FWTM and the locations of the points D and E by setting P equal to 0.1. The last line in the preceding code calculates the resolution from the y profile. Note that our function accepts the profiles in row vector format; therefore, we transpose the y profile (which is in column vector format).

A.2.4 Dual or Multiple Line Profile Analysis and Pixel Size Measurement

The intrinsic (i.e., without the collimator in place) resolution of gamma cameras is measured by means of a slit phantom, which comprises of 1-mm-wide parallel slits that are 30 mm apart (see Figure A.2.4 [right]).

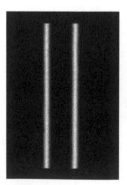 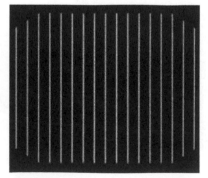

FIGURE A.2.4
Left: Image of a dual-line source acquired by a gamma camera to measure the system spatial resolution without scatter. Right: Image of a slit phantom captured by a gamma camera.

This phantom is mounted on the head of the gamma camera without the collimator in place (hence the name "intrinsic"). The function of the collimator is to collimate the photons coming at the detectors (for a detailed discussion of GCS, see Chapter 1).

Medical physicists in nuclear medicine calculate the intrinsic resolution of gamma cameras from the count profiles of the slits in an image. They also measure the pixel size using the known distance between the slits. In addition to the intrinsic resolution, the slit phantoms are used to calculate another important characteristic of gamma cameras, the linearity. Linearity is defined as the standard deviation of the measured peak locations (denoted by C in Figure A.2.1). Although we will not discuss it here, our resolution function can be used to calculate the linearity as well because it returns the peak location.

Now we will explain how one can calculate the resolution and pixel size from the profile of a dual-line source using simple image processing techniques. However, this can easily be extended to the case of multiple line sources.

First, the profile across the two line sources is thresholded at a level half the maximum count. The locations of the maximum intensities (denoted by the filled stars in Figure A.2.5) within each peak region, which is shown by the gray bar in the same figure, are found. The line-source resolution method described in Section A.2.2 is applied to the points around each peak to compute the center points C_1 and C_2 denoted in Figure A.2.5 and then the distance between them. The pixel size is given by the relation D_A/D_M (mm/pixel), where D_A is the actual distance in millimeter and D_M is the measured distance in pixels.

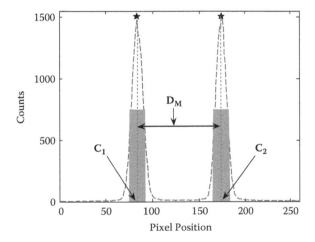

FIGURE A.2.5
Graph demonstrating dual profile analysis and pixel size measurement. The dashed line is the profile across a dual-line-source profile. The solid bars denote the identified peak regions. The vertical dotted lines denote the location of center points, $C_{1,2}$.

Let us demonstrate this on our dual-line-source image shown in Figure A.2.4 (left). Here, the two line sources are exactly 50 mm apart. We assume that our cropped image includes the two line sources perpendicular to the x axis. First, we average three neighboring rows in the middle of the image to reduce the noise, and then find the maximum intensity in the profile. The average profile is thresholded at one quarter of the maximum. Although it is a one-dimensional (1-D) signal or vector, we treat the binary profile as an image and label it using the MATLAB function bwlabel. The outputs of this process are the labeled profile regions and the number of profile regions. So, as we mentioned earlier, this is applicable to multiple line profiles such as the case with the slit phantoms. The following script thresholds and labels the multiple line profiles:

```
linprof = mean(SubImg(midx-numLines:midx+numLines,:),1);
lmax = max(linprof);
bw = linprof > lmax/4;
[L,numR] = bwlabel(bw);
```

The first for loop in the following code finds the locations of the maximum-count pixels in each profile and saves them to the variables V and c to be used later. The second for loop computes the resolution and location of the center point of the profile using the function mipresolution-lineProfile. Note that the variable wsize determines the limits of the window around each center point. This is normally estimated as four times the expected FWHM of the system, which is normally provided by the manufacturer of the GCS as a specification of the system.

```
Da = 50; % in mm
for i = 1:numR
    t1 = ismember(L,i);
    t2 = double(t1).*double(linprof);
    [V,c] = max(t2);
    Locations(i,1) = c;
end

for i = 1:numR
    prof = linprof(c-wsize:c+wsize);
    [FWHMX,FWHMPX,fpeak1] = mipresolutionlineProfile...
        (prof, 0.5);
    centerpos(i) = c-wsize+FWHMP(i,1)-1+(FWHMP(i,2)-...
        FWHMP(i,1))/2;
end
Dm = abs(centerpos(2)-centerpos(1));
pixSize = Da/Dm % in mm
```

The last line in this script computes the pixel size using the number of pixels between the center points and the actual distance between two line sources. We know that the sources are 50 mm apart. As we mentioned, this code does not make any assumption about the number of line sources in the image; therefore, it can be used to compute the resolutions and the pixel size from the image of multiple line-source profiles with slight modification.

Figure A.2.4 shows the image of slit phantom (right) used to calculate the intrinsic resolution, the intrinsic linearity, and the pixel size of gamma cameras. Normally, the resolution values from multiple line profiles are computed across the image and their average is reported as the final result.

A.2.5 SPECT Resolution without Scatter (in Air)

The following test conducted in nuclear medicine measures the SPECT spatial resolution in the absence of scatter. The test phantom consists of three point sources suspended in air. The NEMA guideline clearly specifies the arrangement of the point sources in space. Figure A.2.6 shows the surface-rendered image of the point sources.

After acquiring data in SPECT mode, the reconstructed volumetric image of the point sources is processed to calculate the central, tangential, and peripheral resolutions. The following enumerated list is the pseudo-code for the entire process that has to be carried out to identify the point sources in the volumetric image and to calculate resolutions in terms of the FWHM values. Note that it is not required to calculate the FWTM values.

1. Threshold the volume image.
2. Label the point sources (volume of interest) as separate objects.
3. Calculate the centroid of each point source object.
4. Identify the center point source from the x coordinates of the centroids.
5. Sum slices in transverse, coronal, and sagittal views to obtain slices with the required thicknesses.
6. For each slice
   a. Threshold image
   b. Identify three point sources and extract a square ROI around the maximum intensity of each point source
   c. Calculate the x and y resolutions of the three point sources on each slice using the algorithm described in Section A.2.3
7. Save the results to an Excel file.

Let us now demonstrate the entire process on a SPECT image acquired by a GCS. Note that this is a tomographic image consisting of two-dimensional (2-D) transaxial slices.

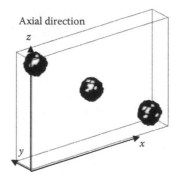

FIGURE A.2.6
Surface-rendered image of the three point sources used to measure the SPECT resolution in air.

In step #1, we threshold the whole volume image to segment three point sources. The threshold is predefined and usually very robust because these images are acquired under controlled conditions and are required to have a high enough number of counts at each point source. In step #2, the binary volume image is labeled to identify the point sources. The following code carries out these two steps:

```
bw = SPECTImg > Threshold;
[L,numObjects] = bwlabeln(bw,18);

if numObjects ~= 3
        warndlg('Number of point sources detected is not 3');
end
```

The warning statement here warns the user if the number of points detected is not three, as we expect to have three point sources. This may also mean that the used threshold has failed to segment the point sources and a different threshold value should be tried. After the identification of the point sources, in step # 3 we locate the center point source to be able to create slices centered at this location. We will compute the centroids of the detected point sources and find the center point source as follows:

```
    S = regionprops(L,'centroid');
xPositions = sort([S(1).Centroid(1),S(2).Centroid(1),...
    S(3).Centroid(1)]);
for i=1:numObjects
    if (S(i).Centroid(1) == xPositions(2))
        XCen=i;
    end
end
```

Now, we need to add transverse, coronal, and sagittal views to create a single slice of a certain thickness in each view. The following code performs this:

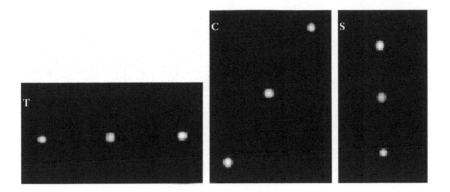

FIGURE A.2.7
Added slices in transverse (T), coronal (C), and sagittal (S) views.

```
% Compute number of transverse slices to add
numS = round(130/(2*SliceThickness));
% Compute the locatioin of the central slice
centS = round(S(XCen).Centroid(3));
% Transaxial slice
TImg = sum(SPECTImg(:,:,centS-numS:centS+numS),3);
% Compute number of coronal slices to add
numS = round(30/(2*PixelSize));
centS = round(S(XCen).Centroid(2));
% Coronal slice
CImg = squeeze(sum(SPECTImg(centS-numS:centS+numS,:,:),1));
% Compute number of sagittal slices to add
numS = round(30/(2*PixelSize));
centS = round(S(XCen).Centroid(1));
% Sagittal slice
SImg = squeeze(sum(SPECTImg(:,centS-numS:centS+numS,:),2));
```

The resultant slices shown in Figure A.2.7 have three point sources from which the resolutions can be calculated in terms of FWHM using the method discussed in Section A.2.3. The final resolution characteristics are defined as the average of the different combinations of x and y resolutions.

A.2.6 Linograms

Linograms can be useful for finding the axial misalignments between the detector pairs in GCSs. We will explain how to generate a linogram from the projections (views) of one or multiple point sources as described in [3]. The generation of a linogram image is in fact rather straightforward. Each

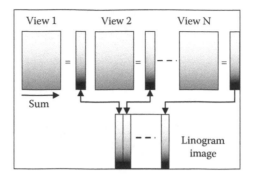

FIGURE A.2.8
Generation of a linogram.

n × m projection or view acquired by a GCS in SPECT mode is summed along its x-axis (or rows) and rearranged as a column of the linogram image. Thus, the final linogram image has n rows and the columns equal to the number of views. Figure A.2.8 illustrates this generation process schematically.

In nuclear medicine, the projections are normally saved as a volume image, a stack of 2-D images in DICOM format, to a single file (see Appendix B to learn more about handling DICOM images). Each view is summed along its rows. The following simple code can generate a linogram image from a given set of projections:

```
z = size(img,3);
for i=1:z
    LinoImg(:,i) =sum(img(:,:,i),2);
end
```

Figure A.2.9 shows one of the projections of the three point sources on the left, and on the right is the linogram image generated from the same projection data. These data were acquired by a dual-head gamma camera. Thus, any axial misalignment between the two heads of the GCS would present itself as a step discontinuity in the middle of the linogram image.

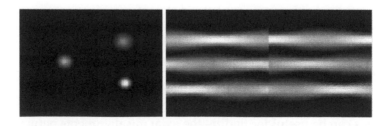

FIGURE A.2.9
Left: One of the projections of the three point sources. Right: Linogram generated from the same projection data set.

A.2.7 Calculation of Modulation Transfer Function (MTF) from a Line-Source and a Point-Source Image

Optical transfer function (OTF) of a medical imaging system can be defined as the Fourier transform of its point spread function. The modulation transfer function (MTF) is the magnitude of the OTF. In practice, to calculate the OTF, the image of a point source is acquired by the imaging system and its Fourier transform is computed. It is also common to acquire the image of a line source oriented along the x and y directions to calculate the MTF along the y and x directions, respectively.

In this section, we will calculate the MTF of a GCS from the image of a pair of line sources acquired under two different conditions: with and without scatter. We already know how the image of a line-source pair looks like (see Figure A.2.4 [left]). Again, the images in DICOM format can be read using

```
ImInfo = dicominfo('filename');
Img = dicomread(ImInfo);
```

TABLE A.2.1

Parameters and their descriptions in MATLAB codes (see also Figure A.2.10 for the graphical illustration) pertaining to the fast Fourier transform of a 1-D signal

Parameter in MATLAB code	Description
y	Signal (e.g., line profile).
Fs	Sampling rate (samples/unit distance)
n = length(y)	Number of sample points
x = (0:n-1)/Fs	Sample positions
Y = fft(y,N)	It refers to the number of sample points in the frequency domain. Hence, it is also called N-point FFT of the signal y. The statement N=2^nextpow2(n) can be used to find N.
dx = 1/Fs	Sample spacing in spatial domain
f = Fs*(0:N/2)/N (0,1/ Ndx,2/Ndx,...,1/2dx)	Frequencies (in unit distance/cycle): $\left(0, \dfrac{1}{Ndx}, \dfrac{2}{Ndx}, \ldots, \dfrac{N/2}{Ndx}\right)$
fn = 1/(2dx)	Maximum frequency or Nyquist frequency. It is also known as the fold-over frequency because the spectrum repeats itself (i.e., periodic).
df = 1/(N*dx)	Sample spacing in the frequency domain
YA = abs(Y)	Amplitude of Y
YP = Y.^2	Power of the signal y

The profiles depending on the orientation of the line sources can be extracted. For a line source perpendicular to the x direction, the profile can be extracted by extracting row 32, for instance:

```
yprof = Img(32,:);
deltay = ImInfo.PixelSpacing(2);
```

From the DICOM header information, we can obtain the pixel sizes or spacing in both x and y directions. We will use the pixel size to calculate the frequency in terms of line pairs per unit length.

Before we start computing MTF from the line profile, let us summarize some of the parameters pertinent to the fast Fourier transform (FFT) of a 1-D signal and how they can be computed in MATLAB. Table A.2.1 presents these parameters in MATLAB codes and their descriptions. Figure A.2.10 hows the graphs of a 1-D signal (e.g., line profile) in the space and frequency domains. It is straightforward to extend the parameters and calculations in Table A.2.1 to 2-D signals (e.g., 2-D images).

The following MATLAB code first finds the value of N to perform N-point FFT and the frequency vector f using deltay, which is the pixel size in x direction. Note that the function nextpow2 returns "the smallest power of two that is greater than or equal to the absolute value of n." The calculated Fourier transform is saved to the array Y.

```
n = length(yprof);
N = 2^nextpow2(n);
Fs = 1/deltay;
f = Fs*linspace(0,1,N/2)/N;
Y = fft(yprof,N);
```

The following code plots Y against the frequency using the MATLAB function stem

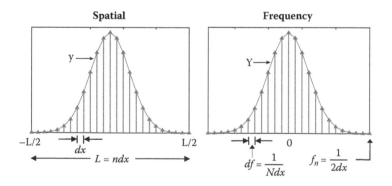

FIGURE A.2.10
A signal (e.g., line profile) in the spatial and frequency domain (see Table A.2.1 for the description of parameters in MATLAB code).

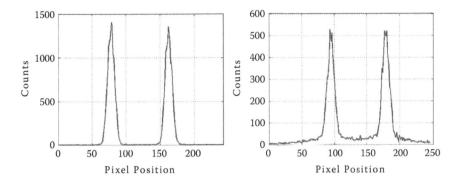

FIGURE A.2.11
Line profiles extracted from the image of a line source in air (left) and in a scattering medium (right).

```
figure;
dunit = 'mm'; % unit of the deltay
h = stem(f,abs(Y(1:N/2))/abs(Y(1)),'fill','-' );
set(get(h,'BaseLine'),'LineStyle',':');
set(h,'MarkerFaceColor','red');
xlabel(['u (line pairs/' dunit ')'],'Fontsize',14);
ylabel('|Y(u)|','Fontsize',14);
set(gca,'FontSize',14)
```

In Figure A.2.11, we have two line profiles extracted from the planar images of a line source, which was scanned suspended in air and in a scattering

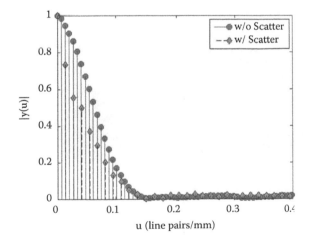

FIGURE A.2.12
The magnitudes of the fast Fourier transform (i.e., MTF) of the line profiles shown in Figure A.2.11.

medium (embedded among the sheets of perpex): left and right graphs, respectively. The graphs in Figure A.2.12 show the FFT of these line profiles. Note the impact of scatter on system resolution. Scatter affects the entire range of the spectrum. Therefore, it will affect the contrast of low-resolution objects as well as high-resolution small objects in the image [4]. As shown in this graph, the MTF of an imaging system even in one direction provides a lot of information about the resolution of the system. However, relating the resolution defined in terms of line pairs per unit length to its real impact on the image may be difficult.

In the following example, we demonstrate the computation of the resolution of a SPECT system with scatter in 2-D. To do this, we will use an axial slice from the tomographic image of the SPECT triple-line-source phantom, shown in Figure A.2.13 (top left), with three line sources inserted into a cylindrical water phantom. In this case, the water in which line sources are immersed mimics a scattering medium. Here, the cross sections of the sources shown in Figure A.2.13 (top left) will be regarded as point sources.

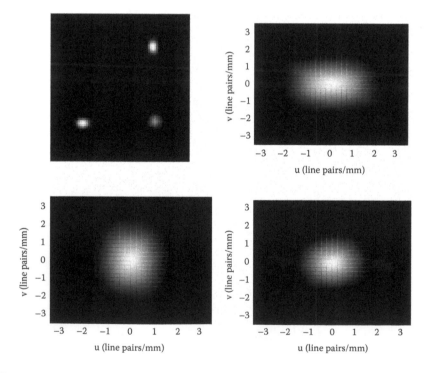

FIGURE A.2.13

Top left: An axial slice from the tomographic image of the SPECT triple-line-source phantom with three line sources inserted into a water phantom. The cross sections of the lines shown in the image are regarded as point sources. Top right: MTF of the top point source. Bottom left: MTF of the bottom left point source. Bottom right: MTF of the bottom right point source.

First, a rectangular ROI is placed around each point source and the ROI region is cropped from the image. The following code reads the transaxial slice (#32) of the triple-line-source image, crops the ROI, and saves it into the array z, and the maximum dimension of the ROI is used to find the sample size N to perform N-point FFT:

```
ImInfo = dicominfo('NM0001.dcm');
img = dicomread(ImInfo);
imagesc(Img(:,:,32);
z = imcrop;
L = size(z);
N = 2^nextpow2(max(L));
```

The parameter N is the nearest (to the maximum dimension of the image) power of 2, that is, $N = 2^p \geq max(L)$. For example, if the largest dimension of our image is 322, then,

```
>> N = 2^nextpow2(322)
N =
512
```

The reason we are trying to find the nearest power of 2 is that FFT operations can be performed more efficiently when the sample size N is an exact power of 2. The delta in the following script is the pixel size and is equal in both dimensions. As seen in the code, the calculated FFT in 2-D is saved to the variable Z.

```
delta = ImInfo.PixelSpacing(1);
z = double(z);
Fs = 1./delta;
Z = fft2(z,N,N);
```

The following code then plots the magnitude of the transform using the mesh function:

```
figure;
dunit = 'mm';
[U,V] = meshgrid(Fs*(-N/2:1:N/2-1)/2,Fs*(-N/2:1:N/2-1)/2);
meshc(U,V,abs(fftshift(Z)));
view([0,90]);
set(gca,'FontSize',14)
if ~isempty(dunit)
    xlabel(['u (line pairs/' dunit ')'],'Fontsize',14);
    ylabel(['v (line pairs/' dunit ')'],'Fontsize',14);
else
    xlabel('Frequency (u)','Fontsize',14);
    xlabel('Frequency (v)','Fontsize',14);
end
```

Figure A.2.13 shows our three point sources on the top left corner. The MTF for each point source is given in the same figure. The respective MTFs are shown in the same order as the point sources in the image. Note the top point source and its MTF (top right). The width of the point source in the x direction is narrower than its width in the y direction, whereas the width of the MTF in the x direction is wider in the x direction than it is in the y direction. Note also the circular shape of the MTF of the point source at the bottom right of the original image. This point source was at the center of rotation of the system, so it is fairly circular in shape. As these point sources indicate, the resolution of a SPECT system is not isotropic. This is the reason why we have to define the resolution characteristics of a SPECT system in terms of central, tangential, and radial resolution parameters.

References

1. NEMA, Performance Measurements of Scintillation Gamma Cameras, NU 1-2001 standards, NU 1–2001. National Electrical Manufacturers Association (NEMA) ed., 2001.
2. O. Demirkaya and R. A. Mazrou, Performance test data analysis of gamma cameras, *IEEE Trans.Nucl Sci* 5: 1506–1515, 2007.
3. J. W. Wallis, Use of the selective linogram in cardiac tomography quality control, *J Nucl Cardiol* 2: 303–308, 1995.
4. S. R. Cherry, J. A. Sorenson, and M. E. Phelps, *Physics in Nuclear Medicine*, 3rd ed. Philadelphia, PA: Saunders, 2003.

Application 3

Analysis of Islet Cells Using Automated Color Image Analysis

CONTENTS

A.3.1 Introduction

As islet transplantation and immunosuppressive regimens become increasingly successful, islet transplantation is likely to find widespread clinical application for curing patients with insulin-dependent diabetes mellitus. An important determinant of successful transplantation is the quantity of islets engrafted, with many advocating at least 5000 equivalents per kilogram to be transplanted. The measurement of islet equivalents has been traditionally a manual process. Automated color image analysis is an alternative, objective, and more accurate approach.

In this application, we will demonstrate how color images of islet cells can be segmented and quantified. We will use the functions available in the MATLAB Image Processing Toolbox.

The images of isolated human islets that we will be using here were captured using a ZEISS Axioskop2 plus light microscope in RGB color space and were transformed to the L*a*b color space in the MATLAB programming environment. In RGB images, the dark gray islet cells are surrounded by a light gray background. By transforming to L*a*b space, we intend to reduce the dimension of the problem from 3 (RGB colors) to 2 (colors a and b). The intensities of the a and b color images will be clustered using the well-known K-means clustering algorithm (see Chapter 6 for a detailed discussion). After identifying the pixels that are red (islet cells and some background), a further separation within this class can be performed using the *L* values. The histogram of the *L* values of these pixels will be computed first. A histogram-based thresholding algorithm will then be applied to find a threshold to separate the truly reddish pixels from the surrounding background.

A.3.2 Transformation to L*a*b Space

The original image was captured in RGB color space. Transforming images from one color space to another is widely done to facilitate processing and analysis of images. If one desires to perform an image segmentation or pixel clustering, the characteristics or features of objects of interest may appear better separated in a certain color space than in others. Therefore, in this application we will transform the RGB color image to another color space known as L*a*b to reduce the color dimension, and in turn to have a better separation between the intensity clusters. The L*a*b color space is originally derived from the CIE XYZ tristimulus values. The L*a*b space consists of a luminosity layer *L*, and a chromaticity layers *a* and *b*. All of the color information is contained in the *a* and *b* layers or the channels. Note that transforming images from RGB to L*a*b space reduces the dimension of the problem from 3 (RGB colors) to 2 (colors *a* and *b*) for color analysis purposes, and therefore, color analysis may be facilitated.

To perform the transformation in MATLAB, we first create a color transformation matrix to convert from sRGB, which is similar to RGB, to the L*a*b color space, using the MATLAB function makecform. We then apply the color transformation using the MATLAB function applycform to the original image to create the image in the L*a*b color space. The following script performs these two steps:

```
% Transform image into L*a*b space
cform = makecform('srgb2lab');
Img_lab = applycform(Img,cform);
```

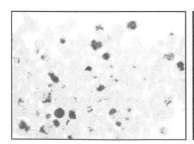 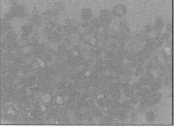

FIGURE A 3.1
Left: Original islet cell in RGB format. Right: Image transformed to L*a*b space.

Figure A.3.1 shows the original image in RGB format on the left and the transformed image on the right. As seen in this figure, both images have the three distinct gray levels corresponding to three different colors in the RGB image, although they are different.

A3.3   Segmentation of Islet Cells

Following the color transformation, the pixels belonging to islet cells are identified in two steps: (1) K-means clustering using the chromaticity information, and (2) further separation using the luminosity information.

The intensities of the color bands are clustered into different groups using the well-known K-means clustering algorithm, as implemented in the MATLAB Image Processing Toolbox. For a detailed discussion of this segmentation technique, the reader can refer to Chapter 6. As seen in Figure A.3.1, there are three distinct gray levels referring to the colors exiting in the original image: the light gray and dark gray. Therefore, we will assume that there are three classes or groups to be separated with the K-means clustering algorithm. The only input parameter that is essential and critical for function K-means is the number of clusters to be determined. The color image of the islet cells can be downloaded from the Web site of the book (see Appendix D).

A.3.3.1   K-Means Clustering

We will first separate *a* and *b* components of the image because all the color information is contained in *these* components. The *L* component of the image carries only the luminance information. The following code separates *a* and *b* components first and reduces the 2-D image into a long 2-D matrix with the reshape function available in MATLAB (see Chapter 2 for the discussion of reshape). We set the number of clusters to 3.

```
ab = double(Img_lab(:,:,2:3));
[nrows,ncols,cc] = size(ab);
ab = reshape(ab,nrows*ncols,2);
nColors = 3;

% repeat the clustering 3 times to avoid local minima
[cluster_indx cluster_centers] = kmeans...
  (ab,nColors,'distance', 'sqEuclidean','Replicates',3);
pixel_labels = reshape(cluster_indx,nrows,ncols);
```

This script performs the clustering with the options seen in the statement. Note that the Euclidian distance is used to measure the distance

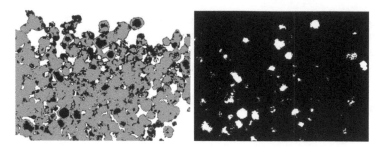

FIGURE A 3.2
Left: The original image whose pixels are assigned with the pixel indices. Right: Islet cells are denoted by white color after the second stage of the segmentation.

between the color features and cluster centers. The output variables are cluster indices saved in `cluster _ indx` and the cluster centers saved in `cluster _ centers`. The last line in the code generates an image whose pixels are assigned with the pixel indices.

A.3.3.2 Further Separation Using the Luminosity Component

As we have seen in Figure A.3.2, the color segmentation by itself using the clustering algorithm could not identify pixels belonging to the islet cells only. Some of their surrounding pixels are also identified as being part of the islet cells. We will now show that a further and better separation within this class can be achieved using the luminosity component. We first compute the histogram of the L values of these pixels that are

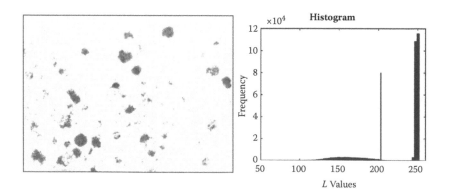

FIGURE A 3.3
Left: Luminosity band of the L*a*b image. Right: Histogram of the L values of pixels indicated by triangles in the ab space shown in A 3.4, and the computed threshold (T = 203) to separate cells and cell fragments from their surrounding background.

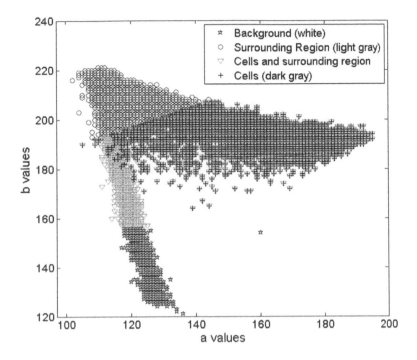

FIGURE A 3.4
Left: Scatter plot of the a and b values. The L values above the threshold shown are denoted by "+" sign marker in the left plot.

identified in the first stage. We then apply the histogram-based thresholding algorithm, the between-class variance, which is discussed in detail in Chapter 6, to find a threshold to separate the true islet cells pixels from their surrounding pixels much more accurately.

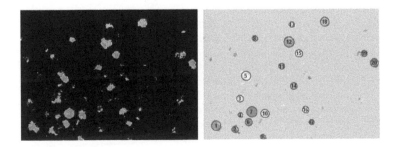

FIGURE A 3.5
Left: Segmented islet cells identified using the binary mask image in Figure A.3.2 (right). Dark areas refer to the noncell areas. Right: Cells are labeled with pseudocolors and of certain sizes are labeled with a circle and a number.

```
% Finding reddish areas
mean_cluster_val = zeros(3,1);
for k = 1:nColors
    mean_cluster_val(k) = mean(cluster_center(k));
end
[mean_cluster_val,idx] = sort(mean_cluster_val);
islet_cluster_num = idx(2);
```

A.3.4 Analysis of Cell Features

Now we have a binary image, where the cell pixels are assigned 1, and the rest are assigned 0. First, we perform connected-component labeling to identify islet cells, labeling each cell with the same label. Then, each labeled cell will be analyzed to extract features such as the location of the cell centroid, area, and minor and major axes of the ellipse, which fits the convex hull of the cell. Before doing any of this, a size threshold can be used to separate cells from the cell fragments. The rmdebris function can remove fragments smaller than a certain size.

```
pixel_size = 0.74396; % micrometer
se = strel('disk',3);
bw_labels = repmat(bw,[1 1 3]);
simg(bw_labels~=1) = 0;
bw = bwfill(bw,'holes');
bw2 = rmdebris(bw,50);
L = bwlabel(bw2);
stats = regionprops(L,'all');
RGB_label = label2rgb(L, @spring, 'c', 'shuffle');
imlook(RGB_label);hold on
numofspots = size(stats,1);
count = 1;
for snum = 1:numofspots
    ediam = stats(snum).EquivDiameter;
    avdiam = (stats(snum).MajorAxisLength+stats(snum)....
        MinorAxisLength)/2;
    ldiam = stats(snum).MajorAxisLength;
    sdiam = stats(snum).MinorAxisLength;
    if ldiam > 40 & sdiam > 40
        txt = num2str(count,'%2d');
        x = stats(snum).Centroid(1);
        y = stats(snum).Centroid(2);
        text(x,y,txt,'fontsize',10,'fontweight','bold',
            'color',... 'k','horiz','center');
        circle(ediam/2,x,y,'b');
        v(count,1) = pixel_size*pixel_size*stats(snum).Area;
        v(count,2) = pixel_size*stats(snum).EquivDiameter;
        v(count,3) = pixel_size*stats(snum).MajorAxisLength;
        v(count,4) = pixel_size*stats(snum).MinorAxisLength;
```

```
        v(count,5) = pixel_size*(stats(snum).
            MajorAxisLength+stats(snum).MinorAxisLength)/2;
        count = count+1;
    end
 end
```

The above MATLAB script performs the processes described above. This entire process can be automated (i.e., can be run without user interaction) and can be executed in batch mode to process multiple images.

The original image, shown in Figure A.3.1, shows the cross section of the entire specimen at a certain optical depth. The 2-D image of an actual volumetric cell can be problematic in quantification. The fragments we see in the image may in fact be the cross sections of cells sliced through at a different depth. It is possible to acquire the images of cells in 3-D using an optical sectioning technique. The optical sectioning technique allows the reconstruction of thick biological specimens into a 3-D image. The acquired images (i.e., optical slices) may then be processed to remove the out-of-focus information contributed by the structures lying in the above and below neighboring planes. This process is generally known as deconvolution process.

Appendix A

Notation

Images can be scalar-valued or vector-valued. In a scalar-valued image each pixel or voxel is assigned a single value (feature), whereas pixels or voxels in a vector-valued image have one or more features assigned to them. An n-D scalar-valued image I is defined as a function or mapping, $I : \mathbb{R}^n \to \mathbb{R}$. In medical imaging, most imaging modalities such as CT, MRI, and PET generate scalar-valued images; however, there are also modalities producing vector-valued images such MRI diffusion tensor imaging. This imaging technique measures the diffusion of water in nerve tissue. This anisotropic, orientation-dependent diffusion, is described by a diffusion tensor, which is generally represented by a matrix. A color image is another typical example of a vector-valued image in which each pixel is represented by a vector $\mathbf{v} = [R\ G\ B]^T$, where R, G, and B refer to the three primary color components: red, green, and blue, respectively. Then, an n-D color image I can be defined as $I : \mathbb{R}^n \to \mathbb{R}^3$. The vector valued-images are also known as multivalued images. The latter naming is perhaps more appropriate as image elements may be represented by vectors or matrices.

To generalize, an n-D vector-valued image can be defined as a mapping $I : \mathbb{R}^n \to \mathbb{R}^m$, where n and m represent the dimensions of the image and the feature vector that is assigned to each pixel or voxel. Each component of a multivalued image is a mapping $I_i : \mathbb{R}^n \to \mathbb{R}$, $i = 1, 2, \cdots, m$, E^3 denotes the 3-D Euclidian space. Throughout the book, we will frequently refer 2-D images as surfaces in E^3. This representation is also known as the topographical representation of 2-D images.

The following list of notations is used throughout the book unless stated otherwise elsewhere in the book:

2-D and 3-D: Refer to 2-D and 3-D image spaces

$\mathbb{R}$: The real numbers

$|A|$: Length of matrix A

$\|A\|$: Norm of matrix A

A^T: Transpose of A

A^{-1}: Inverse of A

Corr : Correlation coefficient

Cov : Covariance

∂X: Boundary of X

I: Identity matrix or a digital image

κ, K, H: Curvature of a curve, Gaussian curvature, and mean curvature, respectively.

∇: del, derivative operator

∇I: Gradient of I

$\dfrac{\partial I}{\partial x} = I_x$: Partial derivative in x

Δ or ∇^2: Laplacian operator

ΔI or $\nabla^2 I$: Laplacian of I

div: divergence operator

Π: Product

Σ: Sum

v: Vectors are usually denoted by bold and italic Roman or Greek letters.

σ, σ^2: Standard deviation and variance

$\dfrac{\partial f}{\partial x_i} = f_{x_i}$: Partial derivative with respect to x_i; $\dfrac{\partial^2 f}{\partial x^2} = f_{xx}$; denotes the second partial derivative of function f

$f^{(k)}$: kth derivative of f

sgn(x): Signum function

$\delta(x)$: Direct delta

$*, \oplus$: Convolution

Table A.1 shows Greek letters that may be used as symbols in the book. Therefore, a familiarity with these letters will help readers understand the topics.

TABLE A.1

Greek letters used in the book as symbols in equations

Letter	Name	Letter	Name
A, α	Alpha	Λ, λ	Lambda
B, β	Beta	N, ν	Nu
Γ, γ	Gamma	$\Sigma\,\zeta\,\sigma$	Sigma
Δ, δ	Delta	Φ, ϕ, φ	Phi
E, ε, ϵ	Epsilon	Y, υ	Upsilon
H η	Eta	$\Psi\,\psi$	Psi
Θ, θ	Theta	$\Omega\,\omega$	Omega
K, κ	Kappa	$\Xi\,\xi$	Xi

Appendix B

Working with DICOM Images

DICOM is the acronym for Digital Image Communication in Medicine. It is a standard for storing, printing, and transferring medical information in general and images in particular. It comprises a file format definition and a communication protocol. This standard was developed by the American College of Radiology (ACR) and the National Electrical Manufacturers Association (NEMA). The first version of the ACR-NEMA standards was published in 1985. DICOM, which is the most widely used medical imaging format, enables the sharing of medical information and the integration of different medical devices from different vendors through the Picture Archiving and Communication System (PACS). Here, we will discuss only its file format specifications and how the DICOM images generated by different imaging modalities can be read or processed in the MATLAB programming environment.

It should be noted that DICOM standards used by different vendors may have slight variations. This is the reason why every vendor will have a DICOM conformance statement in which they specify which DICOM classes or services they support. These services may include storage commitment, query/retrieve, modality work list, etc. The vendors also provide information about their DICOM file format specifications. These DICOM conformance statements are usually publicly available in the vendors' Web sites. It should also be noted that the images produced by different modalities may differ.

In this Appendix, we will also present the fields (attributes) that users are required to notice when working with these images. Our 3-D image display tool, imlook3d, is capable of reading images from three main modalities, namely, computer tomography (CT), magnetic resonance (MR), and positron emission tomography (PET) images. It can also read nuclear medicine images. Some of the scripts or codes that we present here can be found in our imlook3d program, which can be downloaded from the MATLAB file exchange.

The MATLAB Image Processing Toolbox has four functions pertinent to handling DICOM files. These are dicominfo, dicomread, dicomwrite, and dicomdict. The dicominfo and dicomread functions are particularly important as they are used to read the image header and image data, respectively. The dicominfo function reads the DICOM header and returns the header in a structure. The dicomread function reads the image from the file whose name is specified as an input argument, which can also be the DICOM header structure returned by dicominfo. For more information about these functions, we refer the reader to MATLAB help pages. Table B.1 shows some of the important image attributes common to PET, CT, MRI, and nuclear medicine (NM) modalities.

TABLE B.1

Some of the important header information common to PET, CT, MRI, and SPECT modalities

Field name	Description
FileModDate	Modification date of the file
FileSize	Size of the file
Format	File format
FormatVersion	Version
Width	Width of the image
Height	Height of the image
BitDepth	Bit depth, e.g., 8, 16 bits
ColorType	Graylevel or color image
Rows	Same as the image height
Columns	Same as the image width
PixelSpacing	A vector of pixel sizes [x , y] in actual units
SliceThickness	Slice thickness
NumberOfFrames	Number of slices in a 3-D image saved into a single file, e.g., SPECT
NumberOfSlices	Number of slices in a 3-D image, e.g., CT and MR. It can be useful while reading a 3-D image to know how many slices the 3-D image comprise.
Modality	Indicates the modality by which the image is produced. For PET, for example, dh.Modality ='PT', where dh is the header structure returned by dicominfo function.

3-D volumetric images in DICOM format may be saved in two different ways: (1) all the slices are saved into a single file (e.g., SPECT images or raw projection data in nuclear medicine),, (2) each slice is saved into a separate file(e.g., MR, CT, and PET images). We will discuss how we can read these images saved in two different ways.

The following script can read a volumetric image consisting of multiple slices, each being saved into separate files:

```
[filename, pathname] = uigetfile,'Image');
if isequal(filename,0)|isequal(pathname,0)
    setstatus('File not found');
else
    cd(pathname)
    k = findstr(filename,'.');
```

```
        fnames = dir([filename(1:2) '*']);
        dh = dicominfo(filename);
        r = dh.Width;
        c = dh.Height;
        numSlices = length(fnames);
        nimg = zeros([r,c,numSlices]);
        hw = waitbar(0,'Reading volume image, please wait...');
        for i=1:numSlices
            dh = dicominfo(fnames(i).name);
            nimg(:,:,i) = dicomread(dh);
            waitbar(i/numSlices,hw);
        end
    end
```

This script allows the user to pick up the first file from the directory, and it reads the rest of the files (slices) itself. At the end, all the slices are put into a 3-D array. The script also has a waitbar showing the progress during the reading process. Note that the names of the files for slices are read using the dir function. Before we start reading the slices, we allocate a 3-D array for the entire image as we already know the dimensions (i.e., rows, columns, and the number of slices) of the image. The fnames variable holds all the files existing in the directory.

When we read images of different modalities, we should consider several important issues. In some modalities, the image intensities in the DICOM file may be mapped to a new range or they may be normalized during its creation. In such a case, it is necessary to perform a reverse mapping to obtain the original intensity values before any processing is performed. There are two pertinent parameters in the DICOM header structure. These are RescaleSlope and RescaleIntercept. The following script reads the header of a CT slice and displays these two parameters:

```
>> dh = dicominfo('CT002001109.dcm');
>> dh.RescaleSlope
ans = 1
>> dh.RescaleIntercept
ans = 0
```

The values indicate that no mapping was applied to this slice, as the slope and intercept are 1 and 0, respectively. The following statement shows how these two parameters are used to remap the intensity values back to their original values:

```
nimg = dh.RescaleSlope*dicomread(dh) +
    dh.RescaleIntercept;
```

The image intensities are first multiplied by dh.RescaleSlope, and then dh.RescaleIntercept is added to obtain the original intensities.

Here, the `dicomread(dh)` reads the image whose header is returned to the structure dh. If the image intensities are not scaled or mapped during the creation, the header structure may not have these two variables. In this case, during an automated reading process, similar to the earlier script , MATLAB will give error messages and interrupt the reading process. We can use the following script to avoid such an error or interruption during a reading process:

```
if (isfield(dh,'RescaleSlope')
    rslope = dh.RescaleSlope
else
    rslope = 1;
end
if (isfield(dh,'RescaleIntercept')
    rintercept = dh.RescaleIntercept
else
    rintercept = 0;
end
```

Note that we are checking the existence of these fields and are using them if they exist. This has to be performed for every slice that is read, as every slice will have its own rescale and intercept parameters.

Another important issue while reading volumetric images, whose slices are saved into individual files, is the slice order. The file number, which is a suffix attached to the file name (e.g., 'CT002001109.dcm'), may not match the actual anatomical order of the slice. This may happen especially in PET whole-body imaging (see Chapter 1) where multiple axial fields of view (each is a volume image by itself) are acquired in a step-and-shoot mode, and subsequently the individual volumes are assembled together. In such a case, the image index information is read from the DICOM header to find the correct slice location before the image array is read. The slice is then stacked in the correct order using the image index information. The following loop illustrates how to extract the image index and stack the slices in correct order:

```
for i=1:numSlices
    dh = dicominfo(fnames(i).name);
    idx = dh.ImageIndex;
    nimg(:,:,idx) = dh.RescaleSlope*dicomread(dh)+...
        dh.RescaleIntercept;
    waitbar(i/numSlices,hw);
end
```

The variable dh.ImageIndex denotes the correct axial order of the slice. Note that the 3-D array that holds the image slices is created beforehand. Figure B.1 shows the coronal views of a whole-body PET image. The slice

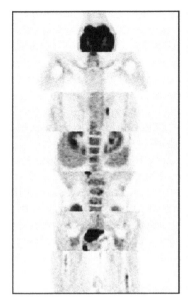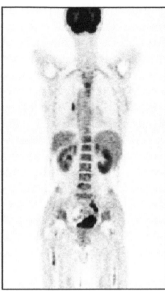

FIGURE B.1
Coronal views of a whole-body PET image. The left image is read with disregard to the image index in the DICOM header, whereas the right image is read using the image index information.

order problem is particularly obvious in coronal or sagittal views. The image on the left is read with disregard to the image index information in the header, whereas the image on the right is stacked using the image index information. Obviously, the slice order in the left image is mixed.

In general, CT and MR DICOM images are saved into multiple files in the order of anatomical location. In other words, the file number 1 holds the first slice, the file number 2, the second slice, and so on.

B.1 Working with PET DICOM Images for Quantification

PET images are originally acquired as transaxial slices. When saved in DICOM, each slice is saved into a separate file. PET DICOM headers have many fields that the user should pay attention to, especially if he is interested in quantitative analysis. The values in PET images are stored in a certain unit. The following field of the PET header dh indicates the unit the intensities are stored in:

```
dh.Units: 'BQML'
```

The Becquerel/milliliter (Bq/ml) is a common unit. If one requires converting these values to some other unit such as the standard uptake values (SUVs), extra processing has to be done. SUVs denote the activity distribution within the tissue normalized by the injected activity, normalized to body weight. For further details about the SUV, the reader can refer to the Chapter 1. We will discuss how we can convert the image intensities saved in 'BQML' to SUVs. The following discussion applies to the DICOM images produced by a GE PET scanner. The reader has to be careful if it can be applied to those from other vendors.

PET images have header fields that carry information about the radiopharmaceutical injected to the patient. The measurement and injection time of the radiopharmaceutical are important parameters used in calculating SUVs. To convert to SUV, we first require the net injected activity that is decay corrected to the start of the scan, which is the reference time point used in GE DICOM if the values are decay corrected. The structure in the header

```
dh.RadiopharmaceuticalInformationSequence.Item_1
```

carries the information about the radiopharmaceutical injected into the subject. The table below shows the parameters saved in this structure.

Radiopharmaceutical	FDG — fluorodeoxyglucose
RadiopharmaceuticalStartTime	105200.00
RadionuclideTotalDose	495239648
RadionuclideHalfLife	6588
RadionuclidePositronFraction	0.9700

The following script extracts the injected dose, half-life of the isotope, and the time of the measurement:

```
tracerAct =
info.RadiopharmaceuticalInformationSequence.Item_1.
  RadionuclideTotalDose;
halfLife =
info.RadiopharmaceuticalInformationSequence.Item_1.
  RadionuclideHalfLife;
measuredT =
info.RadiopharmaceuticalInformationSequence.Item_1.
  RadiopharmaceuticalStartTime;
```

The following script calculates the elapsed time from the time of injection until the time of scan. Note how the date and time information is concatenated together to compute the elapsed time, which is the difference between the time of injection and the time of acquisition, or study time, using etime.

```
% Calcualte the ellapsed time
studyD = [str2num(info.StudyDate(1:4)),...
    str2num(info.StudyDate(5:6)),...
    str2num(info.StudyDate(7:8))];
seriesD = [str2num(info.SeriesDate(1:4)),...
    str2num(info.SeriesDate(5:6)),...
    str2num(info.SeriesDate(7:8))];
studyT = [str2num(info.StudyTime(1:2)),...
    str2num(info.StudyTime(3:4)),...
    str2num(info.StudyTime(5:6))];
seriesT = [str2num(info.SeriesTime(1:2)),...
    str2num(info.SeriesTime(3:4)),...
    str2num(info.SeriesTime(5:6))];
measT = [str2num(measuredT(1:2)),...
    str2num(measuredT(3:4)),...
    str2num(measuredT(5:6))];
 acqTime = info.AcquisitionTime;
 acqT = [str2num(acqTime(1:2)),...
    str2num(acqTime(3:4)),...
    str2num(acqTime(5:6))];
% compute the ellapsed time in sec
ellapsedTime = etime([seriesD,seriesT],[seriesD measT]);
```

Using the elapsed time, one can compute the decay-corrected activity. In the following statement, the activity is decay corrected for the elapsed time from the measurement of the radiopharmaceutical to the start of the scan:

```
actualActivity = tracerAct*(2^(-ellapsedTime/halfLife));
```

Then, the SUVs can be calculated as follows:

```
WEIGHT = dh.PatientWeight;
suvFactor = WEIGHT*1000/actualActivity;
```

B.2 The Patient-based Coordinate System

DICOM uses a patient-based coordinate system, which is known as the LPS (Left, Posterior, Superior) system. Figure B.2 shows the diagram of this coordinate system. The directions left, posterior, and superior point in the positive x, y, and z directions, respectively. The DICOM fields that provide information about the origin of the image, image orientation, and field-of-views (FOVs) are

ImagePositionPatient[3]	This is a vector with three elements. The first two values provide the origin of the image with respect to the LPS system. The last element is the axial slice location.
ImageOrientationPatient[6]	It is a column vector of six elements. It provides the direction cosines of the first row and first column in the x, y, and z directions. It holds the row values for x, y, and z and the column values for x, y, and z.
FieldOfViewDimensions[2]	It is a vector of two elements. It provides the transaxial and axial FOV sizes, usually in millimeter.

The following statement shows the maximum range of the FOVs of PET. The first number is the diameter of the transaxial FOV, and the second number is the length of the axial FOV all in millimeter.

```
>> dh.FieldOfViewDimensions'
ans =
    700 157
```

The following image orientation information shows that the image has not been rotated, and the rows increase from right to left, and the columns increase from anterior to posterior.

```
>> dh.ImageOrientationPatient'
ans =
    1 0 0 0 1 0
```

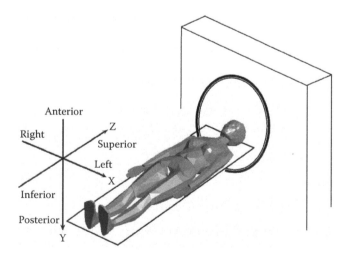

FIGURE B.2
Patient-based LPS coordinate system. The articulated humanoid body (Nancy) used here has been programmed into MATLAB by Walterio Mayol-Cuevas from H-Anim working group, and can be downloaded from the MATLAB Central\File Exchange.

Note that the first three numbers indicate the row direction, and the last three the column direction. The orientation information of a sagittal MR image is

```
>> dh.ImageOrientationPatient'
ans =
    0  1  0  0  0 -1
```

This shows that the rows increase from anterior to posterior, and the columns increase from superior to inferior (−z direction).

Let us see the image position information with respect to the LPS system:

```
>> dh.ImagePositionPatient
ans =
 -297.6563
 -297.6563
 -135.5900
```

The minus signs of the first two numbers indicate that the top left corner of the image is in the right anterior region. The third number is the slice location. This is the image position information from a CT image acquired by a PET/CT scanner:

```
>> dhc.ImagePositionPatient
ans =
 -250.0000
 -250.0000
 -11.7700
```

Note the differences between the PET and CT images acquired by a PET/CT scanner. In the next section, we will demonstrate how some of this information can be used to resample images.

B.3 Resampling PET and CT Images to a Common Pixel Size

Functional imaging modalities such as PET and SPECT do not have high enough resolution to discern anatomical structures. CT or MR, however, has excellent resolution capabilities. To combine the advantages of two different modalities, hybrid systems have been built in the last decades. CT images in SPECT/CT and PET/CT scanners therefore help locate anatomically the functional or molecular activities captured by SPECT or PET. Recently, investigators have been working to combine PET and MR imaging systems.

In hybrid systems such as PET/CT, both PET and CT images are acquired and registered to a common coordinate system. This type of registration is called hardware registration. Although both images lie in this common coordinate system, each image is saved at a different pixel size due to their resolution limitations. In a whole-body PET/CT, PET transaxial images are normally reconstructed into a matrix of 128 × 128, whereas CT images are reconstructed into a matrix of 512 × 512. Typical pixel sizes are about 4.5 mm in PET and about 1 mm in CT. The slice thicknesses may be the same depending on the CT acquisition parameters. It will be difficult to perform processing or analysis involving both of these images simultaneously because of the different pixel sizes. In this section we will demonstrate how one can resample both images to the same pixel size.

The following function, meshgridPETCT, returns mesh grids for CT and PET images for a specified pixel size, nps. To achieve this, the function uses the image position information as well as the pixel sizes in the DICOM header structure imageInfo.

```
% This function creates mesh grids for PET and CT images
function [Nx,Ny,Ox,Oy] = meshgridPETCT (imageInfo,
modality,nps);
NLS = -230;
NRS = 229;
NT = -150;
NB = 150;
LS = imageInfo.ImagePositionPatient(1);
TS = imageInfo.ImagePositionPatient(2);
Px = imageInfo.PixelSpacing(1);
Py = imageInfo.PixelSpacing(2);
[Nx,Ny] = meshgrid(NLS:nps:NRS, NT:nps:NB);
if modality == 'pt'
    [Ox,Oy] = meshgrid(LS:Px:-LS,TS:Py:-TS);
elseif modality == 'ct'
    [Ox,Oy] = meshgrid(LS:Px:-LS-Px,TS:Py:-TS-Py);
else
end
```

Note that the arbitrary limits of the new rectangular region (see Figure B.3) are hardcoded in the function. We know that the size of the sampled region is 60 × 30 mm, whereas the size of the actual FOV is 60 × 60 mm. This FOV is specified within the image reconstruction protocol.

Let us test our function on a PET image from the PET/CT image set. We will use a pixel size of 2 mm. The PET image has the pixel size of 4.6875, whereas the corresponding CT image pixel size is 0.9766 mm. Thus, the PET image is sampled to a smaller pixel size, whereas the CT image will be sampled to a larger pixel size. The following script shows the sampling of the PET image only. It is straightforward to run the same script for the corresponding CT

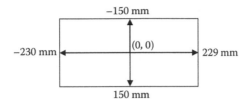

FIGURE B.3
Resampled rectangular region cropped from the full FOV.

image. Note that the `interp2` function is used to resample the PET image, which is specified at the original grid locations `ptgx` and `ptgy`, at the new grid locations `Nx` and `Ny`. Note also that the image is mapped back to its original intensity range using the slope and intercept values in the header.

```
% Create meshes for both PET
nps = 2; % mm
[Nx,Ny,ptgx,ptgy] = meshgridPETCT (petinfo,'pt',nps);
% Read PET header and image
dh = dicominfo('PT050.dcm');
tmpimg = dh.RescaleSlope*dicomread(dh) +
dh.RescaleIntercept;
% Resample PET image
pimg = interp2(ptgx,ptgy,single(tmpimg),Nx,Ny,'cubic');
```

Figure B.4 shows the resampled PET and CT, and the fused images.

B.3.1 An Example Application from PET/CT

Here we will show an example application in which we are required to sample both images to the same pixel size in order to perform a quantitative analysis. In this example, we wish to find bony lesions (cancer in the bone), and quantify the uptake and CT values within the lesion region. Subsequent to resampling, we first segment the entire bone in the CT image using a simple threshold of 150 HU (Hounsfield unit). Then, using

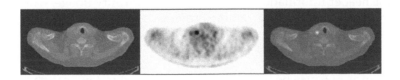

FIGURE B.4
PET and CT images resampled to a pixel size of 2 mm. Left: CT. Middle: PET. Right: Fused PET/CT.

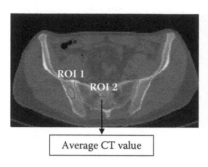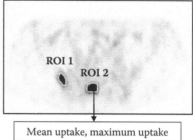

FIGURE B.5
CT and PET images from a PET/CT scan. ROIs defined on PET are overlaid on both PET and CT images.

the binary bone image as a mask, we find the pixel with maximum uptake in the PET image within the mask.

Afterwards we compute the ROIs centered at the maximum uptake pixel using the isoline of 0.5* (the maximum intensity) (see Chapter 2). The isoline is the contour along which the intensity values are larger or equal to a constant value of 50% of the maximum intensity. This percentage is somewhat arbitrary and can be modified.

Figure B.5 shows the PET and CT images with the ROI boundaries superimposed. The same ROIs can be used to extract the average CT value from the CT, and the mean and the maximum uptake values from the PET.

B.4   Working with Nuclear Medicine Images

In this section, we will discuss the peculiarities of nuclear medicine images that may be required by clinical scientists, engineers, and physicists working in the field.

In nuclear medicine, the planar images, projection views, and the reconstructed SPECT images are all saved into a single file. Thereby, it is easier to read nuclear medicine (NM) images than those of PET, CT, and MRI. In MATLAB, it requires only one statement to read these images. Let us read the header information of a flood field uniformity image, which is a planar image, acquired by a gamma camera.

```
dh = dicominfo('NM001.dcm');
```

For instance, one may be interested in the energy window information of the camera during the acquisition:

```
>>dh.EnergyWindowInformationSequence.Item_1.
EnergyWindowRangeSequence.Item_1
```

```
ans =

    EnergyWindowLowerLimit: 126
    EnergyWindowUpperLimit: 154
```

It holds the lower and upper limits of the energy window, normally in kiloelectronvolt. The information about the used radiopharmaceutical is saved in

```
>> dh.RadiopharmaceuticalInformationSequence.Item_1

ans =

            Radiopharmaceutical: 'MDP'
       RadiopharmaceuticalVolume: ''
    RadiopharmaceuticalStartTime: ''
           RadionuclideTotalDose: ''
        RadionuclideCodeSequence: [1x1 struct]
```

The following field holds the number of detectors in the gamma camera system:

```
>> dh.NumberOfDetectors

ans =

     1
```

Apparently, this is an image acquired by a single head gamma camera. The detector information sequence field holds the following information about the detectors:

```
>> dh.DetectorInformationSequence.Item_1

ans =

           CollimatorGridName: 'None'
              CollimatorType: 'NONE'
               FocalDistance: ''
         ImagePositionPatient: [3x1 double]
      ImageOrientationPatient: [6x1 double]
```

In the case of a SPECT image, this header structure will have more and different fields. This example is from a SPECT image header:

```
>> dh.DetectorInformationSequence.Item_1

ans =
```

```
          GantryDetectorTilt:  0
     CenterOfRotationOffset:  0
          FieldOfViewShape:  'RECTANGLE'
     FieldOfViewDimensions:  [2x1 double]
         CollimatorGridName:  'VXHR'
            CollimatorType:  'PARA'
             FocalDistance:  0
              XFocusCenter:  0
              YFocusCenter:  0
      ImagePositionPatient:  [3x1 double]
   ImageOrientationPatient:  [6x1 double]
                ZoomFactor:  [2x1 double]
```

FieldOfViewDimensions may be particularly useful if one is interested in extracting the useful field-of-view (FOV), which is usually smaller than the full FOV of the camera. As seen in the preceding structure, some of the fields are vectors that hold a number of values such the FieldOfViewDimensions that holds the width and the height of the FOV.

In this appendix, we have provided a glimpse of the information stored in the DICOM header. For more information on the DICOM file format, the reader can refer to the following references:

1. http://www.nmr.mgh.harvard.edu/~tosa/#imageformat
2. http://www.vtk.org/Wiki/Proposals:Orientation
3. The DICOM Standard in PDF: http://medical.nema.org/dicom/
4. In particular, Part 3: Information Object Definitions from the link: http://medical.nema.org/dicom/2004.html

Appendix C

Medical Image Processing Toolbox

In this appendix we list the functions of the Medical Image Processing Toolbox, some of which are also provided in the chapters. The functions used in each chapter are listed in tables in order of appearance.

This toolbox can be downloaded from the following link:
http://www.biomedimaging.org

TABLE C.1

Chapter 1: Medical imaging systems

Function	Description
mipconstants	Provides/returns the commonly used constants in the basic sciences.
mipmapCTwindow	Performs windowing on CT images.

TABLE C.2

Chapter 2: Fundamental tools for image processing and analysis

Function	Description
mipimoverlay	Overlays a binary image on a gray-level image and returns the overlaid image.
miporthogonal	Creates orthogonal views from a 3-D image.
mipremoveundefinedNums	Removes undefined numbers such infs and nans.
mipimbin	Bins (by summing) image pixels rowwise or columnwise to create a smaller image.
miphisto2d	Computes 2-D histograms.
mipjhist	Computes 2-D histogram of the joint distribution of two images.
mipcorrimage	Simulates an image with correlated pixels.
mipdiskimage	Creates a disk image of a given radius.
mipsphereimage	Creates a sphere of known size.
mipsigmoid2d	Creates a 2-D sigmoid function.
mipsigmoidoned	Creates a 1-D sigmoid function.
mipshereshell	Creates a spherical shell.
miprmdebrisn	Removes small objects from a binary 2-D or 3-D image.

(Continued)

421

TABLE C.2 (CONTINUED)

Chapter 2: Fundamental tools for image processing and analysis

Function	Description
`mipcorrcoef3d`	Computes the 3-D correlation coefficient.
`mipboundingboxe3d`	Computes the bounding box of a 3-D object.
`mipneighborhood2d`	Gets the intensities of the 2-D neighborhood 4-pixel or 8-pixel.
`mipneighborhood3d`	The 3-D version of `mipneighborhood2d`
`mipforwarddiff,` `mipbackwarddiff,` `mipcentraldiff`	Compute forward, backward and central differences of an image.
`mipgauss`	Creates 1-, 2-D and 3-D Gaussian functions of a given size sigma.
`mipdog`	Computes and returns the derivative of a 1-D Gaussian.
`mipsdog`	Computes and returns the second derivative of a 1-D Gaussian.
`mipstructuretensor`	Computes the structure tensor of an image.
`miphexagon`	Simulates a hexagon image.
`mipimgauss`	Adds Gaussian noise to an existing image.

TABLE C.3

Chapter 5: Nonlinear anisotropic diffusion filtering

Function	Description
`mipadfoned`	Performs 1-D Perona–Malik diffusion.
`miplinoned`	Performs 1-D linear filtering using the Laplacian.
`miptvdiffusion`	Performs total-variation–based diffusion.
`mipseconderiv`	Computes the second derivative I_{xx} or I_{yy} of an image I.
`mipsecondpartialderiv`	Compute the second partial derivative I_{xy} or I_{yx}
`mipaffinecurvaturemove`	Performs affine curvature motion diffusion.
`mipisodiffusion2d`	Performs 2-D nonlinear scalar diffusion, in which the noise threshold is determined automatically using the method proposed by Canny in his seminal edge detection paper. It has also the Gaussian and median regularization options.
`mipisodiffusion3d`	Performs 3-D nonlinear scalar diffusion. It is the 3-D version of the function `mipisodiffusion2d`.

TABLE C.4

Chapter 6: Image segmentation by thresholding

Function	Description
mipimhist	Computes the histogram.
mipcmean	Computes the mean from a histogram for a range of intensities.
mipcvar	Computes the variance from a histogram for a range of intensities.
mipbcv	Computes the between-class variance, the optimal threshold based on its maximization.
mipkurita	Computes the Kurita's criterion function and the optimal thresholds based on its maximization.
mipminerror	Computes the minimum error function criterion and the optimal thresholds based on its minimization.
mipbcviterative	This is the iterative version of the mipbcv for three regions; thus it returns two thresholds.
mipUnivarGMixFit_Segment	Segments images via Gaussian/normal mixture modeling.
mipentropy_th	This function computes an optimal threshold using the entropy-based criterion function.
mipsahoo_thresh	This function returns the optimal threshold value using the 2-D Tsallis entropy method.
mipbrink_thresh	This function returns the optimal threshold value using the 2-D Shannon entropy method.
mipfcmSegmentation	Segments the input image by fuzzy C-means algorithm and returns the multilevel image at the output. It requires number of regions as the input.
mipkmeansSegmentation	Segments the input image by K-means clustering algorithm and returns the multilevel image at the output. It requires number of regions as the input.

TABLE C.5

Chapter 7: Image segmentation by Markov random field modeling

Function	Description
mipTotalEnergy	Computes the total energy.
mipregionstats	Computes the statistics of regions given a gray-level and a binary image in which each region is labeled with a different label.
mipicm2d2r	The ICM algorithm for 2-D images with two regions (2r)
mipicm2dmr	The ICM algorithm for 2-D images with multiple regions (mr)
mipgray2multilevel	Converts a gray-level image to multilevel images of n regions, which take on values from 1 to n, using the thresholds $t_1,...,t_{n-1}$.
mipicmvectorized2dmr	This is the vectorized version of the ICM algorithm that updates every pixel in parallel.

(Continued)

TABLE C.5 (CONTINUED)

Chapter 7: Image segmentation by Markov random field modeling

Function	Description
mipmetropolis2d2r	This implements the segmentation by MRF using the Metropolis algorithm for 2-D images with two regions only.
mipmetropolis2dmr	This implements the segmentation by MRF using the Metropolis algorithm for 2-D images with multiple regions only.
mipsample_discretedist	This function draws samples from a discrete probability distribution of any form.
mipgibbs2d2r	This implements the segmentation by MRF using the Gibbs sampling for 2-D images with two regions.
mipgibbs2dmr	This function implements the segmentation by MRF using the Gibbs sampling for 2-D images with multiples regions.
mipicm3d	This function is the ICM algorithm extended to 3-D.

TABLE C.6

Chapter 9: Image analysis and feature extraction

Function	Description
mipcircularity	Calculates the circularity.
mipvolprop	Calculates the volume properties.
mipcircconv	Performs circular convolution on closed boundaries.
mipnormscattermat	Computes the scatter matrix.
miparcshapeindex	Computes both the eigenvalues and the shape index for an arc consisting of set of points.
mipcurvature	Computes the curvature of boundary points.
mipfitellipse	This is Fitzgibbon's algorithm that fits ellipse to a set of boundary points. The algorithm is provided as it is in his Web site except that it is renamed mipfitellipse.
miphoughcircle	Implements the Hough transform for circle detection, that is, generates the Hough transform accumulator array for a given radius range.
mipaddcircle	This function does the circle search for a given (single) radius in the Hough transform accumulator array.
mipextractcircles	This function detects the possible circles in the Hough transform matrix by checking its local maxima.
mipcelldetect	Cell detection demo on embryo images using the Hough transform.

TABLE C.7

Chapter 10: Applications

Function	Description
mipresolutionlineProfile	Calculates the resolution parameters FWHM and FWTM from a line source.

Appendix D

Description of Image Data

In this appendix we list image data and their characteristics. These images can be downloaded from the following Web site:

http://www.biomedimaging.org

After the Medical Image Processing Toolbox is installed, the image data can be saved into a directory named ".../miptoolbox/images". The user has to make sure that the miptoolbox directory along with its subdirectories are included in the path. If the user saves the miptoolbox into the directory "D:/miptoolbox", one can add the toolbox and its subdirectories to the path using the following statements:

```
mipdir = 'D:/miptoolbox';
addpath(genpath(mipdir));
```

Once the directory in which the images are saved is in the path, then the statements given below can be used to read the individual images. Our image database includes more images than those used in the book so that the readers can try our or their own methods on a range of images. These images can also be read using the GUI imlook3d (see Chapter 2).

Image	Description
Brain	Sagittal view of the MR brain image used in image segmentation examples. To read: `>> img = imread('brain.png');`

(Continued)

(CONTINUED)

Image	Description
GFP 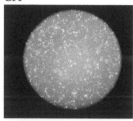	Color image of green fluorescent cells in RGB format. Image courtesy of Dr. Abu Al-Khabar. They can be used in image segmentation and correction of the nonuniform background. It is used in Application 1. To read: `>> img = imread('gfp.png');`
Retina 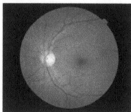	Color image of retina in RGB format captured by a fundus camera. These images can be used to test various image processing algorithms. To read: `>> img = imread('leftretina.tif);`
Embryo 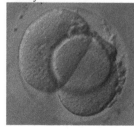	Gray-level image of an embryo. To read: `>> img = imread('embryo.tif);`
Islet Cells 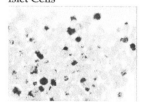	Color image of islet cells in RGB format. To read: `>> img = imread('isletcells.png);`
CT Slice 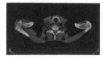	CT slice from a whole-body image at the abdomen level saved in DICOM format. To read: `>> img = imread('CTabdomen.dcm);`

(Continued)

(CONTINUED)

Image	Description
CT Slice 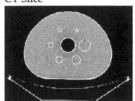	CT slice from the image of the NEMA image quality phantom in DICOM format. It shows a cross section through the middle of small hollow spheres inside the phantom. To read: `>> img = dicomread('CTnemaiq.dcm);`
Knee X-ray 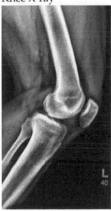	X-ray image of a left knee To read: `>> img = imread('knee.tif);`
Uniformity 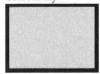	Flood-field uniformity captured by a gamma camera system and saved in DICOM format. A similar image was used in Chapter 2 to demonstrate the pixel binning operations. To read: `>> img = dicomread('gcuniformity.dcm);`

Dual Line source 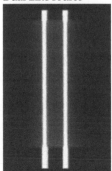	These are planar images of a dual line source with and without a scattering medium. They were acquired by a gamma camera to test its extrinsic resolution. We have used similar images in Application 2.
	To read the images:
	`>> img = dicomread('duallinesource_woscatter.dcm);`
	`>> img = dicomread('duallinesource_wscatter.dcm);`

Image	Description

SPECT Resolution images	The reconstructed SPECT images of a triple-point and triple-line source phantoms acquired by a gamma camera system. The former is used to measure the resolution of a SPECT system on air while the latter is used to calculate the resolution with scatter.
	To read the images:
	`>> img = dicomread('SPECTresolution_`
	`onair.dcm);`
	`>> img = dicomread('SPECTresolution_`
	`wscatter.dcm);`

Glomeruli 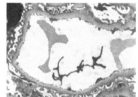	Image of kidney glomeruli captured by an electron microscope and scanned from a hardcopy. Image courtesy of Dr. Abdulgani Thabakhi. To read the image: `>> dh = imread('glomeruli.tif);`
Mammogram 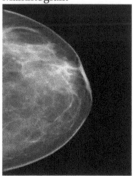	The image of a mammogram image saved in TIF format. To read: `>> img = imread('mammogram.tif);`

Microarray 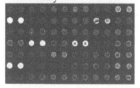	Image of a cDNA microarray slide.
	To read:
	`>> cy3 = imread('GeneExpressionCy3.`
	`TIF');`
	`>> cy5 =`
	`imread('GeneExpressionCy5.TIF');`

Index

A

Absolute quantification (AQ), 42
Acceptance testing, 379
Accumulator array, 355, 359
ACFs, *see* Attenuation correction factors
Acquisition modes, 37
ACR, *see* American College of Radiology
ADF, *see* Anisotropic diffusion filtering
AEC algorithms, *see* Automatic exposure control algorithms
Aequorea victoria, 371
Affine invariant curvature motion (AICM), 215
AICM, *see* Affine invariant curvature motion
American College of Radiology (ACR), 407
Anisotropic diffusion filtering (ADF), 192
Antiferromagnetic material, 280
Antiferromagnetism, 281
Apodizing windows, 183
AQ, *see* Absolute quantification
Ascending aorta MR image, 312, 317
Attenuation correction factors (ACFs), 42
Automatic exposure control (AEC) algorithms, 10

B

Bayesian information criterion (BIC), 267
Bayes' theorem, 118–121
BCV, *see* Between-class variance
Bernoulli distribution, 130–131
Beta distribution, 138, 140
Between-class variance (BCV), 224–236
  BCV as image bimodality measure, 231–233
  bimodality threshold for normal distribution, 232–233
  bimodality threshold for uniform distribution, 232
  criterion functions equivalent to BCV, 228–230
  iterative implementation of BCV for trimodal images, 233–236
BGO, *see* Bismuth germinate
BIC, *see* Bayesian information criterion
Bismuth germinate (BGO), 36

Brain image
  CT, 215
  data, 425
  edge functional, 324
  mixture modeling based segmentation results, 273
  MRI, 80, 213, 305, 306
  noisy MR, 324
  segmented, 259, 305, 306
Brain imaging, static, 43
Brownian motion, 144

C

Canny edge detector, 311
CDF, *see* Cumulative distribution function
cDNA microarray image, 238
Charvat–Havrda–Tsallis entropy, 247, 250
City-block distance, 100
Clique patterns, image segmentation, 286
Cobb–Douglas distribution, 144
Color image analysis, automated, analysis of islet cells using, 397–403
  analysis of cell features, 402–403
  deconvolution process, 403
  insulin-dependent diabetes mellitus, 397
  RGB colors, 397
  RGB images, 397
  segmentation of islet cells, 399–403
    further separation using luminosity component, 400–401
    K-means clustering, 399–400
    transformation to L*a*b space, 398–399
    ZEISS Axioskop2 plus light microscope, 397
Compton scattering, 41
Computed tomography (CT), 4–17, 51, 407
  advantages of, 4
  axial sequences, 10–11
  brain image, 215
  contrast scale, 6
  CT fluoroscopy, 14
  image(s)
    quality, 16–17
    spinal vertebral bone, 342
  modulation transfer function, 17
  multislice CT scanners, 14–16